International Review of Neuro
VOLUME 37

SELECTIONISM

and the

BRAIN

Editorial Board

SELECTIONISM
and the
BRAIN

Edited by OLAF SPORNS
GIULIO TONONI

The Neurosciences Institute
La Jolla, California

International Review of Neurobiology
VOLUME 37

ACADEMIC PRESS

San Diego   New York   Boston   London   Sydney   Tokyo   Toronto

Copyright © 1994 by ACADEMIC PRESS, INC.

Academic Press, Inc.
A Division of Harcourt Brace & Company
525 B Street, Suite 1900, San Diego, California 92101-4495

United Kingdom Edition published by
Academic Press Limited
24-28 Oval Road, London NW1 7DX

International Standard Serial Number: 0074-7742

International Standard Book Number: 0-12-366837-9 (casebound)

International Standard Book Number: 0-12-658110-X (paperback)

PRINTED IN THE UNITED STATES OF AMERICA
94   95   96   97   98   99   BB   9   8   7   6   5   4   3   2   1

CONTENTS

SECTION I
SELECTIONIST IDEAS AND NEUROBIOLOGY

Selectionist and Instructionist Ideas in Neuroscience
OLAF SPORNS

Population Thinking and Neuronal Selection: Metaphors or Concepts?
ERNST MAYR

Selection and the Origin of Information
MANFRED EIGEN

SECTION II
DEVELOPMENT AND NEURONAL POPULATIONS

Morphoregulatory Molecules and Selectional Dynamics during Development
KATHRYN L. CROSSIN

Exploration and Selection in the Early Acquisition of Skill
ESTHER THELEN AND DANIELA CORBETTA

Population Activity in the Control of Movement
APOSTOLOS P. GEORGOPOULOS

SECTION III
FUNCTIONAL SEGREGATION AND INTEGRATION IN THE BRAIN

Reentry and the Problem of Cortical Integration
GIULIO TONONI

Coherence as an Organizing Principle of Cortical Functions
WOLF SINGER

Temporal Mechanisms in Perception
ERNST PÖPPEL

SECTION IV
MEMORY AND MODELS

Selection versus Instruction: Use of Computer Models to Compare Brain Theories

GEORGE N. REEKE, JR.

Memory and Forgetting: Long-Term and Gradual Changes in Memory Storage

LARRY R. SQUIRE

Implicit Knowledge: New Perspectives on Unconscious Processes

DANIEL L. SCHACTER

SECTION V
PSYCHOPHYSICS, PSYCHOANALYSIS, AND NEUROPSYCHOLOGY

Phantom Limbs, Neglect Syndromes, Repressed Memories, and Freudian Psychology

V. S. RAMACHANDRAN

Neural Darwinism and a Conceptual Crisis in Psychoanalysis

ARNOLD H. MODELL

A New Vision of the Mind

OLIVER SACKS

CONTRIBUTORS

Numbers in parentheses indicate the pages on which the authors' contributions begin.

Daniela Corbetta (75), Department of Psychology, Indiana University, Bloomington, Indiana 47405

Kathryn L. Crossin (53), Department of Neurobiology, The Scripps Research Institute, La Jolla, California 92037

Manfred Eigen (35), Max-Planck-Institut für Biophysikalische Chemie, D-37077 Göttingen, Germany

Apostolos P. Georgopoulos (103), Brain Sciences Center, Veterans Affairs Medical Center, Minneapolis, Minnesota 55417

Ernst Mayr (27), The Museum of Comparative Zoology, The Agassiz Museum, Harvard University, Cambridge, Massachusetts 02138

Arnold H. Modell (335), Harvard University, Cambridge, Massachusetts 02168

Ernst Pöppel (185), Forschungszentrum Jülich GmbH, D-52425 Jülich, Germany

V. S. Ramachandran (291), Brain and Perception Laboratory, Psychology Department and Neuroscience Program, University of California, San Diego, La Jolla, California 92093

George N. Reeke, Jr. (211), The Rockefeller University, New York, New York 10021

Oliver Sacks (347), Albert Einstein College of Medicine, New York, New York 10014

Daniel L. Schacter (271), Department of Psychology, Harvard University, Cambridge, Massachusetts 02138

Wolf Singer (153), Max-Planck-Institut für Hirnforschung, D-60528 Frankfurt, Germany

Olaf Sporns (3), The Neurosciences Institute, La Jolla, California 92037

Larry R. Squire (243), Veterans Administration Medical Center, and Departments of Psychiatry and Neurosciences, University of California School of Medicine, San Diego, California 92161

Esther Thelen (75), Department of Psychology, Indiana University, Bloomington, Indiana 47405

Giulio Tononi (127), The Neurosciences Institute, La Jolla, California 92037

PREFACE

A tremendous explosion of research activity in the neurosciences has occurred in the past two decades. Our understanding of how the nervous system functions has been broadened by a variety of approaches ranging from classical anatomy and physiology to new and emerging molecular and imaging techniques. However, many fundamental questions remain. How does the specific structure of the brain originate during development, apparently without a fixed blueprint? How do organisms adapt to ever-changing environments? How does human memory work? What is the neural basis of consciousness? A wealth of empirical results providing a basis for answering these questions is now available. What is needed is to organize these results into a global theoretical framework relating biology to psychology.

Theories of brain function have accompanied neuroscience since its very beginnings without ever really becoming an integral part of it. Prior to the recent research explosion, most global theories were derived from philosophical or psychological theories of the mind. Very few theoreticians have striven for a global theory based directly on the biology of the brain, its evolution, and its development. This book attempts a synthesis of the emerging empirical evidence and new concepts of brain organization. The central focus of this synthesis is a particular set of theoretical ideas that consider the brain as a selective system. The term "selectionism" as we use it here is meant to highlight this focus. Our choice is motivated by the belief that selectionism offers the most promising avenue toward a comprehensive, explanatory, and predictive theory of the brain. Alternative proposals, such as those based on instructionism and information processing, have received and continue to receive much attention, especially from workers in the fields of cognitive science and artificial intelligence. They are discussed in this volume only insofar as they directly relate to and contrast with selectionist concepts.

The strength of a theory lies not only in how well it matches available empirical evidence, but also in how it covers phenomena from a wide range of fields and subfields to provide explanatory links between them. A particular strength of theories based on selectionism is that—as the term itself suggests—they firmly embed brain function within the context of development and Darwinian evolution, something that information-processing theories generally fail to do (or actively avoid doing). We have made a strong effort to encourage the authors of the chapters in this volume to stress these explanatory links.

A necessary adjunct of a global brain theory is a set of precisely defined models designed to address specific questions and help guide ongoing research. This has become a special responsibility of the neural theoretician, one that is all the more realizable as powerful computational methods for both studying and modeling the nervous system have become available. Computational neuroscience has thus provided an additional stimulus for furthering our theoretical understanding of brain function. Often the successful application of computational modeling has been used as evidence for the notion that the brain itself is a computational system, an interpretation we consider to be misleading. Several chapters in this volume demonstrate that the use of computational methods does not contradict the adoption of an essentially noncomputational view of brain function.

In order to increase the coherency of the volume and to allow the reader to identify and grasp some of the central theoretical issues more quickly, the editors have provided the interested reader with brief summaries and short discussions linking the various contributions. These discussions attempt to capture and highlight some of the more relevant or controversial theoretical ideas that emerge from an author's contribution; they also reflect a number of direct exchanges at various meetings held at The Neurosciences Institute. We hasten to add that the authors represented in this book were not chosen according to their unflagging support for selectionist theories of the brain. Rather, as their contributions demonstrate, they were chosen because their research is of particular importance for building theories of the brain. We also point out that this volume does not attempt to be exhaustive; not everybody who has expressed selectionist ideas related to the brain (or has rejected them) has been included. Moreover, due to the highly interdisciplinary character of most of the contributions, it has proven impossible to avoid duplications and repetitions of some of the material. The editors have tried to keep this to a necessary minimum.

The idea for this book emerged from a wealth of encounters between the research fellows and a number of visiting scientists at The Neurosciences Institute. Since its inception in 1981, The Neurosciences Institute (now located in La Jolla, California) has provided intensive support for interdisciplinary studies of the brain. The institute has been host to over 900 scientists from 24 countries working in fields ranging from molecular biology to psychoanalysis. We feel that the contributions to this volume reflect this range quite well. In addition to its role as a catalyst of discussion and exchange between scientists, reflected here to some degree, the Institute has supported an in-house research program in theoretical neurobiology, devoted to the design of realistic biologically based computational models. It has been a consistent practice at The Neurosciences Institute to embody a set of related selectional models in the so-called Darwin series of automata, whose construction anticipated some important recent developments in autonomous systems and robot design. These artifacts afford the theoretician an unprecedented opportunity to link events ranging from the molecular level to the level of brain dynamics during particular sequences of behavior. While they are not, strictly speaking, machines, we may consider that they provide a unique opportunity to study "machine psychology." A more distant goal of this line of research is to progress from such initial embodiments of selectional models to the realization of a conscious automaton. That one may even begin to consider the possibility of a conscious artifact, however far off, follows from the mounting conviction that consciousness is indeed a scientifically addressable (and solvable) problem.

Not all the visiting scientists and research fellows at The Neurosciences Institute are part of this volume; we thank all of them for their various intellectual contributions. The Institute's success in bringing together scientists from different disciplines and fields and in creating an intellectual atmosphere conducive to a free exchange of ideas is largely the result of the efforts of the Institute's research director, W. Einar Gall; we are grateful for his help in preparing this volume. In many ways this book is a tribute to Gerald Edelman, who, as a perusal of this volume will show, has pioneered many of the theoretical ideas discussed and elaborated in individual chapters. Since 1977, he has originated and pursued the most comprehensive set of selectionist ideas so far applied to the brain. His intellectual energy and keen interest in all matters relating to the brain have been the driving forces behind many of the Institute's activities. Without his support, this volume would not have been possible.

Olaf Sporns
Giulio Tononi

SECTION I
SELECTIONIST IDEAS AND NEUROBIOLOGY

The first section of this volume addresses some of the general issues that confront selectionist views of the brain. These include the applicability of population thinking, the nature of variation and of differential amplification, the distinction between self-organizing and selectional aspects of neural development, the notion of degeneracy, and the role of some specific concepts that are unique to neurobiology.

In the first chapter, Olaf Sporns compares instructionist and selectionist approaches to brain function. Though selectionist systems may differ widely in terms of mechanisms, as in the case of natural selection and of clonal selection in immunology, they all follow a common set of principles: preexisting variability, frequent encounters with an environment, and differential amplification. After a summary of the evidence suggesting that all three principles are realized in the brain, Sporns considers in detail the theory of neuronal group selection (TNGS), the selectionist theory of brain function proposed by Gerald Edelman. Some of the concepts introduced by the TNGS apply specifically to the brain. Among these are the notion of neuronal groups, local populations of strongly interconnected and cooperative neurons; reentry, the reciprocal and recursive exchange of signals along anatomical paths linking neuronal groups both within and between brain areas; and value, the means by which the saliency of environmental events can globally influence synaptic change within the nervous system. These concepts and the evidence supporting them are discussed at length in this chapter as well as in others throughout this volume.

As Ernst Mayr perceives it, his task here is to determine whether the principles of variation and selection that have been successfully applied to evolution can also be applied appropriately to the functioning of the brain. Mayr distinguishes three views of evolution: saltational, transformational, and variational evolution, and asks the question which of these views applies to the brain. Saltational evolution corresponds to essentialism, the notion that there are immutable classes or natural types and that all variation between exemplars is accidental and irrelevant.

Transformational evolution refers instead to a gradual change representing the unfolding of the intrinsic nature of an organism. An example would be the lawful progression of ontogenetic differentiation and morphogenesis. Variational evolution is the paradigm of selectionism, as exemplified by Darwin's theory of natural selection. Its key notion is that there must be a population of variant individuals that is subject to differential reproduction, resulting in biased survival, or "survival of the fittest." In the end, although Mayr does not offer a definitive choice, he seems to suggest that, until proved otherwise, ontogenetic differentiation is a sufficient characterization of brain development, as it is in any other organ.

The chapter by Manfred Eigen is concerned mainly with the problem of how information is generated in biological systems and with the role of selection in this process. He reviews his studies on the generation of viral quasi-species, distributions of nucleotide sequences in sequence space that cluster around a wild type. Selection, according to Eigen, can be seen as a force that aggregates these clusters around peaks in a fitness landscape and thereby generates information. Eigen then discusses the key relationships between variability (mutation rate), stability, and flexibility of adaptation. Finally, Eigen considers the issue of differential reproduction and selection, suggesting that, in general, mechanisms of differential reproduction require some sort of cyclic structure. As an example (extensively studied by Eigen and his co-workers), he refers to the hypercycle, which contains a self-reproductive template cycle with a superimposed catalytic feedback loop. His final suggestion is that the closure of cyclical processes, which could be achieved in the brain through the process of reentry, might be important for the differential amplification of synaptic circuits.

SELECTIONIST AND INSTRUCTIONIST IDEAS IN NEUROSCIENCE

Olaf Sporns

The Neurosciences Institute
La Jolla, California 92037

Traditionally, competing theories in biology have been either instructionist or selectionist. Whereas instructionist theories postulate a necessary transfer of information from an environment into a biological system or domain, selectionist theories stress principles such as variation and adaptation. The purpose of this article is to take a closer look at these two approaches and discuss some representative biological examples. Selectionist thinking has been extremely successful in biology; in a sense, through the theory of natural selection, all of biology is based on selectionist principles. It is the main argument of this work that selectionism can and should be extended to neural systems. To understand fully the biological basis of mental and psychological phenomena, we need empirical research linking biology to psychology as well as a theoretical framework provided by a global view of brain function. Selectionism can provide such a framework, and there is increasing experimental evidence for selectionist principles operating at various levels in the nervous system.

INTERNATIONAL REVIEW OF
NEUROBIOLOGY, VOL. 37

3

I. Old and New Metaphors of Brain Function

Throughout modern history our view of the brain has been influenced by metaphors, usually borrowed from some of the most advanced technology of the time. Descartes compared nerves to the systems of waterpipes that were used in animated figures. According to Descartes, animals were merely machines, all their actions resulting from mechanical processes. Humans differed in that they possessed an immaterial soul that was not subject to mechanical laws and that interacted with the body. The mechanistic and dualistic viewpoint underlying Descartes' vision provided a tremendous boost to the development of science and remains to this day perhaps the most influential view of how brain and mind work. The building of automata that would replicate human or animal behavior has a long tradition (reviewed in Reeke and Sporns, 1993) that is essentially rooted in Cartesian dualism.

Most recently, the most powerful metaphor to understand brain function and the functions and properties of (human) minds has certainly been the computer. The computer metaphor basically implies that the brain is a piece of specialized hardware, and the mind a kind of software implemented to run on this hardware (Fodor, 1983; Pylyshyn, 1984; Johnson-Laird, 1988). This view forms part of a philosophy of mind called functionalism, which essentially postulates that mental phenomena are rule based or instruction based and computational in nature. As such they are independent of particular material implementations. It should be noted that the use of the computer as an explanatory model for brain function and the underlying philosophy of functionalism have been subject to severe criticism both from neuroscientists and from philosophers of mind (Putnam, 1988; Searle, 1992; Edelman, 1992). Considered from a biological perspective, functionalism runs counter to the general recognition of the importance of evolutionary and developmental constraints on morphology (Reeke and Sporns, 1990).

Abandoning the computer metaphor for nervous function and the machine model of the mind does not imply, though, that computational methods are useless in neuroscience. Increasingly, computers serve as tools to investigate the brain as a complex system by modeling and simulating neurons and neuronal networks. Other articles in this volume contain examples of such studies.

If functionalism must be rejected, what can take its place? Darwinian principles of selection have been enormously successful in providing explanatory and predictive theories in various fields of biology. Indeed, the biological sciences are unique in their use of selection as a fundamental principle. Although biological theories based on instruction have been proposed to account for various systems, they have met with considerably less success than their selectionist counterparts.

II. Instructionism and Selectionism

Instructionist theories in biology stress the transfer of information from one domain (e.g., the environment) to another (e.g., a biological system). The biological system will—by means that differ from case to case—embody or store the information it has received. The system's construction and ongoing operation depend crucially on the transfer of this information from its environment. Selectionist theories, on the other hand, generally do not require such information transfer in their construction. Rather they work on the basis of three principles: (1) preexisting variation among components within the biological system, (2) encounter of the biological system with an environment and polling of the system's components, and (3) differential amplification of those components of the system that meet a threshold criterion after encounter. (The criterion in evolutionary selection is fitness.) Such a system though not containing any structures or fixed rules that are directly transferred from the environment, will behave *ex post facto* as if the system has been instructed. This is a crucial point: after the fact, systems that work according to instruction or selection may appear to perform alike, but acquiring this performance is achieved by very different principles and mechanisms in both cases.

One of the most important distinctions between the two approaches is the relevance of variation among components of the biological system. Because it is based on information transfer, instructionism does not require any preexisting structure within the system (except insofar as it relates to the successful transfer and storage of information): it can do with a tabula rasa. Variation is simply noise and has no functional importance per se except to degrade performance. A selective system, on the other hand, has a repertoire of preexisting variable functional components, in addition to ways of differentially amplifying those that perform best or match to the environment. In this case, variation is centrally important in achieving good adaptive performance of the system. Though variability may be structural or dynamic, structural differences between functional elements can give rise to additional variability in the ensuing dynamics.

There are several established examples of selective systems in biology. All of these examples share selection as a principle, though the mechanisms by which selectional principles work differ in each case (Table I). The theory of natural selection presents a consistent and comprehensive account of the evolution of species. It is based on variability among individual phenotypes, their encounter with a surrounding ecosystem, and differential reproduction. The details of evolutionary theory are under constant investigation and major theoretical questions remain the subject of sometimes fierce debate, but no instructionist counterproposal of any value has been made for quite some time. An instructionist theory of evolution would stress the transmission of adaptive traits from the environment directly to the individual, as seen, for example, in Lamarckian hypotheses. Such goal-directed improvement of adaptive traits is not that far removed from the old "argument from design," the belief that the perfection reached by living organisms, especially humans, requires a designer, i.e., preexisting information.

Another example in which selectionism has prevailed is in the explanation of immunity. To explain the function of the immune system, instructionist as well as selectionist proposals have been made (discussed in Edelman, 1967). The core of the instructionist proposals was that the antigen molecule would "impress" itself on the antibody molecule. The transfer of information in the form of three-dimensional structure from the antigen to the antibody is an example of instruction. Note that no

TABLE I

SELECTIONAL PRINCIPLES AND MECHANISMS OF VARIOUS BIOLOGICAL SYSTEMS

Selectional principles	Selectional mechanisms		
	Evolution	Immune system	Brain
Generation of diversity	Mutation, gene flow, recombination, etc.	Variable region, recombination, and mutation	Structural and dynamic variability as result of developmental processes
Encounter and polling	Behavior in econiche	Exposure and binding to antigen molecules	Sensory inputs, interoceptive signals, motor activity
Differential amplification	Differential reproduction (natural selection)	Clonal selection and expansion	Alteration of synaptic weights

preexisting diversity of antibody molecules is required, and no *differential* amplification is needed given the direct one-to-one transfer of information. This view is no longer tenable: empirical facts resoundingly confirmed the selectionist view, as set forth most extensively by Burnet (1959). Antigen molecules encounter a variable set of antibody molecules that, prior to encounter, differ in the three-dimensional structure of their binding sites and thus their affinity for antigens. High-affinity binding of an antigen to an antibody triggers clonal expansion of the cell bearing that antibody and thereby differential amplification of this antibody species over others that bind less well. All three criteria of selection are fulfilled: variation, encounter with polling, and differential amplification.

It may appear superficially that applying selectionist principles to the brain is straightforward. However, some earlier attempts have not been very successful, some for lack of empirical evidence to formulate clearly basic theoretical notions or substantiate them, and others for failing to take into account the unique multilevel nature of neural, mental, and behavioral phenomena. Most previous attempts to link selection and brain function have been directed toward understanding the shaping of brain structure over the course of evolution. Early conceptual links between selection as a principle and the working of the brain as evident in behavior can be found as early as 1911 in the work of Thorndike. Thorndike's "law of effect" postulated that the association between a stimulus and a response is strengthened or weakened, depending on the amount of reward following the response (Thorndike, 1911). The psychological school of behaviorism came to similar although overall more radical conclusions. The linkage between stimulus and response is the direct result of reinforcement. The potential role of selection in the context of behaviorism was discussed most completely by Skinner (1981). However, certain essential elements of selectionism are missing from this approach. There is no variable population of functional units that interact with an unlabeled world; instead, "selection by consequences" (Skinner's term) bears a strong resemblance to instructionist philosophies in which the environment impresses information on an unstructured brain.

One of the most clearly formulated neurobiologically based proposals was that of Young (1979); the emphasis is put on a selective view of memory. As in other proposals that focus on specific processes, such as the development of muscle innervation (Changeux and Danchin, 1976), the predominant mechanism is eliminative selection, i.e., the use-dependent destabilization of existing synaptic connections. Whereas eliminative selection forms an important component of selective systems, it does not touch on their more "creative" aspects, e.g., the continuing generation of variability by intrinsic activity. Furthermore, none of these proposals addresses the crucial problems of recognition and category formation as related to the population structure of the nervous system. Although these earlier approaches seem be inadequate from our latter-day perspective, they nonetheless open up the possibility of casting major aspects of brain function, from the dynamics of neuronal populations to ongoing behavior and even consciousness, in a comprehensive selectionist framework.

A thoroughly selectionist view of brain function must originate in "population thinking." As Ernst Mayr wrote (1959),

> The populationist stresses the uniqueness of everything in the organic world. . . . All organisms and organic phenomena are composed of unique features and can be described collectively only in statistical terms. . . . The ultimate conclusions of the population thinker and of the typologist are precisely the opposite. For the typologist, the type (*eidos*) is real and the variation an illusion, while for the populationist the type (average) is an abstraction and only the variation is real. No two ways of looking at nature could be more different.

To understand better how selectionist and population thinking can be usefully applied to brain function, we may consider some of the key problems that all theories of brain function must face and answer. As will become evident, these problems cannot be answered from the point of view of instructionism (at least not in accord with existing empirical evidence). They deal with the issue of how a system facing an unlabeled world can develop adaptive perceptual and motor categories and how one can explain the predominance of variability at almost all levels of neural organization.

III. Key Problems for Global Brain Theories

A. CATEGORIZATION

Newborn animals are confronted with a world full of sensory stimuli about which very little is known *a priori*. The partitioning of this stimulus world into meaningful categories will depend on the individual experience of that animal, and in particular on the adaptive value that this partitioning has for the organism. Different organisms, even those belonging to the same species, can and will often differ in their ways of responding to identical sensory stimuli. The evolution of different animal species living in the same habitat will often result in divergent modes of behavior and different adaptive strategies. For an organism lacking extensive experience or prewiring, the world is an "unlabeled place" (Edelman, 1987). For instance, the category membership of even simple objects may be ambiguous and is not intrinsically determined. Categorization of such objects requires exploration and choice, both depending extensively on various criteria of adaptive value, which may be evolutionarily fixed or be subject to modification during experience (Friston *et al.*, 1994). Selectionism opposes essentialism, the postulate that categories exist in the world as an absolute given in the absence of experiential interaction of an observer with this world. Given that the relations between the objects of the world on the one side and the organism with its complicated brain structure on the other side are not predetermined (in fact, not predeterminable), a brain theory is faced with a major explanatory burden. Any proposed solution must be consistent with known ontogenetic mechanisms and neural structures. Modern psychological research has revealed that category structure is experience dependent and highly variable between individuals of the same species (e.g., Mervis and Rosch, 1981); these results are consistent with a selectionist view of category formation. It is interesting to note that there is an analogy between the formation of species in evolution and of perceptual and conceptual categories during adult life.

A problem very similar to the construction of perceptual categories is the formation of movement patterns and synergies during motor development. Motor and sensorimotor coordination develop gradually and most movements are not "given" or hard-wired but depend in their realization on actual performance and experience. The ongoing growth and morphological change of the sensorimotor apparatus of an animal during early as well as adult life demand that the neural structures controlling this apparatus be capable of following changes adaptively by forming and dissolving motor categories when needed. No programmed system would be able to anticipate fully the demands made on an organism by its environment in the course of a lifetime, a key argument for the necessity of somatic selective mechanisms.

Though the world is unlabeled (in the sense of unambiguous informational categories), the nervous system of the organism facing it is not unstructured. Both evolution and development provide any given organism with a huge number of constraints, mainly in the form of specific morphology and anatomy of brain and body. These constraints set boundary conditions for possible modes of interaction with the world, but they do not prescribe the exact parsing of the world into perceptual or motor categories. An important structural constraint is variability of circuits in all parts of the brain.

B. Variability

The indeterminacy of the informational content of world objects and events is matched by the structural variability of animal nervous systems, at many levels of organization. As Karl Lashley pointed out in 1947, "the brain is extremely variable in every character that has been subjected to measurement. . . . Individuals start life with brains differing enormously in structure" (Lashley, 1947, p. 333). Lashley does not offer a theoretical explanation for this effect but ventures to speculate that "such variations . . . cannot be disregarded in any consideration of the causes of individual differences in mental traits" (Lashley, 1947, p. 333). Lashley anticipated the potential influence of structural variability on individual behavior, although he did not see the implications for the potential role of selection in the brain. The structural variability of the brain does not usually affect gross anatomical features that are characteristic for the animal species. But the size and position of cortical areas (Merzenich *et al.*, 1987; Watson *et al.*, 1993), the distribution of neurotransmitters and peptides (Mai *et al.*, 1993), the thickness of fiber tracts, the number of neurons constituting a nucleus (Ahmad and Spear, 1993), the recruitment of muscles during stereotyped behaviors such as locomotion (Loeb, 1993), and particularly the microanatomy of neurons [even in invertebrates; see, e.g., French *et al.* (1993) and other examples in Edelman (1987)] and neuronal circuits vary significantly from individual to individual in virtually all animal species. Structural variability is not genetically coded but represents the result of epigenetic regulatory processes acting during development. Such regulatory processes, for example, involve the adhesion, movement, differentiation, growth, division, and death of cells. The generation of diversity in growing neuronal structures is a necessary outcome of the action of morphoregulatory controls on cellular driving forces that are sensitive to local influence and context during development (Edelman, 1988). The enormous degree of variability within the nervous system that results is irreconcilable with theories of the nervous system based on the manipulation of information (e.g., functionalism); machines specialized for such functions usually require precise wiring at all levels and scales. Indeed, most information-processing theories of the brain perpetuate the erroneous conclusion that complex behaviors must be carried out by precise circuitry.

A last point to be stressed is that structural variability in the brain implies dynamic variability. The cooperative action of functional neuronal elements that vary structurally among themselves gives rise to a dynamics that is highly variable (although, of course, not entirely random). Dynamic variability is essential in the generation of motor actions in response to sensory stimuli. Variable actions can form a repertoire from which adaptive or value-linked behaviors (and their corresponding neural elements) can be selected. This forms the basis for a recent proposal to address the problem of motor development and the acquisition of motor skills in the context of selection (Sporns and Edelman, 1993).

IV. Theory of Neuronal Group Selection

The theory of neuronal group selection provides a comprehensive view of brain function from the standpoint of selectionism. It is at present the most completely worked out global selectionist theory of brain function. First proposed in 1978 (Edelman, 1978), it has since undergone several revisions and extensions (Edelman, 1987, 1988, 1989, 1992). It is a basic tenet of this theory that selection can resolve the apparent contrast between highly variable neuronal circuits facing an "unlabeled world" and the reproducible and adaptive behavior that they produce. The theory proposes that selectional mechanisms govern the formation, adaptation, and interactions of local collections of hundreds to thousands of strongly interconnected neurons called neuronal groups. These mechanisms can be divided into developmental selection, experiential selection, and reentrant mapping.

A. DEVELOPMENTAL SELECTION

Developmental processes generate not only the well-defined macroscopic anatomical order of the nervous system that is characteristic for each animal species, but also lead to the formation of highly variant local neuronal circuitry. Nonselective systems usually need to be protected against variance in their structural components; such variance tends to increase the amount of noise and requires redundancy to restore reliable function. However, in a selective system, a certain degree of variability is mandatory and thus might constitute an adaptive trait in evolution. Developmental mechanisms that give rise to variable structures during epigenesis may thus be actively preserved and refined during evolution.

B. EXPERIENTIAL SELECTION

Postnatally, after much of the meshwork of anatomical connections has been laid down, synaptic mechanisms become important agents of plasticity and adaptation. Synaptic selection guides the formation and the dynamics of the variable functional circuitry of neurons as they respond during experience. These experiential selectional processes are also responsible for the formation of neuronal groups as distinct entities under competition for incoming and outgoing signaling pathways. Some of these synaptic mechanisms also act in the developmental formation of the network, and activity-dependent processes continue to shape the morphology of neurons postnatally, such that a clear temporal border between the developmental and experiential phases cannot be drawn. It therefore must be understood that developmental and experiential selection do not occur in separate stages but rather represent two overlapping and mutually interdependent sets of mechanisms.

For somatic selection to operate in the nervous system, the variable functional units must be exposed (either directly or through intermediate units) to a sufficient sample of the afferent sensory signals to permit the units to respond differentially to various objects and events in the environment. Moreover, units undergoing selection must be able to contribute, through the output signals they emit, to some aspect of the behavior of the organism. Finally, the units must have the capacity to change their responses according to the relative success of the behaviors to which they contribute. (The term "success" can only be broadly defined and is not always directly related to the survival of the organism.) The significance or saliency of behaviors or events in the environment is sensed by value systems (Reeke et al., 1990; Friston et al., 1994), components of the nervous sytem that have certain properties: they are responsive to evolutionarily or experientially salient cues, they are able to broadcast their responses to wide areas of the brain and release substances that can modulate changes in synaptic strength, and they show transient responses to sustained input, inasmuch as it is changes in the environment that are important for successful adaptation. Candidates for such systems in the vertebrate brain are the aminergic and cholinergic neuromodulatory systems. Value systems deliver global signals that modulate synaptic changes to reinforce adaptive behaviors. Their action biases the distribution of firing or activation patterns toward such patterns that contribute to such behaviors. In some sense, value is analogous to adaptive fitness in evolution; rather than affecting the distribution of individual phenotypes in a population, value affects the likelihood of recurrence of adaptive or maladaptive neural or behavioral events. Value-dependent mechanisms are an important ingredient in selectional theories of the brain.

C. REENTRANT MAPPING

In order to assure that comparison and association of neuronal responses registered in separate cortical maps take place, neuronal responses must become correlated with each other. This correlation or conjunction is brought about by reentry, the ongoing and recurrent exchange of signals between maps along massively parallel anatomical connections. Reentry may occur in connections running backward from a "higher" to a "lower" area, as well as laterally, between areas at the same hierarchical level but in different pathways. Reentry is typically reciprocal, involving the exchange of signals in both directions between two areas. Often, these areas are located in different sensory pathways (modalities). A striking example of a densely interconnected distributed system is provided by the multiple functionally segregated and reentrantly linked areas of the visual system. In this system, reentry may provide a mechanism for the correlation of responses to different aspects (i.e., form and color) of the same object in the environment (Tononi *et al.*, 1992), solving the so-called binding problem.

Reentry can also provide a structural and functional basis for associative memory, in that the responses of reentrantly activated groups often reflect the existence of stimulus correlations having potential significance (Reeke *et al.*, 1990). The modification of synapses involved in these responses, biased according to the strength of the reentrant response, provides the physical substrate for this form of memory. Functionally, such memory appears as the facilitation of those categorical responses that have previously been selected in response to similar stimuli in the past; such facilitated responses are of course modified according to the current context. According to this view, memory is a process of recategorization rather than a replicative recall from storage of discrete data. Associations are developed across appropriate reentrant signaling pathways through the same mechanisms of synaptic modification that are used elsewhere to stabilize initial categorical responses. Frequently, these associations are formed between neuronal maps and reflect different aspects of a stimulus complex.

V. Empirical Evidence for Selection in the Nervous System

There are many lines of argument that support selectionist theories of brain function. Ultimately, however, any global theory of brain function must be put to the test vis-à-vis empirical evidence. The evidence for adaptive and experience-dependent formation of categories, for individual differences in neural structures, and for the importance of spontaneous exploration in motor development has been briefly mentioned. The rest of this paper will be devoted to a discussion of recent evidence that directly concerns developmental and reorganizational processes as well as the existence of neuronal groups and the action of reentry.

A. DEVELOPMENTAL AND EXPERIENCE-DEPENDENT PROCESSES

We have already mentioned evidence for the existence of variability in the structure and function of the nervous system. This variability is the result of developmental processes leading to the formation of basic neuronal circuitry, which is subsequently modified in a variety of activity- or experience-dependent processes. To review the multitude of effects that have been observed within the limits of this chapter is an impossible task. Instead, I want to focus on several apparently disparate phenomena: the profound changes in synaptic density in the developing and postnatal monkey cortex, selectional events in the formation of intracortical circuitry in the cat visual cortex, the importance of behavioral evaluation in some types of synaptic modification, and the experience-dependent shaping of motor categories.

Synaptic density is only one among many relevant parameters that are indicators of neural development, particularly the elaboration of neural circuitry. Rakic and co-workers measured the synaptic density in the prefrontal cortex of the macaque (Bourgeois and Rakic, 1993) and rhesus monkey (Bourgeois et al., 1994) over the entire life span of the organism. In the rhesus monkey, they found an early rapid phase of synaptogenesis (between 2 months prenatal to 2 months postnatal), followed by a plateau period (lasting until 3 years) and a progressive decline thereafter. In the macaque monkey, this decline amounts to the loss of about 5000 synapses per second in the visual cortex alone between 2.7 and 5 years (Bourgeois and Rakic, 1993). Even though the overall synaptic density does not take into account synaptic turnover and the ongoing remodeling of cortical circuits (see below), these measurements give an impression of the major structural fluctuations that the cortical system undergoes in somatic time. It is obvious in the light of this evidence that a population-based account of cortical function seems more likely to succeed than others that use single cells as functional units and that require precise point-to-point wiring.

The experience-dependent formation of intracortical circuitry has been studied extensively in the primary visual cortex of several species. The system of tangential connections in area 17 of the cat develops mainly after birth (e.g., Callaway and Katz, 1991). Selectivity of the connection pattern (preferential connectivity between groups of neurons that have similar response properties) is achieved after pruning (elimination) of inappropriate connections. Löwel and Singer (1992) reported that the criterion for the selection of tangential connections during visual experience is correlated neural activity. Such use-dependent selection based on correlations provides a general mechanism for the generation of functional anatomical connectivity throughout the cortex. Succinctly stated, "neurons wire together if they fire together." Other studies by Singer and co-workers suggest that while temporal correlations between neuronal groups serve to stabilize cortical circuitry selectively, the same correlations play an important role (after the connectivity has been laid down) in several visual functions (see below, and Singer, in Section III, this volume).

Though these early morphological changes in intracortical connectivity patterns require visual experience, the modification of the functional interaction between at least some cortical neurons appears to depend on behavioral context. A study by Ahissar et al. (1992) on auditory cortical neurons in the awake behaving monkey revealed that the functional connection between two neurons (derived from their cross-correlation) is strengthened most effectively if conditioning is associated with behavior. This relevance of behavioral performance in addition to the dependency of synaptic modification on temporal correlation points to the potential role of value systems in transmitting global signals related to the saliency of stimuli and events to large regions of cortex. The association of cellular changes and behavioral outcome fits well within the context of selectional models of learning and memory.

Another example of developmental plasticity and experience-dependent change is the development of motor behavior in many animal species. Human neonates (as shown in studies by Thelen and colleagues; see Thelen, Section II, this volume) are not born with a fixed and hard-wired set of movements; instead the ability to move within an environment develops over time. Individuals differ significantly in their movement patterns. The progression from a set of simple "synergies" to well-adapted movements can be viewed as a process of selection of movements from a repertoire (Sporns and Edelman, 1993). During ongoing experience and interaction with the environment, appropriate movements are selected and others are eliminated, in response to global value signals related to the salience of these movements to the organism. A selectionist view of motor development avoids typical pitfalls of proposals based on instruction: How can the musculoskeletal system undergoing continuous morphological changes during embryonic development and postnatal life be effectively controlled by a nervous system undergoing equally profound changes in an environment that confronts the organism with a multitude of often unpredictable challenges? The problem of simultaneously controlling many degrees of freedom (Bernstein, 1967) presents insurmountable problems to an instructionist system.

These examples are intended to show that developmental and experience-dependent processes are of central importance in a selectionist theoretical framework and that many lines of evidence are at least consistent with if not directly supportive of such views. In all cases mentioned here, instructive theories provide alternative modes of explanation that are either less parsimonious or simply impossible to realize.

B. EVIDENCE FOR NEURONAL GROUPS

Neuronal groups are central components for any population-based selectional theory of brain function. Such groups may sometimes correspond to regions of strong anatomical connectivity. It is possible, however, that their borders will not coincide with any anatomically distinguishable entity. In general, cells in a group will tend to share their response properties and receptive field structure. Furthermore, they will respond to incoming excitatory signals in a temporally correlated fashion. Such correlations serve both to strengthen the interactions of neurons within a group via synaptic mechanisms and to contribute to their response characteristics. The selectivity of neurons within a group thus results from the specificity of their input fibers as well as from their dynamic interactions. Ongoing interactions of neurons both within and between groups continually increase or decrease as a result of selective changes occurring in response to changes in the patterns of their inputs. Thus, the set of neurons that constitutes a particular group can vary over time, but at any one time, neighboring groups will be nonoverlapping, spatially distinct, and separated by borders.

Group organization has several advantages for the nervous system: it reduces the need for specific point-to-point wiring in map formation by providing spatially extended targets for large afferent arborizations, reentrant or otherwise; it permits units with fixed anatomy to undergo functional reorganization as required by the changing needs and growth of the organism [this point has been demonstrated in a model by Pearson *et al.* (1987), based on experiments of cortical reorganization in the so-matosensory cortex]; it permits essential reciprocal mappings between distant cortical areas to be maintained during such reorganization; it permits signals reflecting sensory context to have consistent effects on units with related function by placing those units in close spatial proxim-ity; it permits selective changes in synaptic efficacy to be coordinated across collections of neurons with related function; and it fosters the long-term stability of connections receiving common patterns of corre-lated input, reducing the danger that useful outputs will be disrupted by uncoordinated synaptic changes induced by any unusual strong inputs.

The general importance of groups in the nervous system is attested to by the widespread occurrence of grouplike local structures such as ocular dominance columns, blobs, slabs, barrels, fractured somatotopies, etc. In any event, the dense interconnections throughout the nervous system make it most unlikely that cells could ever function as individuals. The opposite point of view argues for the autonomous function of single cells at many or all levels of the nervous system. Central to these theories is the notion that local cooperative effects between neurons tend to be ignored or are considered to be of negative impact.

Perhaps the most critical empirical question that the theory of neu-ronal group selection faces is the existence of neuronal groups. If the functional units of the nervous system, in particular of the cerebral cortex, turned out to be single neurons, the theory, being essentially based on population thinking, would have to be discarded. The anatomy of local cortical circuits and axonal arborizations provides the first, still somewhat circumstantial, argument for the existence of local neuronal populations as the basic functional unit. Given the dense plexus of synap-tic endings formed by most cortico-cortical and thalamo-cortical axons and the tendency of cortical neurons to produce a patch of connections with their immediate neighbors (Amir *et al.*, 1993), local interactions are expected to be cooperative, producing correlated activity within local groups of cells. Such dynamic cooperative effects are consonant with the observation that many inputs arriving in a temporally correlated fashion are needed to elicit a response from cortical pyramidal cells (e.g., Abeles, 1991). The advantages of a functional organization of neurons into groups are increased reliability both locally (system performance does not rely on the activity of any single neuron) as well as in transmitting signals to other areas of the brain. An open question is how often neu-ronal groups are anatomically defined (i.e., they have relatively fixed locations and borders) or whether their borders and locations fluctuate with ongoing activity. One might speculate that different arrangements exist in different brain regions; a more anatomical segregation of groups might predominate in primary sensory areas (exemplified by columns in the visual system and barrels in the somatosensory cortex) whereas functionally defined groups may be found more frequently in "higher" areas.

The anatomical argument for groups is supplemented by some fairly direct physiological evidence. In many areas of the brain neurons located in close proximity show similar response properties. Presumably, such clustering reflects the local overlap of cortico-cortical projections as well as local interconnectivty. More direct evidence comes from multiunit recordings in the cat primary visual cortex (Gray and Singer, 1989). Orientation-selective neurons that are recorded with the same electrode and are in close spatial proximity tend to discharge in temporal synchrony when an optimally oriented light bar is present in their receptive fields. Thus, neurons located within the same local region tend to show similar receptive field properties as well as correlated activity. At the same time, these neurons maintain a high degree of variability both in their responses to stimuli and in their temporal discharge patterns (Gray *et al.*, 1992). Models of such groups have demonstrated that locally variable intragroup connectivity can lead to a significant dispersion of their temporal frequencies, an effect that is essential to ensure proper function of neuronal groups in sensory segmentation (Sporns *et al.*, 1989, 1991b). Analogous to the formation of specific cortico-cortical connections (Löwel and Singer, 1992), temporal correlations may not just be an indicator of the existence of neuronal groups, but also a mechanism for their generation during development. Studies (Yuste *et al.*, 1992; Peinado *et al.*, 1993) indicate that intercellular communication through gap junctions involving adjacent neurons may serve to synchronize their electrical activity. The domains formed by this interaction are potential precursors of functional neuronal groups.

C. Dynamic Reorganization of Cortical Maps

The topographically ordered mapping between the body surface and the surface of the somatosensory cortex is not fixed and anatomically hardwired even in the adult animal, but is capable of dynamically readjusting to unpredictable changes in the input. Merzenich *et al.* (1984) have shown that after amputation of a digit of the hand the cortical region previously responsive to that digit does not turn into a "blank" nonresponsive area, but becomes responsive to neighboring digits. This was originally observed within 2 months of amputation. Extensive stimulation of one digit results in an enlarged representation of this digit on the cortical surface, and conjoint stimulation of two adjacent digits results in neurons whose receptive fields include parts of both digits. The time-course of reorganization appears to be relatively fast in almost all cases; in experiments similar to those of Merzenich *et al.*, Calford and Tweedale (1990) observe effects within 20 minutes. A few hours of intracortical microstimulation was found to be sufficient to induce changes in the pattern of cortical representation (Recanzone *et al.*, 1992; Dinse *et al.*, 1993), leading to enlargement as well as shifting of areal and modality borders (Spengler and Dinse, 1992). Correlated neural activity is crucial for these effects, pointing to the importance of functionally coupled neuronal groups in the formation and maintenance of cortical representations.

More recently, Pons *et al.* (1991) found that cortical reorganization can extend over several millimeters, up to 1 cm and more of cortical surface. Several years after amputation of an upper limb the cortical area corresponding to that limb becomes responsive to sensory inputs from the face. Ramachandran has investigated the perceptual correlates of this cortical reorganization (1993, and Section V, this volume), finding that in humans a perceptual response consistent with cortical reorganization can be obtained as early as 4 weeks after loss of an arm.

The dynamic reorganization of cortical properties is not limited to somatosensory or motor cortices; the same kind of plasticity can be found in the visual cortex. Conditioning with certain kinds of visual stimuli can produce rapid changes in the receptive field properties of visual cortical neurons (Pettet and Gilbert, 1992); after masking parts of the visual field receptive field, sizes of neurons can increase severalfold over a short time (about 10 minutes). An intriguing set of hypotheses, quite open to experimental testing, suggests that some of these phenomena are the result of competitive interactions between neuronal groups and of the unmasking of local reentrant circuits within the visual cortex that allow cells to access remote "nonclassical" regions of their receptive fields.

D. Evidence for Reentry

Evidence supporting the role of reentry as a key process of brain function comes from multiple sources. Anatomical studies have demonstrated the abundance and rich patterns of reciprocal connectivity linking neuronal populations both within and between brain areas. Neurophysiology has offered several examples, some of them linked to actual behavioral performance, of how reciprocal interconnectivity can give rise to local modifications in the response properties of neurons or to temporal correlations.

Most cortical areas appear to contain long-range lateral connections linking neurons or neuronal populations within that area (Lund *et al.*, 1993). The best-studied example is the system of lateral, or horizontal, connections in the primary visual cortex. These connections, emitted by pyramidal cells, are most likely excitatory and are characterized by widespread axonal branching (over several millimeters) (Gilbert and Wiesel, 1983), anatomical and functional specificity (Gilbert and Wiesel, 1989), and termination in spatially distinct patches (LeVay, 1988). The reciprocal nature of this connectivity was demonstrated by Kisvarday and Eysel (1992), who used small focal injections of biocytin and subsequent three-dimensional reconstruction to characterize the pattern of interconnectivity. They found mutually overlapping axons between remote sources, indicative of reciprocal functional coupling (reentry) between these cells. That cells are functionally interrelated over distances of several millimeters has been shown in cross-correlation studies (Nelson and Frost, 1985; Ts'o *et al.*, 1986); these relationships tend to be orientation specific. Taken together, the functional anatomy of intraareal connections in the primary visual cortex suggests that reentrant interactions play an important role in defining the tuning properties and cross-correlation structure of neurons in that area. It is possible that these connections play an important role in setting up "nonclassical" receptive fields and contribute to several dynamic effects (for review, see Gilbert, 1992).

Reciprocal pathways are the rule, not the exception, in the macroanatomy of the cortex. A survey by Felleman and Van Essen (1991) of the interconnectivity of visual cortical areas in the macaque monkey revealed that of 305 pathways studied, the vast majority were reciprocal. Similar patterns exist in the human cortex (Burkhalter and Bernardo, 1989) as well as in the cortices of various other mammals. Some investigators have stressed the nonsymmetrical nature of many reciprocal pathways. For example, Zeki and Shipp (1988) have pointed out that projections from a hierarchically lower to a hierarchically higher area tend to be more specific and less diffuse than their reverse projections. What dynamic consequences such reentrant architectures might have is largely an open question; some initial steps have been made using computer simulations of interacting cortical maps. These studies (reviewed in Section III by Tononi and in Section IV by Reeke) have helped to identify at least two distinct, although not rigidly separable, functional modes of reentry: constructive and correlative.

1. *Constructive Mode*

The local response properties of neurons (their receptive fields and tuning characteristics) can be modified as a result of inputs arriving from reentrantly coupled neurons within the same or a different area (constructive mode of reentry). In the cat visual system, it has been shown that area 18 has distinct influences on the responses of neurons located in area 17, often thought to be at a lower hierarchical level of processing. Reversible inactivation by cooling (Sandell and Schiller, 1982) as well as by drug-induced focal blockade of parts of area 18 (Alonso et al., 1993) had an effect on the orientation tuning of cells in area 17. These effects may be mediated by anatomical projections linking area 18 to area 17. In studies of the transcallosal projections linking the visual cortices of the two hemispheres, it was shown (Payne et al., 1991) that reversible cooling of one hemisphere results in profound modifications of the response characteristics of many neurons in the other hemisphere. In other work, blocking or disinhibiting transcallosal inputs by application of γ-aminobutyric acid or its antagonist, bicuculline, results in marked changes in neuronal response properties (Sun et al., 1994).

The involvement of specific reentrant pathways in perceptual or cognitive tasks is sometimes hard to prove. Finkel and Edelman (1989) suggested in a computer model of the visual cortex that certain illusions may depend on reentry. Tononi et al. (1992) predicted that neuronal responses related to the detection of form-from-motion boundaries may depend on reentrant influences of area V5 on area V1. Lesion studies in monkeys (Marcar and Cowey, 1992), as well as transcranial magnetic stimulation (Beckers and Hömberg, 1992) and positron emission tomography studies in humans (Zeki, 1993), provide preliminary evidence that such reentrant activation of V1 by V5 actually takes place. The V1/V5 system is only one example; it is not unreasonable to predict that constructive influences of one area onto another are common within the cortex.

2. *Correlative Mode*

A second consequence of reentrant neuronal interactions is the emergence of temporal correlations. Such correlations have been extensively studied by Gray and Singer in the cat visual cortex (see their contributions in Section III). In some cases it could be shown that the existence of correlations between two cortical regions depends on the integrity of the cortico-cortical connections linking these points (Engel et al., 1991). These cross-correlations have interesting temporal properties that point to the highly dynamic nature of reentrant interactions. Groups of neurons are synchronized for relatively brief periods of time (100–500 msec) (Gray et al., 1992) and both synchronization and desynchronization are fast processes. Based on computer modeling studies, we suggested that the onset and offset of synchrony might be related to fast synaptic changes occurring in reentrant fibers (Sporns et al., 1991a). Cross-correlations between areas 17 and 18 of the cat visual cortex have been observed (Eckhorn *et al.*, 1988) and classified into several classes (Nelson *et al.*, 1992). Coupled neurons tend to have overlapping receptive fields, mirroring the fact that such neurons tend also to be anatomically interconnected. In other experiments, the task-related patterns of widespread correlations between sensory and motor areas of the macaque monkey observed by Bressler *et al.* (1993) are most likely due to reciprocal cortico-cortical interconnectivity linking these areas. In correspondence to results obtained from multielectrode recordings, they found that coherent episodes last several tens to hundreds of milliseconds and that both synchronization and desynchronization occur fast. Taken together, this and other evidence point to a distinct role for reentry in the establishment of temporal correlations.

VI. Outlook

Since its inception, the theory of neuronal group selection has sparked critical evaluations and counterproposals from a number of scientists. Until to date, no alternative *comprehensive* theory has been proposed that is rigorously based on evolution and development and ranges in scope from neuronal populations all the way to consciousness. Most recent theoretical efforts aim at the formulation of mechanistic or computational hypotheses geared toward explaining specific functions of the brain, an occupation that is indispensable for making progress in empirical research. Though reductionism can be extremely fruitful as an operational attitude, in view of the complexity and multilevel nature of the nervous system it hardly suffices as a global theoretical framework. Reductionism on a grand scale as exemplified by several recent *opera* of Francis Crick appears to aim at making difficult problems look simple rather than explain them. Crick's criticism of selectionism has been severe (Crick, 1989), but recent indications are (Crick, 1994) that even this staunch exponent of mechanistic reductionism begins to cast a favorable eye on selectionist concepts such as reentry.

Characteristically, most large-scale theoretical frameworks that are incompatible with or run counter to selectionism reside at a "higher" organizational level, usually within linguistics, cognitive science, or artificial intelligence (the functionalist school; see Reeke, Section IV, this volume). This seems to indicate that whereas it is possible (at least for some time) to ignore the action of selective mechanisms at these levels, at "lower" organizational levels (neurons and neuronal populations, maps, and brain regions) the advantages of selectional theories are far more compelling. In fact, in areas such as neuronal population dynamics, cortical integration, motor development, categorization, and consciousness, the prevailing opposition to selectionist theories has not come from well-formulated *instructionist* counterproposals but from a vaguely defined antitheoretical stance. Once you have the data, what good is a theory? The answer is that their explanatory and predictive power makes theories indispensable adjuncts of empirical research in neuroscience. This volume attests to this, and to the promising role played by selectionist and population thinking.

References

Abeles, M. (1991). "Corticonics." Cambridge Univ. Press, Cambridge, UK.

Ahissar, E., Vaadia, E., Ahissar, M., Bergman, H., Arieli, A., and Abeles, M. (1992). Dependence of cortical plasticity on correlated activity of single neurons and on behavioral context. *Science* **257**, 1412–1415.

Ahmad, A., and Spear, P. D. (1993). Effects of aging on the size, density, and number of rhesus monkey lateral geniculate nucleus. *J. Comp. Neurol.* **334**, 631–643.

Alonso, J. M., Cudeiro, J., Perez, R., Gonzalez, F., and Acuna, C. (1993). Orientational influences of layer V of visual area 18 upon cells in layer V of area 17 in the cat cortex. *Exp. Brain Res.* **96**, 212–220.

Amir, Y., Harel, M., and Malach, R. (1993). Cortical hierarchy reflected in the organization of intrinsic connections in macaque monkey visual cortex. *J. Comp. Neurol.* **334**, 19–46.

Beckers, G., and Hömberg, V. (1992). Cerebral visual motion blindness: Transitory akinetopsia induced by transcranial magnetic stimulation of human area V5. *Proc. R. Soc. London Ser. B* **249**, 173–178.

Bernstein, N. (1967). "The Coordination and Regulation of Movements." Pergamon, Oxford.

Bourgeois, J.-P., and Rakic, P. (1993). Changes of synaptic density in the primary visual cortex of the macaque monkey from fetal to adult stage. *J. Neurosci.* **13**, 2801–2820.

Bourgeois, J.-P., Goldman-Rakic, P. S., and Rakic, P. (1994). Synaptogenesis in the prefrontal cortex of rhesus monkeys. *Cereb. Cortex* **4**, 78–96.

Bressler, S. L., Coppola, R., and Nakamura, R. (1993). Episodic multiregional cortical coherence at multiple frequencies during visual task performance. *Nature (London)* **366**, 153–156.

Burkhalter, A., and Bernardo, K. L. (1989). Organization of corticocortical connections in human visual cortex. *Proc. Natl. Acad. Sci. U.S.A.* **86**, 1071–1075.

Burnet, F. M. (1959). "The Clonal Selection Theory of Acquired Immunity." Vanderbilt Univ. Press, Nashville, TN.

Calford, M. B., and Tweedale, R. (1990). Interhemispheric transfer of plasticity in the cerebral cortex. *Science* **249**, 805–807.

Callaway, E. M., and Katz, L. C. (1991). Effects of binocular deprivation on the development of clustered horizontal connections in cat striate cortex. *Proc. Natl. Acad. Sci. U.S.A.* **88**, 745–749.

Changeux, J.-P., and Danchin, A. (1976). Selective stabilization of developing synapses as a mechanism for the specification of neuronal networks. *Nature (London)* **264,** 705–711.

Crick, F. H. C. (1989). Neural Edelmanism. *Trends Neurosci.* **12,** 240–248.

Crick, F. H. C. (1994). "The Astonishing Hypothesis." Charles Scribners & Sons, New York.

Dinse, H. R., Recanzone, G. H., and Merzenich, M. M. (1993). Alterations in correlated activity parallel ICMS-induced representational plasticity. *NeuroReport* **5,** 173–176.

Eckhorn, R., Bauer, R., Jordan, W., Brosch, M., Kruse, W., Munk, M., and Reitboeck, H. J. (1988). Coherent oscillations: A mechanism of feature linking in the visual cortex? Multiple electrode and correlation analyses in the cat. *Biol. Cybernet.* **60,** 121–130.

Edelman, G. M. (1967). Antibody structure and diversity: Implications for theories of antibody synthesis. *In* "The Neurosciences. A Study Program" (G. C. Quarton, T. Melnechuk, and F. O. Schmitt, eds.), pp. 188–200. Rockefeller Univ. Press, New York.

Edelman, G. M. (1978). Group selection and phasic re-entrant signalling: A theory of higher brain function. *In* "The Mindful Brain" (G. M. Edelman and V. B. Mountcastle, eds.), pp. 51–100. MIT Press, Cambridge, MA.

Edelman, G. M. (1987). "Neural Darwinism: The Theory of Neuronal Group Selection." Basic Books, New York.

Edelman, G. M. (1988). "Topobiology: An Introduction to Molecular Embryology." Basic Books, New York.

Edelman, G. M. (1989). "The Remembered Present: A Biological Theory of Consciousness." Basic Books, New York.

Edelman, G. M. (1992). "Bright Air, Brilliant Fire: on the Matter of the Mind." Basic Books, New York.

Engel, A. K., König, P., Kreiter, A. K., and Singer, W. (1991). Interhemispheric synchronization of oscillatory neuronal responses in cat visual cortex. *Science* **252,** 1177–1179.

Felleman, D. J., and Van Essen, D. C. (1991). Distributed hierarchical processing in the primate cerebral cortex. *Cereb. Cortex* **1,** 1–47.

Finkel, L. H., and Edelman, G. M. (1989). The integration of distributed cortical systems by reentry: A computer simulation of interactive functionally segregated visual areas. *J. Neurosci.* **9,** 3188–3208.

Fodor, J. A. (1983). "The Modularity of Mind." MIT Press, Cambridge, MA.

French, A. S., Klimaszewski, A. R., and Stockbridge, L. L. (1993). The morphology of the sensory neuron in the cockroach femoral tactile spine. *J. Neurophysiol.* **69,** 669–673.

Friston, K. J., Tononi, G., Reeke, G. N., Jr., Sporns, O., and Edelman, G. M. (1994). Value-dependent selection in the brain: Simulation in a synthetic neural model. *Neuroscience* **59,** 229–243.

Gilbert, C. D. (1992). Horizontal integration and cortical dynamics. *Neuron* **9,** 1–13.

Gilbert, C. D., and Wiesel, T. N. (1989). Columnar specificity of intrinsic horizontal and cortico-cortical connections in cat visual cortex. *J. Neurosci.* **9,** 2432–2442.

Gilbert, C. D., and Wiesel, T. N. (1989). Columnar specificity of intrinsic horizontal and cortico-cortical connections in cat visual cortex. *J. Neurosci.* **9,** 2432–2442.

Gray, C. M., and Singer, W. (1989). Stimulus-specific neuronal oscillations in orientation columns of cat visual cortex. *Proc. Natl. Acad. Sci. U.S.A.* **86,** 1698–1702.

Gray, C. M., Engel, A. K., König, P., and Singer, W. (1992). Synchronization of oscillatory neuronal responses in cat striate cortex: Temporal properties. *Visual Neurosci.* **8,** 337–347.

Johnson-Laird, P. N. (1988). "The Computer and the Mind." MIT Press, Cambridge, MA.

Kisvarday, Z. F., and Eysel, U. T. (1992). Cellular organization of reciprocal patchy networks in layer III of cat visual cortex (area 17). *Neuroscience* **46,** 275–286.

Lashley, K. S. (1947). Structural variation in the nervous system in relation to behavior. *Psychol. Rev.* **54**, 325–334.

LeVay, S. (1988). Patchy intrinsic projections in visual cortex, area 18, of the cat: Morphological and immunohistochemical evidence for an excitatory function. *J. Comp. Neurol.* **269**, 265–274.

Loeb, G. E. (1993). The distal hindlimb musculature of the cat—Interanimal variability of locomotor-activity and cutaneous reflexes. *Exp. Brain Res.* **96**, 125–140.

Löwel, S., and Singer, W. (1992). Selection of intrinsic horizontal connections in the visual cortex by correlated neuronal activity. *Science* **255**, 209–212.

Lund, J. S., Yoshioka, T., and Levitt, J. B. (1993). Comparison of intrinsic connectivity in different areas of macaque monkey cerebral cortex. *Cereb. Cortex* **3**, 148–162.

Mai, J. K., Berger, K., and Sofroniew, M. V. (1993). Morphometric evaluation of neurophysin-immunoreactvity in the human brain—Pronounced interindividual variability and evidence for altered staining patterns in schizophrenia. *J. Hirnforsch.* **34**, 133–154.

Marcar, V. L., and Cowey, A. (1992). The effect of removing superior temporal cortical motion areas in the macaque monkey. II. Motion discrimination using random dot displays. *Eur. J. Neurosci.* **4**, 1228–1238.

Mayr, E. (1959). Darwin and the evolutionary theory in biology. *In* "Evolution and Anthropology: A Centennial Appraisal" (B. J. Meggers, ed.), pp. 1–10. Anthropol. Soc. Washington, Washington, DC.

Mervis, C. B., and Rosch, E. (1981). Categorization of natural objects. *Annu. Rev. Psychol.* **32**, 89–115.

Merzenich, M. M., Nelson, R. J., Stryker, M. P., Cynader, M., Schoppman, A., and Zook, J. M. (1984). Somatosensory cortical map changes following digit amputation in adult monkeys. *J. Comp. Neurol.* **224**, 591–605.

Merzenich, M. M., Nelson, R. J., Kaas, J. H., Stryker, M. P., Jenkins, W. M., Zook, J. H., Cynader, M. S., and Schoppmann, A. (1987). Variability in hand surface representations in areas 3b and 1 in adult owl and squirrel monkeys. *J. Comp. Neurol.* **258**, 281–296.

Nelson, J. I., and Frost, B. J. (1985). Intracortical facilitation among co-oriented, co-axially aligned simple cells in the cat striate cortex. *Exp. Brain Res.* **61**, 54–61.

Nelson, J. I., Salin, P. A., Munk, M. H.-J., Arzi, M., and Bullier, J. (1992). Spatial and temporal coherence in cortico-cortical connections: A cross-correlation study in areas 17 and 18 in the cat. *Visual Neurosci.* **9**, 21–37.

Payne, B. R., Siwek, D. F., and Lomber, S. G. (1991). Complex transcallosal interactions in visual cortex. *Visual Neurosci.* **6**, 283–289.

Pearson, J. C., Finkel, L. H., and Edelman, G. M. (1987). Plasticity in the organization of adult cortical maps: A computer model based on neuronal group selection. *J. Neurosci.* **7**, 4209–4223.

Peinado, A., Yuste, R., and Katz, L. C. (1993). Gap junctional communication and the development of local circuits in neocortex. *Cereb. Cortex* **3**, 488–498.

Pettet, M. W., and Gilbert, C. D. (1992). Dynamic changes in receptive-field size in cat primary visual cortex. *Proc. Natl. Acad. Sci. U.S.A.* **89**, 8366–8370.

Pons, T., Preston, E., Garraghty, A. K., Kaas, J., and Mishkin, M. (1991). Massive cortical reorganization in primates. *Science* **252**, 1857–1860.

Putnam, H. (1988). "Representation and Reality." MIT Press, Cambridge, MA.

Pylyshyn, Z. W. (1984). "Computation and Cognition: Toward a Foundation for Cognitive Science." MIT Press, Cambridge, MA.

Ramachandran, V. S. (1993). Behavioral and magnetoencephalic correlates of plasticity in the adult human brain. *Proc. Natl. Acad. Sci. U.S.A.* **90**, 10413–10420.

Recanzone, G. H., Merzenich, M. M., and Dinse, H. R. (1992). Expansion of the cortical representation of a specific skin field in primary somatosensory cortex by intracortical microstimulation. *Cereb. Cortex* **2**, 181–196.

Reeke, G. N., Jr., and Sporns, O. (1990). Selectionist models of perceptual and motor systems and implications for functionalist theories of brain function. *Physica D (Amsterdam)* **42**, 347–364.

Reeke, G. N., Jr., and Sporns, O. (1993). Behaviorally based modeling and computational approaches to neuroscience. *Annu. Rev. Neurosci.* **16**, 597–623.

Reeke, G. N., Jr., Finkel, L. H., Sporns, O., and Edelman, G. M. (1990). Synthetic neural modelling: A multi-level approach to brain complexity. *In* "Signal and Sense: Local and Global Order in Perceptual Maps" (G. M. Edelman, W. E. Gall, and W. M. Cowan, eds.), pp. 607–707. Wiley, New York.

Sandell, J. H., and Schiller, P. H. (1982). Effect of cooling area 18 on striate cortex cells in the squirrel monkey. *J. Neurophysiol.* **48**, 38–48.

Searle, J. R. (1992). "The Rediscovery of the Mind." MIT Press, Cambridge, MA.

Skinner, B. F. (1981). Selection by consequences. *Science* **215**, 501–504.

Spengler, F., and Dinse, H. R. (1992). ICMS induced emergence of new skin field representations in rat somatosensory cortex. *Soc. Neurosci. Abstr.* **22**, 345.

Sporns, O., and Edelman, G. M. (1993). Solving Bernstein's problem: A proposal for the development of coordinated movement by selection. *Child Dev.* **64**, 960–981.

Sporns, O., Gally, J. A., Reeke, G. N., Jr., and Edelman, G. M. (1989). Reentrant signaling among simulated neuronal groups leads to coherency in their oscillatory activity. *Proc. Natl. Acad. Sci. U.S.A.* **86**, 7265–7269.

Sporns, O., Tononi, G., and Edelman, G. M. (1991a). Modeling perceptual grouping and figure-ground segregation by means of active reentrant connections. *Proc. Natl. Acad. Sci. U.S.A.* **88**, 129–133.

Sporns, O., Tononi, G., and Edelman, G. M. (1991b). Dynamic interactions of neuronal groups and the problem of cortical integration. *In* "Nonlinear Dynamics and Neural Networks" (H. G. Schuster, ed.), pp. 205–240. Verlag Chemie, Weinheim.

Sun, J.-S., Li, B., Ma, M. H., and Diao, Y. C. (1994). Transcallosal circuitry revealed by blocking and disinhibiting callosal input in the cat. *Visual Neurosci.* **11**, 189–197.

Thorndike, E. L. (1911). "Animal Intelligence." New York: Macmillan,

Tononi, G., Sporns, O., and Edelman, G. M. (1992). Reentry and the problem of integrating multiple cortical areas: Simulation of dynamic integration in the visual system. *Cereb. Cortex* **2**, 310–335.

Ts'o, D. Y., Gilbert, C. D., and Wiesel, T. N. (1986). Relationships between horizontal interactions and functional architecture in cat striate cortex as revealed by cross-correlation analysis. *J. Neurosci.* **6**, 1160–1170.

Watson, J. D. G., Myers, R., Frackowiak, R. S. J., Hajnal, J. V., Woods, R. P., Mazziotta, J. C., Shipp, S., and Zeki, S. (1993). Area V5 of the human brain: Evidence from a combined study using positron emission tomography and magnetic resonance imaging. *Cereb. Cortex* **3**, 79–94.

Young, J. Z. (1979). Learning as a process of selection and amplification. *J. R. Soc. Med.* **72**, 801–814.

Yuste, R., Peinado, A., and Katz, L. C. (1992). Neuronal domains in developing neocortex. *Science* **257**, 665–669.

Zeki, S. (1993). "A Vision of the Brain." Blackwell Scientific, Cambridge, MA.

Zeki, S., and Shipp, S. (1988). The functional logic of cortical connections. *Nature (London)* **335**, 311–317.

POPULATION THINKING AND NEURONAL SELECTION: METAPHORS OR CONCEPTS?

Ernst Mayr

The Museum of Comparative Zoology
The Agassiz Museum
Harvard University
Cambridge, Massachusetts 02138

As many of you know, I have devoted the past 22 years of my life to an analysis of biological concepts. In this pursuit perhaps nothing has impressed me more than the frequency of controversies caused by the differential use of the same term by different authors. I have shown this for the terms *teleological, evolution, reduction, speciation, species,* and many other terms. There is no hope for mutual understanding, no hope for the resolution of a controversy, as long as opposing authors use the same term but give it different meanings. It is owing to this interest of mine that I was invited to give this paper.

The task that has been assigned to me is to discuss whether the evolutionary terms that Edelman has introduced into neurobiology were introduced legitimately. The question is whether he has used these terms in the same sense in neurobiology in which they are used in evolutionary biology or, more broadly, whether the neurophysiological phenomena and processes to which Edelman applies these terms are truly analogous to the seemingly equivalent evolutionary phenomena.

The editor of this volume, when they invited me, understood that I know virtually nothing about neurobiology, and so they instructed me to discuss the basic meaning of the evolutionary phenomena and theories that were the donors of the new neural metaphors. It is on these terms that I accepted their invitation. I therefore consider it as my task to serve as an interpreter of evolutionary thought and terminology.

Let me begin by pointing out an important source of misunderstanding. There is not one but there are actually three different concepts of evolution or organic change. The differences among the three have to be understood fully before neuronal differentiation can be assigned to one of them, if to any of them.

First, saltational evolution: this is the concept that the world and the phenomena in it are essentially constant and that a novelty can be produced only by a major saltation or mutation, which adds a new kind of entity to the previously existing ones. All authors, from the Greeks up to nearly the end of the eighteenth century, if they supported changes in the world, believed in such saltational evolution. It is indeed the only kind of change possible if one adopts essentialism, and this was, during that time period, more or less true for everybody.

According to the philosophy of essentialism, which goes back to Plato and the Pythagoreans, each phenomenon of nature (each entity) belongs to a class (natural kind). All members of the class are identical and conform to the definition of the class. All seeming variation is accidental and evolutionarily irrelevant. The definition (essence) of a class is constant. Evolution can take place only by the sudden and instantaneous production of a new essence, giving rise to a new species (class).

Because essentialism had a powerful hold on the thinking of the Western world, saltationist evolutionary theories continued to be proposed even after 1859 and were upheld by the early Mendelians (Bateson, DeVries) and a few authors up to about 1950. It is totally inapplicable to neuronal development and shall not occupy us any longer.

Second, transformational evolution: this term refers to the gradual change of an organism or any other object, which does not lose its basic identity in spite of the change. Indeed, the term *evolution* was introduced in the late eighteenth century for a particular theory (the Preformation Theory) of ontogeny. It referred to the development of an individual animal from the fertilized egg to adulthood. Lamarck's theory of evolution was transformational.

All evolutionary changes in inanimate nature, such as of stars or mountains, are transformational. On the whole, all ontogenetic changes are transformational. They have always been considered to be transformational and it will be up to the reader of this contribution to decide whether this is also true for neuronal development. Those who accepted transformational change for organic evolution, like Lamarck, postulated that the changes were caused by extrinsic factors *and* that they could be transmitted to future generations by an inheritance of acquired characters.

The study of the factors that control the differentiation of the fertilized egg into the adult is the concern of developmental biology. It is at the present time an area of intense activity. Perhaps the most important questions raised by the developmental biologists are these: To what extent is this differentiation directly controlled by the genetic program and to what extent do earlier stages in the differentiation (one might call this a somatic program) make a contribution toward the determination of subsequent stages? The study of the interaction between nuclear genes and the cellular and tissue environments is the core area of modern developmental biology.

Someone, like myself, coming to the problem of neuronal differentiation would automatically assume that the nervous system follows the same processes as other developing body tissues. It is this assumption that has been challenged by Gerald Edelman. He thinks that selectionist processes take place during differentiation, which differ in nature from the instruction by the genetic program, and that these selection processes facilitate understanding the complex processes of brain development. Selection belongs to a concept of evolution that is entirely different from transformational evolution, and this requires a discussion of the third of the three basic concepts of organic change: variational evolution, as proposed by Darwin.

Everyone knows that in 1859 Darwin demonstrated the occurrence of evolution with such overwhelming documentation that it was soon almost universally accepted. What *not* everyone knows, however, is that on that occasion Darwin introduced a number of other scientific and philosophical concepts that have been of far-reaching importance ever since. These concepts, population thinking and selection, owing to their total originality, had to overcome enormous resistance. One might think that among the many hundreds of philosophers who had developed ideas about change, beginning with the Ionians, Plato and Aristotle, the scholastics, the philosophers of the Enlightenment, Descartes, Locke, Hume, Leibniz, Kant, and the numerous philosophers of the first half of the nineteenth century, that there would have been at least one or two to have seen the enormous heuristic power of that combination of variation and selection. But the answer is no. To a modern, who sees the manifestations of variation and selection wherever he looks, this seems quite unbelievable, but it is a historical fact.

Let me explain in more detail the contrast between transformational evolution and Darwin's variational evolution. In transformational evolution, a given object, a given entity, gradually changes over time without losing its essential identity. In Darwinian variational evolution, there is a continuous alteration of the two steps of Darwin's selection process. During the first step in every generation, an immense amount of new variation is produced, resulting in the origin of a new population, consisting of unique individuals. No such concept of a population of unique individuals existed when essentialism was the ruling philosophy, because in essentialism a class consists of members all of whom are in principle identical, whereas in a Darwinian population every individual is unique, and gradual evolution is the result of the changing composition of populations from generation to generation. Because all evolution takes place through the change of populations, all evolution by necessity is gradual. Darwinian evolution is a strictly antiessentialistic concept.

Can the concept *population* be employed in neurobiology? How similar to Darwinian populations are neuronal groups? Are neuronal groups unique, and if so, why? To what extent, if at all, are they composed of unique neurons? These and similar questions must be asked by the neurologist if he wants to use the term *population*. This much is certain, there cannot be any neuronal selection if there is not at least a considerable amount of variation.

Variation, in the case of organic evolution, is produced by mutation and genetic recombination. What are the corresponding causal factors responsible for neuronal variation? Indeed, how much neuronal variation is there? Furthermore, how much (if any) of this variation is genetically controlled and how much of it is acquired during differentiation? These are the questions the neurophysiologist is asking.

What is of special interest to Edelman is how variation is acquired during differentiation. Each neuron is potentially affected by the vicinity of other neurons and affected by the establishment of new patterns of synapses. Furthermore, Edelman postulates that neurons respond to signals and that a positive response reinforces the capacity of this neuron to respond to this particular kind of signal. Here we come to the most crucial point of Edelman's theory. He posits that owing to the freedom in the response of the neurons, the subsequent change in the neuron is selectionist and not instructionist, as I understand it. As he realizes, this leaves many open questions. Why do certain neurons or neuronal groups respond to a given signal whereas others do not? Were they genetically different? Did they have an inherited propensity for transmitting certain signals?

The dendritic patterns of no two neurons are exactly the same in the finest details, which leads to the question: What part of this variation is merely developmental "noise" and what part is controlled by an innate propensity for such a development? A nonspecialist like myself is perplexed by the unerring directness by which certain neurons seem to go to certain target tissues and at the same time the remarkable adaptability of neuronal groups as revealed by transplantation experiments. How can we ever determine what part of the behavior of a neuron has a genetic component?

Variation, as I said, is the first step in selection. It is responsible for the populational structure of neuronal groups and of assemblages of neuronal groups. The study of the causes of neuronal variation is one of the most important and yet most difficult areas of neurophysiology.

But let me now turn from variation to the second component of this paradigm: selection. Here we are facing even greater difficulties. When Darwin understood that the survival of a few individuals in every generation was the mechanism that generated evolutionary change, he had to propose some technical term to characterize this process. Being well acquainted with the procedure of animal breeding, wherein the breeder selects certain individuals as the sires and dams to produce the next generation, Darwin chose the metaphor selection. He said nature selects the fittest individuals to produce the next generation. His critics at once attacked the formulation "nature selects," by claiming that this did not differ in any way from saying, "God selects." As much as Darwin defended himself against this insinuation, he was stuck with the word *selection*, which inevitably led to the question, "Who or what selects?"

This dilemma has stayed with the evolutionists right up to this day. For this reason, Alfred Russel Wallace, the codiscoverer of the principle of natural selection, suggested to Darwin to adopt instead Herbert Spencer's metaphor "the survival of the fittest." However, this term was criticized even more severely than the term natural selection, and even though a number of philosophers have now shown that this metaphor is not circular, it has not been possible to displace the term natural selection, even though, in some ways, survival of the fittest *is* a more realistic terminology. Ironically, while everybody became more or less reconciled to the term natural selection, and its use spread into history, literature, and almost any field of human thinking that deals with change, the evolutionists realized increasingly how misleading the term selection actually is. What is called selection is only an *a posteriori* designation of the fact that the progenitors of a new generation of animals or plants are the few survivors among the hundreds, or millions, of offspring produced by a set of parents.

Why do only so few (to be exact, on the average, only two individuals of opposite sex) survive among the enormous number of offspring of the parents? There are scores of reasons. Some were caught by a predator; some failed to find enough food and starved to death; some succumbed to diseases; and some failed to find a mate, to mention only some of the more prominent causes. The reason I bother you with all this detail is that I want to make a very specific and important point: there is no special selection force! In evolutionary biology we bracket together all the factors that prevent survival and successful reproduction and designate them as adverse selection. And this includes a lot of chance processes. Successful survival then is simply not to have succumbed to the multitude of biotic and abiotic factors that prevented the survival of your brothers and sisters.

I hope I have made it clear to you how basically inappropriate the term selection really is in evolutionary biology, and this forces me, in the case of neuronal selection, to question what it means to say a neuronal group is selected: Who or what is doing any selecting? Does selection mean being targeted by signals? Were certain neurons preadapted to respond preferentially to certain signals? Are only some, many, or all neurons of a neuronal group preadapted similarly? If there are different sets of preadaptations, to what extent do these differences have a genetic basis? These are only a few of the numerous questions one must ask about neuronal selection. To judge from the literature seen by me, it is too early to answer most of these questions. Yet to pose such questions, and to attempt to answer them, is actually the best way to advance our understanding. If I had to make a guess, my answer, in the case of neuronal selection, would be the same as that in the case of evolutionary selection, that is, the word *selection* simply means biased survival. However, in the case of neurons it is not a survival in the literal sense, but rather a survival in the service of a particular function, of a particular performance. If one wanted to use a perhaps more neutral term one would not say they had been selected but simply that they are the ones that had prevailed.

Let me take a short aside with respect to the term *degenerate neurons.* J. Z. Young and Victor Hamburger have stressed the redundancy of neuronal networks and I am a little puzzled why Edelman does not accept their term *redundant* and instead uses degenerate. I did not succeed in understanding this explanation. The term *degenerate* comes from the field of mathematics and was introduced into biology in connection with the redundancy of the genetic code, called degeneracy by those who solved the problem of the genetic code. I never thought it was a happy terminology, because to anyone unaware of the background in mathematics, degenerate simply means pathological. Speaking of degenerate neurons means pathological neurons. Why not simply say redundant neurons? Is Edelman perhaps opposed to the term redundant because it was introduced into the literature in an instructionist context? Frankly, I do not feel that this would be a sufficient justification for such an unfortunate term.

Edelman's theory of neuronal group selection was, of course, not the first theory attempting to explain the development of the complexity of the central nervous system. However, says Edelman, all the earlier theories, including those of Hebb (1949), are instructionist whereas "my theory is selectionist." He explains the difference between the alternatives in "Neural Darwinism" (Edelman, 1987, particularly pp. 20 and 21). Not being a neurobiologist, I must confess, I did not fully understand the differences. I shall therefore not attempt to discuss them.

Most or all neuronal selection, if I understand Edelman correctly, takes place during ontogenetic development. In order to avoid equivocation, as far as possible, we must not only formulate precise definitions, but also sharp demarcations. This is more true for the demarcation between neuronal selection and ontogenetic differentiation than for any other terminological discrimination I have to deal with. And, frankly, I have not quite succeeded in achieving such a demarcation. Both processes involve sources of diversification that lead to variation. The entities in both processes interact with their cellular context as well as with other aspects of the internal and external environment. Up to this point, I cannot see any real demarcation between neuronal selection and ontogenetic differentiation. Edelman, however, postulates that neuronal selection "requires a means of differential amplification . . . of those variants in a population that have greater adaptive value." This is part of his neuronal selection theory, but it seems to me that the same is described by developmental biologists for processes of differentiation in nonneural tissues. In other words, I am not sure that even a single aspect of change in neuronal groups has so far been described that one could *not* simply ascribe to normal processes of differentiation taking place also in nonneural tissues. I wonder how Edelman would defend himself if someone would claim that all neuronal selection was nothing but a process of developmental differentiation? This question is an evident consequence of what I have said at the very beginning, which is that all technical terms we are using are potentially equivocal and we must make very clear at all times what, in a given context, the exact meaning of a term is.

Neuronal selection is a somatic process. It takes place within a single genotype. Even if neuronal selection should succeed in producing a very superior phenotype, it still would leave us with the great problem how to transmit this superior phenotype to the next generation. This cannot be done directly because, according to the unbreakable central dogma of molecular biology, no information of the proteins can be transferred back to the nucleic acids. The only solution I see is that natural selection can favor an individual that has a genotype with the propensity to be exceptionally susceptible to neuronal selection. In other words, no specifics in neural connections and synapses can be transmitted as such but only a propensity for certain developmental phenomena that lead to particularly well-adapted phenotypes. This hypothesis in turn leads to the further assumption that the propensity to be able to respond to signals must have a genetic basis. Furthermore, and this takes us right back to Darwinian thinking, there must be a premium on a high variability of developmental propensities among neuronal groups, and it is the differential survival, or perhaps one should say more simply the differential success, of such neuronal groups that can be translated into evolutionary change and ultimately and more specifically into the evolution of nervous systems with even greater complexity and even greater capacity.

I may not have firmly answered many questions, but I hope to have articulated more concisely the questions that the neurophysiologist should attempt to answer.

The first concerns the nature of neuronal variation: To what extent (if at all) do differences among neurons and neuronal groups have a genetic basis? Where such differences are acquired during ontogeny, the question is whether the difference is acquired by instruction, by selection, or by both.

The second question deals with the nature of selection: What is the exact nature of the process called by Edelman neuronal selection? Is it a process to be considered a normal part of embryonic differentiation or is it a process distinct from differentiation and perhaps superimposed on it? Is it a process that is clearly noninstructionist?

And finally, what is the relation between *neuronal* selection and *natural* selection? Because acquired properties of the phenotype, according to the central dogma of molecular biology, cannot be translated into the nucleic acids of a genotype, they cannot, as such, be inherited. However, a genetically based propensity of the genotype for phenotypic flexibility and for a capacity to respond to neuronal selection can indeed be selected for. In this case, what is selected is not the end product, the fully differentiated phenotype, but only the capacity of the genotype to produce such phenotypes.

References

Edelman, G. M. (1987). "Neural Darwinism: The Theory of Neuronal Group Section." Basic Books, New York.
Hebb, D. O. (1949). "The Organization of Behavior." Wiley, New York.

SELECTION AND THE ORIGIN OF INFORMATION

Manfred Eigen

Max Planck Institut für Biophysikalische Chemie
D-37077 Göttingen, Germany

The topic of this volume is selectionism and the brain; instead of trying to define selectionism, however, I will try to answer the question: What is selection? In fact, the title of my contribution should be "Selection as a Principle: How to Generate Information." Implicit in this title is the link between selection and the brain as an information-generating (and -processing) system.

I. What Is Information?

Before we can begin to define the nature and characteristics of selection we must first answer the question: What is information? Classical information theory, as pioneered by Shannon (Shannon and Weaver, 1949), links information to the concept of entropy. Entropy is derived from the probability distribution of a set of system states. Such system states, for example, can be combinations of nucleotides forming genes, or combinations of genes forming a genome. Each system state i occurs with a certain probability p_i. The quantity H (the letter was chosen in reference to Boltzmann's concept of entropy) is of positive sign and is often called "information" (Brillouin, 1962).

$$H = -K \sum_i p_i \log p_i \quad \text{with} \quad 0 \le p_i \le 1 \quad \text{and} \quad \sum_i p_i = 1$$

Figure 1 compiles the relations of this probabilistic concept of information. In fact, it would be more appropriate to call H an "information capacity." It does not refer to any individual state that can be associated with an information-carrying message, but rather to a weighted average

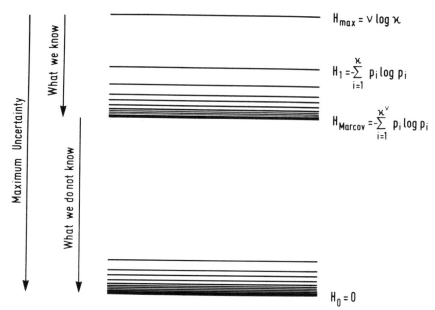

FIG. 1. Information as a quantitative measure of uncertainty. Given a sequence of length ν made of an alphabet of κ symbols, if all sequences are equally probable, the maximum uncertainty is $H_{max} = \nu \log \kappa$. For a binary alphabet ($\kappa = 2$ and $\log_2 2 = 1$), the required information is ν bits. If symbols appear with different probabilities (p_1, $p_2, \ldots, p_\kappa$), $0 \leqslant p_i \leqslant 1$, and $\sum_{i=1}^{\kappa} p_i = 1$, the required information is lowered to H_1. Any additional constraint (e.g., unequal probabilities of symbol combinations) lowers the Shannon entropy H, until (convergently) the Marcov entropy H_{Marcov} is reached, in which all sequences are weighted by individual probabilities. The difference $H_{max} - H_{Marcov}$ is what is known and H_{Marcov} is what we want to know in order to make a unique assignment of a given sequence of symbols. In Shannon's theory, H_{Marcov} essentially determines the limiting value to which the channel capacity has to be matched, in order to guarantee an error-free transmission of messages. In generating "information" we need an irreversible process that reduces H_{Marcov} to zero. The multitude of sequences allowed for by H_{Marcov} thereby is reduced to one unique sequence (or to a consensus sequence in a spectrum of mutants, characterized by a small uncertainty near $H_0 = 0$).

of the possible multitude of messages that could be combined from the the symbols involved. One therefore calls H a quantitative measure of information. It does not address any semantic aspect that we usually associate with the word information, nor does it refer to any evaluation of all the symbol combinations with respect to their possible usefulness.

In the framework of Shannon's theory, every individual state having a finite probability could represent information. The theory tells us what requirements—on average—have to be fulfilled in order to preserve any such defined state. It does not tell us anything about the quality of the information. This is adequate for communication in which the quality or semantic content of the exchanged messages does not matter. Therefore the theory, as Shannon has stated, should be called communication theory rather than information theory.

A defined stationary probability distribution exists only when a system is in some reproducible state of dynamic equilibrium, which also is a state of (locally) maximal entropy. At equilibrium, the system responds to small perturbations by returning to the equilibrated probability distribution. Therefore information cannot arise in systems at thermodynamic equilibrium. Typically, when being in a state of equilibrium, a system has lost all information about any individual state or states occurring before equilibrium was reached. How, then, does information, i.e., a state that involves semantic value, originate?

Information that refers to a given state i (e.g., a message containing semantic information) is connected with the question of representation: "to be or not to be." However, we relate this question often to another question, " to know or not to know," and thereby associate it with our brain, with our capacity of knowing, with the existence of knowledge about a certain state. In this context, information may mean how many binary decisions are necessary to identify a given state. Implicit in those decisions are semantic criteria that are hard to define quantitatively. Information in this respect has nothing to do with the state i as such, but rather with our knowledge about state i (which may be a microstate in an equilibrated distribution). The state as such does not represent information. Rather, our knowledge about the state represents information. How can we get away from this anthropomorphic aspect of information in order to be able to answer the question: How does information originate? After all, genetic information originated before brains came into existence.

One possible hint about how to generate information can be found in classical information theory. If the quantity H referring to a given probability distribution $P = (p_1, p_2, \ldots, p_N)$ is to be narrowed down to zero in order to identify a given state of maximum semantic value, one has to change the probability distribution in some irreversible way. Classical theory has defined the "gain of information" (δH) by substituting a distribution $P = (p_1, p_2, \ldots, p_N)$ by $P' = (p'_1, p'_2, \ldots, P'_N)$ as

$$\delta H = \sum_{i=1}^{N} p'_i \log p'_i / p_i$$

This quantity is always positive. In order to narrow down the information capacity one must in addition suppose that $H(P') < H(P)$, i.e., some introduction of additional constraints. However, as long as these are intrinsically associated with a new equilibrium state, P' and P refer again to our knowledge about the system. In other words, there is only generation of information in what we perceive, not in the system itself (cf. Fig. 1).

Classical statistical theory does not address the question of how to generate information, because it does not deal with how to get from one intrinsic probability distribution P to another probability distribution P'. Changes in probability distributions require irreversible dynamical events, such as bifurcations, instabilities, catastrophes, etc., and these events are not the subject of information theory. But they lead to the issue of "natural selection," which is an issue of nonlinear dynamic theory.

II. What Is Natural Selection?

Natural selection is a result of internal self-organization rather than of external interference, e.g., by some "selector." As such it has to be conceived as the reverse of equipartition or equilibration, requiring far-from-equilibrium conditions and some feedback enhancement as, for instance, effected by self- or complementary reproduction or by cyclic catalysis. In replicator systems two kinds of selection can be distinguished: (1) deterministic selection of the best adapted mutant, i.e., "survival of the fittest," and (2) random appearance of neutral mutants, i.e., "survival of the luckiest" (Kimura, 1983). In principle, a value scheme guiding selection can deal with both cases, as is shown below with the quasi-species model (Eigen *et al.*, 1988).

Natural selection is the basis of generation of information, the primary semantics of which is "to be or not to be." Information characterizes a complex system. Consider the case of genetic information. For any gene the number of possible alternative states is enormous. Given the four nucleotide bases, a sequence of 1000 nucleotides has $4^{1000} \approx 10^{600}$ possible states. Such a number is beyond our imagination. If we ask how many hydrogen atoms, densely packed, would fit into our universe (i.e., a sphere with a radius of about 10 billion light years), the answer is about 10^{107}. In fact, the total amount of matter in our universe is not much larger than 10^{81} hydrogen masses. Even a tiny fraction of all possible gene sequences of length 1000 by far outweighs the material reserves of our universe.

If we want to understand evolution from the point of view of changes in the sequences of nucleic acids, it is useful to define a sequence space that is adapted to the problem of complexity. In such a sequence space individual sequences (molecular states) occupy points, and evolution can be viewed as a trajectory linking such points, from an initial point that has very little information to a final point that has information related to a well-adapted function. A sequence space has to fulfill two requirements. First, it has to be composed of a sufficiently large number of cells or points, such that every possible sequence can be uniquely assigned to one and only one cell or point. Second, all points representing individual sequences have to be ordered such that the ordering correctly reflects the kinships (or similarities) between the sequences. For example, sequences differing in only one position must have a distance of 1. How to construct such a sequence space is shown in Fig. 2. One important property of such a sequence space is that the number of points increases exponentially with the length of the sequence, while, at the same time, the distance (the closest connection between two points) remains short. For a gene with 1000 nucleotides the number of points is $4^{1000} = 2^{2000}$, but the distance between any two sequences is no greater than 2000. (We have to keep in mind that the sequence space of genes is quarternary, i.e., there are four possible nucleotides at each position.)

Though faithful reproduction guarantees conservation of information, errors or mutations allow for a change (gain or loss) in the information content. Error-prone reproduction is a system property, which applies to every sequence of the system and defines an inherent autocatalytic trend. Reproduction causes selection and the generation of new information. If there were no variation within a population of individual sequences, these sequences would all occupy a single point in sequence space. This corresponds to the classical definition of the "wild type." However, if reproduction occurs with a certain (low) error rate (i.e., mutations are allowed), the population will occupy a more or less diffuse region distributed around a center of gravity that now defines the wild type. The wild-type sequence and its neighbors share a high degree of similarity (embodied by the consensus sequence), but are not identical and have slightly different fitness values. If, in an extreme case, reproduction would be occurring at random with no limit to the number of errors made at each step (i.e., the offspring of each sequence are other sequences produced essentially *de novo*), the entire sequence space would be filled. Such an "ideal gas" type of distribution corresponds to a state of minimal information.

III. The Quasi-Species Model

A distribution of sequences around a wild-type configuration is called a quasi-species. The quasi-species is usually characterized by a defined

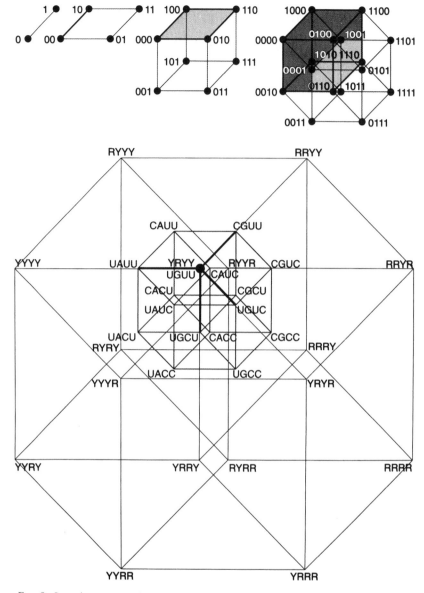

FIG. 2. Iterative construction of sequence space. Starting with one position (occupied by 0 or 1) of a binary sequence, positions are iteratively added, resulting in a doubling of the preceding diagram in which corresponding points are connected by lines. The binary sequence space is a hypercube, each corner representing one of the 2^ν possible binary sequences of length ν (ν is the number of binary symbols, 0 or 1, that comprise the total sequence). The lines connect nearest neighbors, i.e., mutants that differ in only one position. For nucleic acids the quaternary sequence space can be constructed by assigning first only purines (R) and pyrimidines (Y), yielding a binary hypercube. Each point represents one sequence in R and Y notations. Assigning for any sequence the two purines (A or G) and pyrimidines [U (T) or C] yields at each point of the binary R,Y hypercube another hypercube as subspace. This is shown in the lower diagram for the sequence YRYY.

consensus sequence. It nevertheless comprises a huge number of different individual sequences that might differ in quite a number of positions and that might show nearly neutral fitness values. This distribution is the target of selection. Quasi-species have been investigated experimentally by Charles Weissmann and his co-workers (Domingo *et al.*, 1987) as well as by our group, especially by Christof Biebricher (Eigen and Biebricher, 1988). Viruses are prominent examples of quasi-species (Eigen, 1993).

Mathematically, a quasi-species can be represented by an eigenvector that belongs to a maximal eigenvalue. Physically, a quasi-species is a localized population distribution in sequence space that forms and dissolves by phase transitions. Chemically, it is a huge multitude of different but related macromolecules with one or several degenerate consensus sequences.

As we have already mentioned, evolution is guided by a fitness landscape in which the peaks and ridges are densely populated, while valleys and planes are avoided. An error threshold determines the stability of the population distribution centered around the consensus sequence. It acts like a melting or boiling point, above which the population becomes unstable and disintegrates. Evolution can be understood as a punctuated evaporation and condensation of information in sequence space that is shaped by a fitness landscape. There is a relationship between the error rate and the information content of the sequence. A distribution is stable only if the error rate lies below a certain threshold value that is inversely proportional to the number of information-bearing symbols in the sequence. As a consequence, the longer a sequence, the more accurate its reproduction must be; otherwise errors accumulate in successive generations and the original information is lost. For example, the genome of the $Q\beta$ virus contains 4200 symbols and its error rate *in vivo* is about 3×10^{-4}. It turns out that many viruses have mutation rates that are six orders of magnitude higher than for autonomous microorganisms (e.g., bacteria). It is established that these viruses operate very close to their error threshold, keeping the system as a whole stable while attaining the highest possible rate of evolution and flexibility to changes in the environment. (examples are to be found in Table I). Typically, the wild type is contained only at low concentration, but we see many mutants at fairly large distances in sequence space (such as 10- or 15-error mutants). These mutants are almost as well adapted as the wild type and they populate the periphery of the population distribution forming the quasi-species. If environmental conditions change, one of these mutants may gain a selective advantage over the previously dominant sequence. As a result, the original wild-type distribution collapses while a new population

TABLE I

ERROR RATES OF VIRUSES AS COMPARED TO AUTONOMOUS ORGANISMS[a]

Virus/organism	Genome size n (number of bases or base pairs)	Error rate $1 - q$ (per replication round and per base)	Error rate $n(1 - q)$ (per replication round and per genome)
RNA			
Bacteriophage Qβ	4200	3×10^{-4}	1.3
Polio-1 virus	7400	3×10^{-5}	0.2
Vesicular stomatitis virus	11,000	1×10^{-4}	1.1
Foot and mouth disease virus	8400	1×10^{-4}	0.8
Influenza A virus	14,000	6×10^{-5}	0.8
Sendai virus	15,000	3×10^{-5}	0.5
HIV-1 (AIDS virus)	10,000	1×10^{-4}	1.0
Avian myeloblastosis virus	7000	5×10^{-5}	0.4
DNA			
Bacteriophage M13	6400	7×10^{-7}	4.6×10^{-3}
Bacteriophage λ	48,500	8×10^{-8}	3.8×10^{-3}
Bacteriophage T$_4$	166,000	2×10^{-8}	3.3×10^{-3}
Escherichia coli	4.7 million	7×10^{-10}	3.3×10^{-3}
Yeast (*Saccharomyces cerevisiae*)	13.8 million	3×10^{-10}	3.8×10^{-3}
Neurospora crassa	41.9 million	1×10^{-10}	4.2×10^{-3}
Human	3 billion	$\sim 10^{-12}$	$\sim 3 \times 10^{-3}$

[a] Critical error rate: logarithm of average superiority/number of nucleotides in genome. Here q is the fidelity of replication per nucleotide, i.e., the (normalized) probability for inclusion of the correct (complementary) nucleotide; $1 - q$ then is the error rate per nucleotide and per replication round. There is an error threshold relation (Eigen *et al.*, 1988) according to which the product $n(1 - q)$ has to remain below a threshold value, ln σ, where σ rates the fitness of the best adapted mutant relative to its competitors in the quasi-species. For RNA viruses, σ is sufficiently larger than one as to yield ln $\sigma \approx 1$, whereas for DNA genomes of autonomous organisms, σ is only slightly larger than one as to yield ln $\sigma \approx 10^{-2}-10^{-3}$.

builds up around the selected mutant. This results in a kind of punctuated motion in sequence space, in which populations "evaporate" and "condense," sometimes moving over fairly long distances. Such processes have been observed in populations of RNA molecules studied by Biebricher (1987). So far we have stated that information originates by selection and that selection is based on reproduction. But what is meant by reproduction? Different mechanisms of reproduction can be distinguished, depending on the nature of the system under consideration. There is self-reproduction, as in the mechanism of semiconservative replication of DNA molecules. There is complementary reproduction, as in template-instructed RNA replication. And there may be cyclic reproduction, as in a cycle of enzyme-catalyzed reactions (cf. Fig. 3). In general, mechanisms of reproduction require feedback and cyclicity. An example that has been studied experimentally (Eigen *et al.*, 1991) is represented in Fig. 4. It involves both replication and translation. We call such a system a "hypercycle" (Eigen and Schuster, 1979). It involves a feedback loop that is superimposed to the replication cycle and that allows for a selective evolution of translation products. The genotype–phenotype dichotomy in information-generating systems requires reaction networks such as that represented by the hypercycle (Eigen *et al.*, 1991).

IV. Generalization and Conclusion

There are several types of information-generating systems in biology. Genetic information is generated by selection based on the replication of nucleic acid molecules involving a certain error rate. In the differentiation of cells during development we have cell reproduction involving a regulation of expression and guidance by an internal microenvironment (which is fixed unless subject to perturbation). In the immune system there is clonal selection, multiplication of cells, and fine-tuning through somatic mutations. Turning to the nervous system, we see that although individual mechanisms may differ from all the other cases, selection as a principle may well apply. The elementary processes of the nervous system include the firing of neurons (a threshold phenomenon) and the state-dependent tuning of synaptic connections (for example, according to Hebb's rule). Selection processes may involve groups of neurons connected by strong synaptic connections as well as feedback of activity in cyclic (perhaps reentrant) loops. The details of the neuronal processes and arrangements involved are dealt with in other chapters of this volume.

Our general question remains: How does information originate? More specifically, how is it generated in the case of the brain? When attempting to answer this question we must take into account that the human brain is a composite organ subserving many different tasks, including the mapping of the environment, the storage of information after evaluation, perception, motor activity, memory, learning, and thinking, to mention just a few. There are many open questions. What is the unit of information in the nervous system? How is the issue of information linked to the existence of neuronal groups and networks of such groups? What are the organizing principles of neuronal networks? If selection is based on reproduction, and the brain is a selective system,

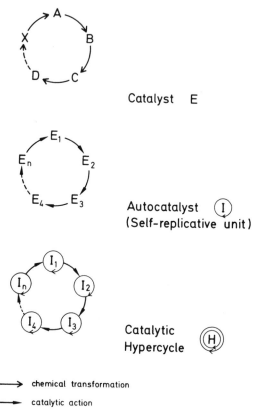

Catalyst   E

Autocatalyst (Ⓘ)
(Self-replicative unit)

Catalytic   Ⓗ
Hypercycle

⟶ chemical transformation

⟶ catalytic action

Fig. 3. Hierarchy of cyclic reaction networks. A catalytic (e.g., enzymatic) reaction represents the simplest reaction cycle. The catalyst and its intermediate states are preserved while substrates flow in and reaction products flow out of the system. Examples of multistep catalytic reactions are the Bethe–von Weizsäcker and the Krebs cycles, the latter including several enzymatic reactions. If the catalyst is not only preserved but also is produced by the catalytic cycle, we call it autocatalytic. Template-instructed RNA synthesis is a multistep autocatalytic reaction, where the template plus and minus strands play the role of autocatalysts. If, in addition, the polymerizing enzyme is produced in the cyclic network, we speak of a hypercycle. A typical hypercycle is shown in Fig. 4. It contains, in addition to the self-reproductive template cycle, a superimposed catalytic feedback loop.

then what does reproduction mean in the context of the nervous system? What are candidates for evaluation and reinforcement? We are only in the very beginning of finding answers to these questions. We know that neurons do not replicate; their numbers are relatively fixed during adult life. But if there is mutual enhancement of linked neurons (forming, for example, neuronal groups), any cyclic closure may define a "self-

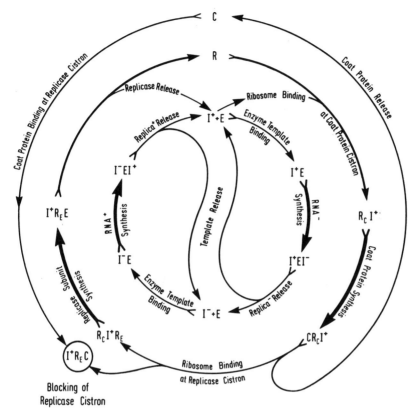

FIG. 4. Hypercyclic reaction scheme of the infection cycle of a bacterial plus-strand virus Qβ. I^+, RNA plus strand; I^-, RNA minus strand; E, replicating enzyme; C, coat protein; R, ribosome; $R_E I^+$, ribosome bound at replicase cistron of I^+; $R_C I^+$, ribosome bound at coat protein cistron of I^+; I^+E, I^-E, I^+EI^-, I^+R_EE, I^+R_EC, and $R_C I^+E$ are complexes among plus strands, minus strands (both being either template or replica), ribosomes, replicating enzyme, and coat proteins.

reproductive" firing unit. This self-reproductive unit may represent a "template," but not in the sense that it leads to multiplication of such circuits (e.g., groups). There must be a property that can grow, analogous to population growth. This property may involve synaptic strength (i.e., quantity or quality of synaptic linkage). We know that synapses can change in strength and can grow and decompose. The phenotype of synaptic linkage in a cycle may be excitation or firing density (or coherence of firing). Competition may be introduced by limitation of synaptic growth and inhibition. Finally, mutation may correspond to modifications (either structural or dynamic) within such cycles.

Finding answers to these and similar questions will be necessary in order to establish the physical foundation of "neural Darwinism."

References

Biebricher, C. K. (1987). "Replication and evolution of short-chained RNA species replicated by Qβ replicase. *Cold Spring Harbor Symp. Quant. Biol.* **52,** 299–306.

Brilluoin, L. (1962). "Science and Information Theory," 2nd ed. Academic Press, New York.

Domingo, E., Sabo, D., Taniguchi, T., and Weissmann, C. (1987). Nucleotide sequence heterogeneity of an RNA phage population. *Cell (Cambridge, Mass.)* **13,** 735–744.

Eigen, M. (1993). Viral quasispecies. *Sci. Am.* **269**(1), 42–49.

Eigen, M., Biebricher, C. K., Gebinoga, M., and Gardiner, W. C. (1991). The hypercycle. Coupling of RNA and protein biosynthesis in the infection cycle of an RNA bacteriophage. *Biochemistry* **30,** 11005–11018.

Eigen, M., and Schuster, P. (1979). "The Hypercycle—A Principle of Natural Self-Organization." Springer-Verlag, Berlin and New York.

Eigen, M., McCaskill, J., and Schuster, P. (1988). Molecular quasi-species. *J. Phys. Chem.* **92,** 6881–6891.

Eigen, M., Biebricher, C. K., Gebinoga, M., and Gardiner, W. C. (1991). The hypercycle. Coupling of RNA and protein biosynthesis in the infection cycle of an RNA bacteriophage. *Biochemistry* **30,** 11005–11018.

Kimura, M. (1983). "The Neutral Theory of Molecular Evolution." Cambridge Univ. Press, Cambridge, UK.

Shannon, C. E., and Weaver, W. (1949). "The Mathematical Theory of Communication." Univ. of Illinois Press, Urbana.

SECTION I

DISCUSSION

Several key issues were raised in these first three contributions, including the relationship between self-organization and selection, the nature of differential amplification, the notion of degeneracy, and the connection between natural and neural selection.

A first issue concerns the respective roles of *self-organization and selection* in the development and functioning of the brain. Some systems, such as the polynucleotide sequences considered by Eigen, are composed of elements that are able to vary in relative independence one from another. This means that, given sufficient time, all possible arrangements of these components could be generated, at least in principle. Thus, when Eigen finds that, under *in vitro* conditions enforcing some fitness criterion, polynucleotide sequences cluster around a fitness peak, he can conclude that this clustering is due to the action of selective forces.

More commonly, however, one must deal with complex systems composed of heterogeneous, mutually interacting elements. In these, alterations in any one element may preclude or require particular changes in another element. These constraints on changes within the system arising from interactions among system elements may limit the number and kind of variants that could be generated and on which selection can act. The resulting "spontaneous" emergence of order is often considered to be the hallmark of a self-organizing process. The development of a biological organism from a fertilized egg, requiring a particularly highly constrained series of changes provides a striking example of such a process (referred to by Mayr as transformational evolution).

Self-organizing properties may be sufficient to explain the development of an organ such as the liver, or even of an entire simple organism, such as *Caenorhabditis elegans;* in these cases, random variations may be considered as useless and potentially damaging noise, and selective processes may not play any apparent role. The question asked by Mayr is whether the development and functioning of the vertebrate nervous system should be interpreted, not unlike the liver, exclusively in terms of self-organization, or whether neural function is crucially dependent, as in the case of Eigen's quasi-species, on processes of random variation, selection, and differential amplification. The answer to this question lies in the realization that the brain, like the immune system but unlike the liver or any other organ of the body, has evolved to help animals deal with novelty and with signals that change far faster than can be anticipated by organismal evolution. As Sporns points out, the nervous

47

system requires a mechanism that allows it to incorporate novel and unpredictable environmental signals into specific anatomical and physiologic changes. This is demonstrated, for example, by the place-dependent development of functional specialization, which adds to the extreme functional heterogeneity of the brain and clearly sets it apart from other organs of the body.

Thus, although many features of the development of the brain, especially at a macroscopic spatial and temporal scale, are governed by evolutionarily constrained processes of self-organization, the detailed connectivity among its neural elements is relatively unconstrained genetically and developmentally. This is not just because there is an unavoidable degree of noise, but precisely because, if such connectivity were fixed, it could not adapt rapidly enough to a world full of novelty and change. And indeed, as we will see in Section II of this volume, a great deal of evidence has now accumulated suggesting that it is the patterns of neural activity selected by encounters of sensory organs with the world that act to prune, strengthen, and differentially amplify that connectivity to shape the adaptive responses of the overall system. This constant structural and functional reshaping of the brain through the interaction with the environment is the essence of both memory and adaptation.

It has been repeatedly emphasized that the three key requirements that allow the brain, as any other selectionist system, to adapt to an unpredictable environment are an independent source of variation, a way to sample environmental signals, and mechanisms of differential amplification. As discussed in the chapter by Sporns and in Section II of this volume, enormous microscopic diversity arises inevitably in the brain because of the epigenetic and stochastic nature of many developmental processes. It is also clear that the nervous system is ideally poised to sample signals from the environment. A more complex issue concerns what processes would correspond to *differential amplification,* a point taken up particularly by Eigen. In the case of natural selection, a phenotype that happens to be more fit than another with respect to a given environment enjoys higher reproductive success. As a result, the characteristics leading to the fitter phenotype that are inheritable will increase their relative frequency in a population, i.e., they will be differentially amplified.

In the brain, the mechanism subserving differential amplification is not, in most cases, differential reproduction. There are other mechanisms, however, that can provide for differential amplification. Certain patterns of activity will happen to match a given input better than others. To obtain differential amplification, it is sufficient that some mechanisms exist that increase the likelihood and specificity of those activity patterns that match or fit best. The key theoretical requirement, in other words, is that such patterns of activity show an increase in autocorrelation, over a time series, that cannot be accounted for by chance alone. The mechanisms giving rise to differential amplification can be instantiated in a variety of different ways. There can be modifications in the number and location of synapses, in their pre- or postsynaptic efficacy, in the availability and activity of neuromodulators, transmitters, receptors, and second and third messengers, or in a combination of all these factors. An indication that mechanisms leading to the differential amplification of frequent and specific responses are at work in the brain is the ubiquitous anatomical evidence for grouping and segregation of axonal terminals and the physiological evidence for functional specialization. In fact, mechanisms whereby correlated inputs concentrate into local patches of synapses and segregate from less correlated inputs will in general lead to stronger and more specific responses.

Another important question is: what is the *target of selection* in the brain? This has long been a key question, although a rather controversial one, in natural selection. Though many different levels of selection have been suggested or emphasized, there seems to be a general consensus that a crucial level in natural selection is that of the phenotype of the individual animal. As Sporns discusses in his chapter, there are many different levels at which selectional mechanisms can act in the brain. One central level of selection in the brain is that of neuronal groups, collections of tens to thousands of neurons that are strongly interconnected locally and that interact cooperatively in determining the magnitude and direction of local synaptic changes. But neuronal groups do not in general function as independent individuals. In particular, the abundant reentrant interactions among neuronal groups ensure that the sampling of signals leading to differential amplification will not just be local. The ability of reentrant circuits to engage in cooperative interactions within and across areas allows selective events to take place across many different spatial and temporal scales. Taking into account this high degree of connectivity and cooperativity, the targets of selection in brain function appear to be distributed activity patterns of neuronal groups and their sensorimotor correlates (e.g., components of gestural motion). The most immediate results of selection are differential changes in the population distribution of these patterns such that some patterns will occur more frequently than others.

A further point mentioned by Mayr concerns the concept of *degeneracy*. This is a term initially used in geometry and quantum theory, and applied to the genetic code. It was subsequently applied to the brain to indicate functional equivalence despite structural difference. Mayr seems to suggest that the term *redundancy* might be a better choice. Regardless of terminological preferences, it is essential to understand that although different structures, say neuronal groups, may be isofunctional in one context or domain (degeneracy), there will always be some other context or domain in which they will behave differently, i.e., they will not be isofunctional. By contrast, identical (redundant) groups will always perform identically. Given the novelty and unpredictability of the environment, this distinction becomes fundamental for a selective system. Redundancy would leave no room for novelty and new adaptations, whereas degeneracy would.

A final issue, raised especially by Mayr, concerns the *relationship between neural and natural selection.* This is a complex and interesting topic that deserves at least a few comments. If neuronal selection plays a central role in shaping brain functions, it is most likely that, as Mayr points out, its basic mechanisms have been developed and refined during natural selection.

Selectionist mechanisms of local synaptic change that lead to an increased likelihood and specificity of neuronal response to particular signals are present, although with several variations, from invertebrates up to man. As pointed out by Sporns, however, such local mechanisms would not be sufficient to guarantee the convergence toward integrated behavioral patterns that are adaptive in the evolutionary sense. Another selectional mechanism, called *value-dependent learning,* has evolved to allow local synaptic changes to be modulated by global modulatory signals reflecting events of evolutionary significance. Natural selection has endowed certain organisms with several means to sense the adaptive value of their behavior. As discussed by Sporns, evidence suggests that value can be reflected in the activity of specific neural structures. These neural value systems can selectively increase the probability of adaptive behaviors by modulating synaptic changes in the circuits relevant to those behaviors. Neuromodulatory systems in the brain, such as the monoaminergic or cholinergic systems, are well suited to carry out this process. They can respond transiently to cues that are evolutionarily important (innate value), or that have acquired importance during experience (acquired value); they broadcast their responses to widely distributed areas of the brain through diffuse projections; finally, they can release substances that modulate neuronal activity as well as changes in synaptic strength. Thus, although evolutionary processes cannot select directly for valuable neuronal responses, they can nonetheless select for several mechanisms that efficiently subserve and constrain neuronal selection in somatic time.

SECTION II

DEVELOPMENT AND
NEURONAL POPULATIONS

The three chapters in this section highlight the role of development in shaping adult morphology and function. The authors address several key issues, among them the interplay between genetic and epigenetic processes during morphogenesis, the emergence of structural variability, the highly dynamic and cooperative nature of processes occurring during motor development and its selectional character, and the evidence for the involvement of populations of motor cortical neurons in various aspects of adult motor function.

As Crossin points out in her chapter, the view that developmental events are genetically coded is too narrow. Though genes and gene products provide important constraints on how cells behave during development, there is an important additional component: epigenetic processes. The time and place of many developmental events are epigenetically controlled. Particularly important are the formation of cell collectives and their mutual interactions, as well as their interaction with the extracellular environment. Adhesion molecules are gene products that play an important epigenetic role in morphogenesis and morphoregulation. They form a molecular link between mechanical events in the formation of cell collectives and subsequent changes in gene expression, which in turn change the way cell collectives behave. Crossin cites evidence for the morphoregulatory role of various classes of adhesion molecules and outlines recent findings concerning their genetic control.

Thelen and Corbetta remind us that development does not stop with embryogenesis and does not only involve the generation of appropriate morphological structures; the acquisition of adequate sensorimotor functions is a process that takes up much of early childhood and adolescence. Indeed, motor plasticity is retained throughout adult life. As in morphogenesis, motor development is epigenetic. It depends critically on active exploration of the environment by the organism and selection of appropriate behavioral acts. Thelen and Corbetta propose a dynamic systems approach to sensorimotor development based on the dual assumptions that patterns of motor coordination are not symbolically represented or stored anywhere in the nervous system and that motor systems exhibit behavior similar to "nonlinear systems" exhibiting attractor states. The conceptual shift leads away from static "instructional" motor patterns and programs to a view of motor development cast in the language of dynamical systems theory. Thelen and Corbetta present data on the acquisition of motor skills from several human infants that shows the highly individual nature of this process. Different individuals employ quite distinct strategies during skill acquisition, a finding consistent with the operation of selection on variation.

Georgopoulos demonstrates that during mature motor function important spatial characteristics of arm movements are specified by populations of motor cortical neurons acting together. The direction of three-dimensional reaching movements is uniquely specified by the coordinated activity of a population of individually broadly directionally tuned cells. Strikingly, the population vector extracted from the activity pattern of these neurons shows a "rotation" if the task requires a movement rotated 90° away from a reference direction. Georgopoulos argues that the observed rotation of the population vector forms the physiological correlate of the cognitive phenomenon of mental rotation. In the various tasks studied the cooperative and coordinated activity of many cells is required to define adequately critical spatial parameters of reaching movements. This work serves as a key example of population approaches to brain function.

MORPHOREGULATORY MOLECULES AND SELECTIONAL DYNAMICS DURING DEVELOPMENT

Kathryn L. Crossin

Department of Neurobiology
The Scripps Research Institute
La Jolla, California 92037

I. Introduction

The question of how the form of an organism arises from a single cell, the fertilized egg, is one that has challenged biologists ever since Hippocrates and Aristotle examined chicken embryos. After genetics was linked to natural selection, during the modern synthesis (Mayr, 1982), developmental biologists were still faced with the question of how genes actually affect animal shape and thereby generate phenotypes on which natural selection could act. It is clear that development contributes an important constraint on evolution and also that natural selection acts at developmental stages as well as it does later in the life cycle and in the adult organism.

The problem of relating gene control to the generation of animal phenotype has been posed in the form of two questions by Gerald Edelman in his book "Topobiology" (1988). The first question is the developmental genetic question: How does the one-dimensional genetic code specify a three-dimensional animal? The second and related question is the evolutionary question: How may the answer to the developmental genetic question be reconciled with large morphogenetic changes that occur over rather short evolutionary times? The latter morphological

53

question is particularly critical with regard to the evolution of the brain as Rakic (1988) has discussed, considering that the primate cortex has undergone enormous changes in less than 2 million years.

What is the nature of the problem raised by these questions? The genetic code can control only the production of specific mRNAs and proteins. Actual developmental processes are cellular in nature, and they are epigenetic. Genes do not specify the exact position of any given cell in time and space, but clearly the properties of a cell are constrained by the gene products that it expresses, by interactions with its neighboring cells, and by interactions with various extracellular matrix proteins, growth factors, and hormones.

Important insights as to the kinds of genes that may be important in these selectional events may be found by considering the primary cellular processes of development (Needham, 1933), including cell division, cell motion, and cell death, together with cell adhesion, differentiation, and embryonic induction. Cell adhesion is a pivotal process for a number of reasons. First, the mechanisms by which cells recognize and adhere to each other must have evolved prior to the emergence of metazoans, and, second, molecules that mediate cell adhesion clearly serve to regulate mechanical processes that occur among the cells. Among the primary processes of development, the formation of cell collectives and the migration of cells are key events leading to morphogenesis. Finally, such collectives of cells can more readily undergo further changes involving the exchange of signals that lead to inductive or differentiation processes. A good example in brain development is the emergence of particular kinds of maps and the ordering of those maps.

The complexity and connectivity of the mammalian brain have caused many to postulate that its development is dependent on the expression of very large numbers of molecular recognition markers (e.g., Sperry, 1963), much like assembling the interlocking pieces of a jigsaw puzzle. A large body of evidence accumulated over the past 10 years suggests that, in contrast to this aspect of the chemoaffinity hypothesis (Sperry, 1963), much of neural structure depends on the dynamic and differential expression of a relatively limited number (tens to hundreds) of different adhesion molecules that mediate neuron–neuron and neuron–glia adhesion as well as neurite fasciculation and nerve guidance (for reviews see Edelman and Crossin, 1991; Takeichi, 1990).

The gene products that serve to link cell adhesion and cell motion to the other primary processes of development have been designated morphoregulatory molecules (Edelman, 1984, 1988, 1992). These include three types of adhesion molecules: cell–cell adhesion molecules (CAMs), which are membrane proteins in one cell that bind to those in another cell; cell–substratum adhesion molecules (SAMs), which form the extracellular matrix and can be bound by various cell surface receptors; and cell junctional molecules (CJMs), which link cells together at specialized sites, some of which allow the exchange of small molecules between cells.

These morphoregulatory proteins control a variety of mechanical events among interacting cells that lead to the generation of cell collectives. The formation of those collectives via such gene products leads to signals back to the genome that affect the expression of the same or other morphoregulatory genes and possibly historegulatory genes, giving rise to the differentiation of various tissues. The critical component of such a scheme is that it is dynamic and regulative, in contrast to a Lego toy or puzzle type of model for development, in which each particular cell knows who its neighbors are and where exactly it belongs in the embryo. The experimental problems that this scheme poses are to understand (1) the chemistry of the morphoregulatory molecules, (2) the control of their expression at the gene level, (3) their effects on cells, (4) how those cells are bound into collectives, and (5) how the signals from the cell collective feed back to new signals in the genome. As I shall consider in the summary at the end of this paper, these mechanisms contribute to the interplay between constancy and variation that is essential to a selectional mechanism for generating neuroanatomy.

To consider some approaches to these problems, I will briefly review the structure, genetics, and binding properties of various cell adhesion molecules, show some examples of the place-dependent expression of these various proteins, particularly with relation to borders in the developing embryo and its nervous system, show how the perturbation of these various kinds of molecules can lead to changes in morphology, and finally discuss the kinds of regulatory genes that affect the expression of adhesion molecules.

II. CAMs: Structure, Genetics, and Binding

The number of characterized cell adhesion molecules has continued to increase since the first adhesion molecule was described in detail over 10 years ago (Hoffman *et al.*, 1982), and by 1991, the number of reports on cell adhesion was growing exponentially (Edelman and Crossin, 1991). Most CAMs that have been found so far fall into three general classes. The first is a class related to the neural cell adhesion molecule (N-CAM), the members of which all have homology to the immunoglobulin superfamily (Williams and Barclay, 1988). In general, their binding is homophilic and calcium independent. In contrast, members of a large class of calcium- dependent CAMs, which have been termed cadherins (Takeichi, 1990), have internal homologies to one another but are not homologous to immunoglobulin or to any other known adhesion proteins. A third class of adhesion proteins, the selectins, appears to function primarily in the immune system and will not be discussed further here.

Members of the Ig superfamily and the cadherin family are expressed in the nervous system (Table I); some appear to be exclusive to the nervous system, such as the neuron–glia CAM (Ng-CAM) and L1, whereas others are more ubiquitously expressed in many organ systems, such as N-CAM and N-cadherin. N-CAM has five immunoglobulin-like domains and two fibronectin type III-like domains (Cunningham *et al.*, 1987); it is found on both neurons and glial elements of the central and peripheral nervous systems. Amalgam is a *Drosophila* protein found in

TABLE I
NEURAL CELL ADHESION MOLECULES

N-CAM (immunoglobulin) superfamily (calcium independent)	Cadherin (calcium dependent)
N-CAM (Cunningham *et al.*, 1987)	N-cadherin (Takeichi, 1988)/A-CAM(Volk and Geiger, 1986)
	T-cadherin (Ranscht and Dours, 1989)
Ng-CAM (Burgoon *et al.*, 1991)	R-cadherin (Reichardt and Tomaselli, 1991)
Nr-CAM (Grumet *et al.*, 1991)	cadherins 4-11 (Suzuki *et al.*, 1991)
G4(Rathjen and Schachner, 1984)	
L1(Moos *et al.*, 1988)/NILE(Bock *et al.*, 1985)	
Contactin (Ranscht, 1988)/	
TAG-1 (Furley *et al.*, 1990)	
F11 (Brummendorf *et al.*, 1989)	
F3 (Gennarini *et al.*, 1989)	
axonin-1 (Zuellig *et al.*, 1991)	
P_0 (Lemke and Axel, 1985)	
MAG (Arquint *et al.*, 1987; Salzer *et al.*, 1987)	
fasciclin II (Harrelson and Goodman, 1988)	
neuroglian (Bieber *et al.*, 1989)	
amalgam (Seeger *et al.*, 1988)	

nervous tissue and in mesodermal derivatives (Seeger *et al.*, 1988), and MAG (Arquint *et al.*, 1987; Salzer *et al.*, 1987) and P_0 (Lemke and Axel, 1985) are glycoproteins isolated from myelin and found to be important in neuron–glial interactions. Each of these three molecules shows immunoglobulin homology but no fibronectin-like repeats. Among the N-CAM family are a number of CAMs that are restricted primarily to the nervous system and that may play important roles in its morphogenesis. They form two subfamilies of Ig-like CAMs that are more closely related to each other than to other members of the N-CAM family. All contain fibronectin-like homologies in addition to Ig homologies. One subfamily includes Ng-CAM (Burgoon *et al.*, 1991), L1 (Moos *et al.*, 1988), NILE (Bock *et al.*, 1985), G4 (Rathjen and Schachner, 1984), 8D9 antigen (Lagenaur and Lemmon, 1987), the newly discovered Nr-CAM (Grumet *et al.*, 1991), and the insect protein neuroglian (Bieber *et al.*, 1989). These proteins are highly homologous in their primary sequences and in their domain structure, but have the most significant similarity (up to 90% in some comparisons) in their cytoplasmic domains. The second subfamily includes Tag-1 (Furley *et al.*, 1990), axonin-1 (Zullig *et al.*, 1991), contactin (Ranscht, 1988), F11 (Brummendorf *et al.*, 1989), and F3 (Gennarini *et al.*, 1989). These molecules are not transmembrane proteins, but rather are attached to the membrane by phospholipid anchors.

A particularly attractive conclusion to emerge from the studies of cell adhesion, and one that may relate to the process of selection on the embryonically derived phenotype, is that of molecular parsimony. Adhesion molecules exhibit the phenomenon termed local cell surface modulation (Edelman, 1976), in which changes in the amount, chemical nature, or localization of particular molecules on cell surfaces can lead to highly nonlinear changes in their functions. This means that the action of a single kind of molecule can result in a multiplicity of states. For example, depending on modulatory chemical events, adhesion molecules can mediate adhesion more or less well, a phenomenon particularly well-documented in the case of N-CAM, in which the rate of binding is inversely proportional to the amount of α-2,8-linked polysialic acid attached to N-linked carbohydrate cores (Hoffman and Edelman, 1983). In fact, modulation may have important effects on neural pattern formation; in the cerebellum of the *staggerer* mouse mutant, which shows connectional abnormalities, the normal progression of N-CAM from a less adhesive form to a more adhesive one is significantly delayed (Edelman and Chuong, 1982).

A second significant aspect of CAMs is the evolutionary relationship they have revealed among molecules of the two main adhesion superfamilies. Homologs of both the immunoglobulin and cadherin classes of molecules now have been found in insects, which suggests that adhesion molecules have a long evolutionary history. Clearly an evolutionary precursor of N-CAM gave rise to all of the proteins in the immunoglobulin superfamily. Because Ig-like molecules exist in *Drosophila*, a genus that has no Ig-mediated immune system, it appears that a common evolutionary precursor gave rise to molecules involved in immune recognition and cell-to-cell adhesion (Edelman, 1987). The N-CAM-like molecules identified in *Drosophila* mediate cell adhesion, and mutations in their genes lead to distortions in nervous system development. The recent identification on neurons in *Aplysia* of an N-CAM-like molecule (Schacher *et al.*, 1990) that is down-regulated on stimulation and that may have a role in neural interactions during learning further reveals the dynamic aspects of the modulation of CAMs, as well as the fact that vertebrate CAMs are likely to have early evolutionary precursors.

III. Developmental Expression of Primary and Secondary CAMs

In the early chicken embryo, N-CAM and the Ca^{2+}-dependent L-CAM are expressed on all cells in the blastoderm and hence are termed primary CAMs (Thiery *et al.*, 1982; Crossin *et al.*, 1985). At the time of gastrulation, both CAMs are down-regulated as cells begin to migrate to form the three germ layers. Somewhat later, at neurulation, which is the first recognizable pattern-forming event for the nervous system, there is a very strong segregation of cells of the neural tube expressing high levels of N-CAM. These cells lose their L-CAM, whereas the adjacent cells in the somatic ectoderm show high levels of L-CAM and then begin to diminish their expression of N-CAM. These very striking borders between cells expressing different CAMs delineate tissues that ultimately will have quite a different fate.

Similar expression patterns are observed at various levels throughout development for a number of CAMs, particularly in the nervous system. N-CAM is expressed very early on the neurectoderm, and it continues to be expressed on neurons as they differentiate, as well as on neural crest cells as they develop into the peripheral nervous system (Thiery *et al.*, 1982). In contrast, the expression patterns of the neuron–glia CAM occur later in development as neurons begin to differentiate; it is therefore termed a secondary CAM (Thiery *et al.*, 1985). Ng-CAM is concerned with fasciculation of neurites. Its expression is very tightly correlated with a number of different developmental events. For example, Ng-CAM is expressed in the spinal cord as motor tracts begin to develop, somewhat later in the tectum, and at particular times in the development of other regions of the brain (Daniloff *et al.*, 1986a). This suggests that there is tight control of the expression of these molecules at the gene level and that there is a strong correlation between the expression of a variety of CAMs in the nervous system and the development of different neural regions.

IV. CAM-Mediated Cell Sorting

The idea that differential CAM expression may contribute to the formation of anatomical borders in the embryo is supported by several cellular transfection studies. The expression of adhesion molecules in cells that do not normally express them has confirmed that binding of N-CAM, L-CAM, and N-cadherin is homophilic. In addition, such studies have established a link between CAM expression, cell morphology, and the expression of cell junctions, thus linking the functions of two families of morphoregulatory molecules (Mege *et al.*, 1988). The expression of L-CAM or N-cadherin in S180 mouse sarcoma cells (which do not normally produce either of these CAMs) induced a phenotypic change in these cells from a fibroblastic to an epithelioid morphology. This alteration was accompanied by marked increases in the expression of adherens and gap junctions (Mege *et al.*, 1988; Matsuzaki *et al.*, 1990). Both cell types aggregated specifically through the expressed CAM, did not bind to each other, and, when mixed, they separated into distinct homogeneous collectives linked internally by gap junctions. In cells that were doubly transfected with cDNAs for L-CAM and N-cadherin, both molecules were active and accumulated at sites of cell contact.

Transfected cell lines were used to examine the ability of CAMs to allow cell sorting into distinct cell collectives (Friedlander *et al.*, 1989). CAM-transfected cells readily sorted from their untransfected counterparts, and L-CAM transfectants sorted from N-cadherin transfectants. Both of these results indicate that different CAM specificities are sufficient for cell sorting such as occurs, for example, in the segregation of somatic and neural ectoderm. More interestingly, however, was the finding that cells with different levels of the same CAM sorted from one another. This suggests that cell surface modulation leading to both qualitative and quantitative differences in the expression *in vivo* of a relatively small number of CAMs can lead to a large variety of patterns among cell collectives during tissue formation. As shown by experiments on chimeric molecules and molecules in which the cytoplasmic domain was truncated (Jaffe *et al.*, 1990; Nagafuchi and Takeichi, 1988), sorting events depend on interaction with the cytoskeleton.

V. SAMs in Neural Morphogenesis

CAMs play significant roles in embryogenesis and neural histogenesis by bringing cells together and by allowing for cell migration when they are down-regulated. Cell migration, and neurite outgrowth in the nervous system, are guided and constrained by a variety of substrate adhesion molecules. A pair of interactive extracellular matrix molecules, cytotactin (Grumet *et al.*, 1985) [also known as myotendinous antigen (Chiquet and Fambrough, 1984), tenascin (Chiquet-Ehrismann *et al.*, 1986), $Jl_{220/200}$ (Faissner *et al.*, 1988), or hexabrachion (Erickson and Iglesias, 1984) (reviewed in Erickson and Bourdon, 1989)] and a cytotactin-binding chondroitin sulfate proteoglycan called the cytotactin-binding (CTB) proteoglycan (Hoffman and Edelman, 1987), appear to play a role in neural development and neurite outgrowth.

Cytotactin is composed of several structurally related polypeptides (Grumet *et al.*, 1985) that arise from differential splicing of a single gene (Jones *et al.*, 1988, 1989). Sequence analysis of cytotactin cDNAs shows extensive similarity to genes specifying three other proteins (Jones *et al.*, 1988, 1989; Spring *et al.*, 1989). The 5' end encodes 13 epidermal growth factor (EGF)-like repeats; these are followed by 11 fibronectin type III repeats, three of which are included by differential splicing; the 3' end encodes a domain similar to the β and γ chains of fibrinogen and contains a putative calcium-binding site. These domains of the protein can be mapped onto its structure as seen in rotary-shadowed electron microscopic images. The molecule appears as a complex structure with six arms emanating from a central core. The central core is a highly disulfide-bonded region at the amino terminus of cytotactin. The arms are composed of EGF-like repeats and fibronectin type III repeats, with the region of fibrinogen homology forming the terminal knob seen at the end of each arm. In the nervous system, the molecule is made by glia but not neurons and is secreted into the extracellular space (Hoffman and Edelman, 1987; Grumet *et al.*, 1985; Hoffman *et al.*, 1988; Crossin *et al.*, 1989). It is made by various other cells in the body including smooth muscle cells and immature chondrocytes. Cytotactin binds CTB proteoglycan, which is synthesized by central nervous system neurons and, in various forms, also by nonneural cells elsewhere in the body. Cytotactin also binds fibronectin, and it also has been shown to bind directly to neurons and fibroblasts (Hoffman and Edelman, 1987; Hoffman *et al.*, 1988; Friedlander *et al.*, 1988). Cytotactin is involved in glia–neuron adhesion *in vitro* by a mechanism independent from Ng-CAM (Grumet *et al.*, 1985). Exposure to cytotactin causes neuronal and fibroblastic cells in culture to round up, and it also tends to inhibit cellular migration. In the presence of fibronectin, which generally supports cell flattening and migration, the effects of cytotactin are decreased (Friedlander *et al.*, 1988; Tan *et al.*, 1987); thus the two interactive molecules appear to have conjugate effects on cell behavior.

Cytotactin is notable because it appears in a series of cephalocaudal waves of expression during development (Crossin *et al.*, 1986). These waves may reflect temporal growth gradients that are an important part of morphogenesis. A particularly striking example of such a wave is seen in somites. In addition, a correlation between cytotactin and CTB proteoglycan expression occurs in each developing somite (Tan *et al.*, 1987), possibly affecting patterning events in the development of the peripheral nervous system.

Somites are segmental blocks of mesoderm appearing early in vertebrate animal development. They arise in development in craniocaudal sequence from the so-called segmental plate of mesoderm. After such segmentation, which appears to be correlated with N-CAM and N-cadherin expression (Duband *et al.*, 1987), cytotactin appears adjacent to the basement membrane of the posterior portion of each somite in a cephalocaudal sequence (Tan *et al.*, 1987). Somewhat later, a portion of each somite becomes mesenchymal, forming the sclerotome through which neural crest cells migrate. Migration of neural crest cells occurs only through the anterior part of the sclerotome. Neural crest cells that have down-regulated N-CAM and migrated on fibronectin paths enter this region of each somite; they will later reexpress N-CAM and form dorsal root ganglia.

At this time or just before, both fibronectin and CTB proteoglycan are present throughout the sclerotome. Cytotactin appears, however, only in the anterior portion, and after this remarkable segmented appearance, CTB proteoglycan decreases in the anterior half and is seen only in the posterior half; fibronectin remains distributed throughout. This modulated pattern arises even in the absence of neural crest cells. When a portion of the neural tube is removed very early, prior to the emigration of the crest cells, the expression of cytotactin and CTB proteoglycan is still restricted to the anterior and posterior halves of each somite. The concurrent finding that cytotactin alters neural crest shape and movement is consistent with the hypothesis that, in the anterior region of each somite, cytotactin causes cell surface modulation of neural crest cells and that this cytotactin together with its ligand, fibronectin, may differentially change the pattern of motion of these cells.

Clearly, this example suggests a complex regulatory sequence of patterned expression of CAMs and SAMs, showing definite correlation with cell function and distribution and the primary processes of development. The presence of a network of interactive SAMs (e.g., cytotactin, fibronectin, CTB proteoglycan) in different distributions is likely to be significant in the alteration of morphogenetic patterns. Further evidence for the importance of such molecules in CNS development will be discussed below with regard to the function of CAMs and SAMs in selectional aspects of tectal, cerebellar, and cerebral cortical development.

VI. CAMs and SAMs in Neural Development and Regeneration

Studies of a number of systems exemplify the idea that CAMs and cytotactin play dynamic morphogenetic roles, particularly with regard to cell and neurite movement. On disruption of morphology seen during regeneration after nerve injury and in genetic mutants, one observes concomitant changes in CAM and cytotactin expression (Rieger et al., 1986). Moreover, perturbation of CAM or cytotactin binding functions using antibodies resulted in perturbation of morphological development in the optic tectum of the frog (Fraser et al., 1984, 1988) and in in vitro cultures of the chick cerebellum (Chuong et al., 1987). Studies in the developing mouse cerebral cortex indicate the expression of SAMs is dependent on neural activity and that the presence of SAMs may affect the pattern of neurite outgrowth (Crossin et al., 1989). These studies are detailed below.

After establishment of the peripheral nervous system by neural crest cells, a process in which CAMs and SAMs play key roles (for review, see Sanes, 1989; Edelman and Crossin, 1991), these molecules are used again in later pattern formation. Because one may readily observe regenerative effects, and also because of the occurrence of defined interactions of different cell types (Schwann cells, neurons, muscles), structures in the periphery provide an excellent opportunity to test the notion that interactions of cells in different tissues regulate CAM and SAM expression. For example, N-CAM, Ng-CAM, and cytotactin are highly concentrated at nodes of Ranvier in adult peripheral nerve (Rieger et al., 1986). In contrast, unmyelinated axonal fibers are uniformly stained at low levels by specific antibodies to both CAMs, but not by antibodies to cytotactin. Moreover, a developmental analysis has suggested that the interaction between neurons and Schwann cells (which display N-CAM and Ng-CAM at their surfaces) may play a role in establishing the one-dimensional periodic pattern of nodes (Rieger *et al.*, 1986). These findings have led to the hypothesis that surface modulation of neuronal CAMs mediated by signals shared between neurons and glia, together with modulation of expression of glial-derived SAMs, may be necessary for establishing and maintaining the nodes of Ranvier.

Several studies have shown that disrupted morphology or altered morphogenesis can actually lead to changes in CAM and SAM modulation patterns. For example, perturbation *in vivo* of normal cell–cell interactions during degeneration and regeneration has been shown to result in alteration of CAM expression and distribution (Rieger *et al.*, 1985; Covault and Sanes, 1985; Daniloff *et al.*, 1986b). N-CAM is present at the neuromuscular junction of striated muscles but is absent from the rest of the surface of the myofibril (Rieger *et al.*, 1985). After cutting the sciatic nerve, the molecule appears diffusely at the cell surface and in the cytoplasm but returns to normal after regeneration (Rieger *et al.*, 1985; Covault and Sanes, 1985; Daniloff *et al.*, 1986b). These experiments indicate that early events related to regeneration are accompanied by altered CAM modulation. More recent experiments (Daniloff *et al.*, 1986b, 1989) show that both crushing and cutting a nerve have widespread effects on CAM and cytotactin expression, ranging from altered CAM expression in motor neurons of the spinal cord on the affected side to modulatory changes in N-CAM, Ng-CAM, and cytotactin within Schwann cells that are local to the lesion. Genetic perturbations of morphology also result in perturbation of CAM and SAM expression. In two dysmyelinating mutants, trembler and motor end-plate disease, the distribution patterns of N-CAM, Ng-CAM, and cytotactin were found to be disrupted in the myelinated fibers (Rieger *et al.*, 1986). Another study indicates that alterations in the amount of N-CAM are associated with a number of human myopathies (Walsh and Moore, 1985; reviewed in Crossin, 1991). This is in accord with the observations on alteration of CAM expression in muscle degeneration and regeneration.

An early example of the possible importance of CAMs in the formation of morphology required for the establishment of neuronal maps was provided by studies in which alterations were observed in the orderly mapping of the retina to the optic tectum *in vivo* when anti-N-CAM Fab' fragments were introduced into the tectum (Fraser *et al.*, 1984, 1988). In these experiments, antibodies to N-CAM were implanted into a particular point in the right half of the tectum in *Xenopus laevis* tadpoles. The antibodies diffused into the surrounding tissue, and the receptor fields in the left control side of the tectum were compared with the right side where the spike of antibodies to N-CAM was placed. In the treated tectum, the overall topology of the retinal–tectal projection was basically maintained, but the receptive fields were distorted and enlarged. The level of antibody was shown to diminish over time and the enlarged receptor fields returned to normal when this occurred. These results suggest that the formation of maps and their subsequent stabilization may be guided and constrained by the levels of CAMs present in the system.

An example that reveals correlated activities of CAMs and SAMs is seen in cellular migration of external granule cells in the developing cerebellum to form its layered cortical structure. In the developing cerebellum, external granule neurons send out neurites into the subjacent molecular layer and finally translocate on radial glial cells to form the internal granule layer. This process occurs *in vitro* in tissue slices and can be followed by labeling the granule cell with tritiated thymidine; the slice culture system can be perturbed by adding antibodies to various adhesion molecules. The granule cells express both N-CAM and Ng-CAM, and the radial glia synthesize and secrete cytotactin. Perturbation studies (Hoffman *et al.*, 1986; Chuong *et al.*, 1987) indicated that Fab' fragments of antibodies to N-CAM have only slight effects on the migration of external granule cells in cerebellar slices *in vitro*. In contrast, Fab' fragments of anti-Ng-CAM arrested most cells in the external granular layer, while Fab' fragments of anticytotactin arrested most cells in the molecular layer. Analyses of the time course combined with sequential addition of different antibodies in different orders showed that anti-Ng-CAM had a major effect in the early period of culture and a lesser effect in the second part of the culture period. Anticytotactin had essentially no effect at the earlier time but had major effects at a later period. This suggests that these molecules affect two temporally distinct processes of migration previously demonstrated in anatomical studies. The evidence suggests that Ng-CAM may play a role in both early and late events.

Correlation of these effects with the spatiotemporal expression of these different CAM and SAM molecules suggested a dynamic complementary scheme in which temporal expression, different binding roles, and different functional effects on interactions between neurons and Bergmann glia mediated by the CAM and SAM interactions are required for pattern formation in the cerebellar cortex. Inasmuch as each of these molecules appears in a sequence prior to these events, there must be a precise coregulation of signals for their expression as well as coordination of their different binding functions in affecting migration. This will be a fruitful topic for future studies, given the recent isolation of the promoter region of the genes for cytotactin (Jones *et al.*, 1990) and N-CAM (Hirsch *et al.*, 1990).

A final example illustrates the role of SAMs in forming borders during neural development and the potential regulation of their synthesis by neural activity. The developing mouse somatosensory cortex contains a highly structured area, called the barrel field, with a characteristic appearance (resembling stacked wine barrels) composed of axon-rich areas surrounded by cell-rich areas. This area represents the projection from the neurons of the vibrissa on the face of the mouse; the cortical pattern is dependent on this vibrissal input. Cytotactin and CTB proteoglycan are both enriched in the walls of each barrel in the barrel field from its earliest development (Crossin et al., 1989). Their expression in the barrel walls peaks at postnatal day 7 and by day 13 is uniform throughout, suggesting that the transient presence of these molecules is correlated with the critical period (Crossin et al., 1989; Jhaveri et al., 1991). Like the anatomical pattern, the pattern of molecular expression is dependent on peripheral input; when the input is removed by electrocauterization of the whisker follicle, the molecular pattern in the cortex is destroyed. Thus, activity of the thalamocortical axons plays a key role in establishing this molecular pattern, as previously demonstrated for the anatomical barrel pattern. Rather than establishing a prepattern, the coordinate expression of glial cytotactin and neural CTB proteoglycan may serve to facilitate neuronal migration on radial glia and may play a role in inhibiting dendrites of cortical interneurons from traversing these molecular boundaries into adjacent barrels. Recent experiments indicate that both cytotactin (Crossin et al., 1990; Faissner and Kruse, 1990) and CTB proteoglycan (Crossin et al., 1990) inhibit neurite outgrowth in a dose-dependent fashion in in vitro explant cultures and thus the presence of these molecules may serve similar functions in vivo by serving as barriers to neurite outgrowth. Such events serve as strong constraints in selectional events during neurogenesis.

VII. Regulation of Place-Dependent CAM and SAM Gene Expression

A clue to understanding the control of place-dependent expression of CAMs and SAMs has come from studies of the promoter regions of the DNA encoding morphoregulatory proteins. The promoter regions for cytotactin in chicken (Jones et al., 1990) and for N-CAM in mouse (Hirsch et al., 1990) and chicken (Jones et al., 1992b) have been identified and characterized. The morphological studies described above indicate that a number of local signals must affect the expression of CAMs and SAMs to account for their exquisite spatiotemporal regulation. What types of genes are responsible for determining the place-dependent expression of morphoregulatory molecules? It has been shown that there may be a link between the expression of CAM and SAM genes and that of homeobox-containing genes. Homeobox-containing genes were first described in *Drosophila* by means of mutational analysis; mutations in these genes lead to homeotic transformations. A particularly striking example of homeotic transformation was the antennapedia gene mutation, which resulted in a leg substituted in the place of the antenna in the adult fly. As the genes responsible for various homeotic mutant phenotypes were identified, they were shown to be expressed in a highly place-dependent fashion during *Drosophila* development. As these genes were characterized further it became clear that many of them encoded transcription factors containing the homeobox motif. The homeobox is a 183-nucleotide DNA segment that encodes a 61-amino acid protein region, called the homeodomain, which is a helix–turn–helix domain that resembles the DNA-binding regions of a variety of other DNA-binding proteins. In *Drosophila*, and more recently in mammalian systems, the products of homeobox-containing genes have been shown to have unique place-dependent expression at particular times during development. Many of these genes are found in the developing nervous system, where they may play a role in specifying the development of particular structures or specifying boundaries between different regions in the developing nervous system.

Recent analyses of the promoter regions for the genes encoding N-CAM and cytotactin have shown that they contain DNA sequences resembling sequences that are bound by proteins encoded by various homeobox-containing genes. Initial studies were therefore performed to determine whether the products of homeobox-containing genes could effect the expression of N-CAM and cytotactin *in vitro*. For N-CAM (Jones *et al.*, 1992a), it was found that two homeobox-containing genes, *Hox2.5* and *Hox2.4*, can differentially modulate the expression of the N-CAM gene in cotransfection experiments in NIH3T3 cells. These two genes appear to control N-CAM expression *in vitro* in a switchlike fashion, depending on the concentration of each of the two homeodomain proteins. The superexpression of *Hox2.5* activated the N-CAM promoter, whereas increasing amounts of *Hox2.4* mitigated the effect of *Hox2.5*. The effects of these two *Hox* genes were shown to be dependent on a 47-base pair DNA segment in the N-CAM promoter region that contained two potential homeodomain binding sites with TAAT motifs similar to such motifs in the promoter regions of other genes. Mutations in the homeobox sequence motifs abolish the effects of *Hox2.4* and *Hox2.5*.

Similarly, the cytotactin promoter was shown to contain DNA sequences that may be responsive to the products of homeobox-containing genes (Jones *et al.*, 1990). In cotransfection experiments, the activity of the cytotactin promoter was shown to be enhanced in the presence of the homeobox-containing gene *Evx-1* (Jones *et al.*, 1992b). The region of the cytotactin promoter responsible for this activation was shown to contain a TRE-AP1 motif. This motif is a DNA-binding region previously shown to be important in the binding of the products of the *fos* and *jun* gene family of transcription factors and in mediating responsiveness of a variety of genes to growth factor signals. This suggests possible coregulation of gene expression by homeobox-containing transcription factors and by transcription factors activated by the binding of growth factors to their cell surface receptors.

These preliminary experiments represent the first identification of potential targets of homeobox-containing genes in vertebrate animals other than that of other homeobox-containing genes. It will be particularly important to determine whether these various gene products regulate the activity of the N-CAM and cytotactin promoters *in vivo*. If some members of the classes of homeobox-containing gene products are actually found to regulate the expression of these morphoregulatory genes *in vivo*, these findings would provide at least part of an explanation for the place-dependent expression of cell and substrate adhesion molecules. In any case, they provide a framework for an exploration of the gene products that affect the expression of morphoregulatory molecules. Alterations of such signals *in vivo* and their relationship to the expression of the adhesion proteins will be particularly revealing to our understanding of how these various classes of proteins may work *in vivo* to facilitate morphogenesis. Conversely, an understanding of how adhesion systems subsequently feed back and change the expression patterns of various genes would also enhance our understanding of the coordinative role of cell adhesion in morphogenesis.

VIII. Summary and Perspectives: What Are the Implications for Selectional Events during Development?

There is now a well-established correlation between the function of morphoregulatory proteins and the emergence of tissue morphology. These expression patterns are dynamic and they are likely to be under the control of known pattern-forming genes such as *Hox* and *pax*, so we might think of this relationship as forming a loop (Fig. 1): i.e., that *Hox* and *pax* gene products bind to the promoter regions of CAM and SAM genes, which in turn affects the expression of these and possibly other

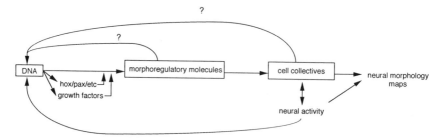

Fig. 1. Morphoregulatory loops involving DNA, the expression of morphoregulatory molecules, and the formation of cell collectives. The evidence to date suggests that growth factors as well as the products of certain *Hox* and *pax* genes can affect the expression of the DNA encoding morphoregulatory molecules. The expression of various morphoregulatory molecules then affects the formation of cell collectives, as well as allowing or inhibiting cell and neurite migration. The reciprocal coordination between cell collectives and neural activity leads to a variety of neural morphologies and to the formation of maps in the nervous system. What is still unknown in this type of morphoregulatory loop is how the formation of cell collectives or how the expression of morphoregulatory molecules feeds back to change the expression of particular kinds of DNA. Nevertheless, such a loop forms a perspective for further studies in understanding the contribution of pattern-forming genes to the formation of neural morphology and neural maps.

morphoregulatory molecules. The resulting cell collectives formed via CAM interactions presumably send signals back to the DNA, and again change the expression patterns of genes for other morphoregulatory proteins. Reiteration of these kinds of loops could serve to guide and constrain developing morphology. In the nervous system, it could lead to rich patterns of neural connectivity that can then be subjected to selection processes based on experience, as discussed by others in this volume.

The dynamic expression of morphoregulatory proteins in such loops of gene expression relates to pattern-forming genes, such as *Hox* and *pax*, and to other genes, such as those related to differentiation and those that are sensitive to neural activity. Such schemes are consistent with selectional modes of neuroanatomy (Changeux and Danchin, 1976; Edelman, 1978). Because of the highly interconnected nature of these loops of gene expression, they are both dynamic and epigenetic. Any variation in the environment, such as a change in neural activity or growth factor expression, could therefore lead to a change in morphology. Coordination of gene expression in such loops necessarily generates diversity, which in turn provides a substrate for selection. This type of scheme couples gene expression to molecular events that lead to changes in cellular interaction or signaling and impact on developing morphology. Constant adjustments involving gene expression and cellular interactions serve to connect a variety of signaling events to neural structure.

Clearly the kinds of gene products I have discussed here are candidates for linking the one-dimensional genetic code to three-dimensional animal form. Indeed, from the levels of control between *Hox* genes and the morphoregulatory proteins, one can imagine, however dimly, how events such as heterochrony in evolution might be viewed in molecular terms from the result of small changes in the timing of expression of the *Hox* genes or of their morphoregulatory molecule targets. This certainly has consequences in thinking both about natural selection on morphological phenotypes during evolution and about the constraints governing the selection of connections in the developing nervous system.

References

Arquint, M., Roder, J., Chia, L.-S., Down, J., Wilkinson, D., Bayley, H., Braun, P., and Dunn, R. (1987). Molecular cloning and primary structure of myelin-associated glycoprotein. *Proc. Natl. Acad. Sci. U.S.A.* **84**, 600–604.

Bieber, A. J., Snow, P. M., Hortsch, M., Patel, N. H., Jacobs, J. R., Traquina, Z. R., Schilling, J., and Goodman, C. S. (1989). *Drosophila* neuroglian: A member of the immunoglobulin superfamily with extensive homology to the vertebrate neural adhesion molecule L1. *Cell (Cambridge, Mass.)* **59**, 447–460.

Bock, E., Richter-Landsberg, C., Faissner, A., and Schachner, M. (1985). Demonstration of immunochemical identity between the nerve growth factor-inducible large external (NILE) glycoprotein and the cell adhesion molecule-L1. *EMBO J.* **4**, 2765–2768.

Brummendorf, T., Wolff, J. M., Frank, R., and Rathjen, F. G. (1989). Neural cell recognition molecule F11: Homology with fibronectin type III and immunoglobulin type C domains. *Neuron* **2**, 1351–1361.

Burgoon, M. P., Grumet, M., Mauro, V., Edelman, G. M., and Cunningham, B. A. (1991). Structure of the chicken neuron-glia cell adhesion molecule, Ng-CAM: Origin of polypeptides and relation to Ig superfamily. *J. Cell Biol.* **112**, 1017–1029.

Changeux, J.-P., and Danchin, A. (1976). Selective stabilization of developing synapses as a mechanism for the specification of neuronal networks. *Nature (London)* **264**, 705–711.

Chiquet, M., and Fambrough, D. M. (1984). Chick myotendinous antigen. I. A monoclonal antibody as a marker for tendon and muscle morphogenesis. *J. Cell Biol.* **98**, 1926–1936.

Chiquet-Ehrismann, R., Mackie, E. J., Pearson, C. A., and Sakakura, T. (1986). Tenascin: An extracellular matrix protein involved in tissue interactions during fetal development and oncogenesis. *Cell (Cambridge, Mass.)* **47**, 131–139.

Chuong, C.-M., Crossin, K. L., and Edelman, G. M. (1987). Sequential expression and differential function of multiple adhesion molecules during the formation of cerebellar cortical layers. *J. Cell Biol.* **104**, 331–342.

Covault, J., and Sanes, J. R. (1985). Neural cell adhesion molecule (N-CAM) accumulates in denervated and paralyzed skeletal muscles. *Proc. Natl. Acad. Sci. U.S.A.* **82**, 4544–4548.

Crossin, K. L. (1991). Cell adhesion molecules in embryogenesis and disease. *Ann. N.Y. Acad. Sci.* **615**, 172–186.

Crossin, K. L., Chuong, C.-M., and Edelman, G. M. (1985). Expression sequences of cell adhesion molecules. *Proc. Natl. Acad. Sci. U.S.A.* **82**, 6942–6946.

Crossin, K. L., Hoffman, S., Grumet, M., Thiery, J.-P., and Edelman, G. M. (1986). Site-restricted expression of cytotactin during development of the chicken embryo. *J. Cell Biol.* **102**, 1917–1930.

Crossin, K. L., Hoffman, S., Tan, S.-S., and Edelman, G. M. (1989). Cytotactin and its proteoglycan ligand mark structural and functional boundaries in somatosensory cortex of the early postnatal mouse. *Dev. Biol.* **136**, 381–392.

Crossin, K. L., Prieto, A. L., Hoffman, S., Jones, F. S., and Friedlander, D. R. (1990). Expression of adhesion molecules and the establishment of boundaries during embryonic and neural development. *Exp. Neurol.* **109**, 6–18.

Cunningham, B. A., Hemperly, J. J., Murray, B. A., Prediger, E. A., Brackenbury, R., and Edelman, G. M. (1987). Neural cell adhesion molecule: Structure, immunoglobulin-like domains, cell surface modulation, and alternative RNA splicing. *Science* **236**, 799–806.

Daniloff, J. K., Chuong, C.-M., Levi, G., and Edelman, G. M. (1986a). Differential distribution of cell adhesion molecules during histogenesis of the chick nervous system. *J. Neurosci.* **6**, 739–758.

Daniloff, J. K., Levi, G., Grumet, M., Rieger, F., and Edelman, G. M. (1986b). Altered expression of neuronal cell adhesion molecules induced by nerve injury and repair. *J. Cell Biol.* **103**, 929–945.

Daniloff, J. K., Crossin, K. L., Pinçon-Raymond, M., Murawsky, M., Rieger, F., and Edelman, G. M. (1989). Expression of cytotactin in the normal and regenerating neuromuscular system. *J. Cell Biol.* **108**, 625–635.

Duband, J.-L., Dufour, S., Hatta, K., Takeichi, M., Edelman, G. M., and Thiery, J.-P. (1987). Adhesion molecules during somitogenesis in the avian embryo. *J. Cell Biol.* **104**, 1361–1374.

Edelman, G. M. (1976). Surface modulation in cell recognition and cell growth. *Science* **192**, 218–226.

Edelman, G. M. (1978). Group selection and phasic reentrant signaling: A theory of higher brain function. *In* "The Mindful Brain" (G. M. Edelman and V. B. Mountcastle, eds.), pp. 51–100. MIT Press, Cambridge, MA.

Edelman, G. M. (1984). Cell adhesion and morphogenesis: The regulator hypothesis. *Proc. Natl. Acad. Sci. U.S.A.* **81**, 1460–1464.

Edelman, G. M. (1987). CAMs and Igs: Cell adhesion and the evolutionary origins of immunity. *Immunol. Rev.* **100**, 11–45.

Edelman, G. M. (1988). "Topobiology: An Introduction to Molecular Embryology." Basic Books, New York.

Edelman, G. M. (1992). Morphoregulation. *Dev. Dyn.* **193**, 2–10.

Edelman, G. M., and Chuong, C.-M. (1982). Embryonic to adult conversion of neural cell adhesion molecules in normal and staggerer mice. *Proc. Natl. Acad. Sci. U.S.A.* **79**, 7036–7040.

Edelman, G. M., and Crossin, K. L. (1991). Cell adhesion molecules: Implications for a molecular histology. *Annu. Rev. Biochem.* **60**, 155–190.

Erickson, H. P., and Bourdon, M. A. (1989). Tenascin: An extracellular matrix protein prominent in specialized embryonic tissues and tumors. *Annu. Rev. Cell Biol.* **5**, 71–92.

Erickson, H. P., and Iglesias, J. L. (1984). A six-armed oligomer isolated from cell surface fibronectin preparations. *Nature (London)* **311**, 267–269.

Faissner, A., and Kruse, J. (1990). J1/tenascin is a repulsive substrate for central nervous system neurons. *Neuron* **5**, 627–637.

Faissner, A., Kruse, J., Chiquet-Ehrismann, R., and Mackie, E. (1988). The high molecular weight J1 glycoproteins are immunochemically related to tenascin. *Differentiation (Berlin)* **37,** 104–114.

Fraser, S. E., Murray, B. A., Chuong, C.-M., and Edelman, G. M. (1984). Alteration of the retinotectal map in *Xenopus* by antibodies to neural cell adhesion molecules. *Proc. Natl. Acad. Sci. U.S.A.* **81,** 4222–4226.

Fraser, S. E., Carhart, M. S., Murray, B. A., Chuong, C.-M., and Edelman, G. M. (1988). Alterations in the *Xenopus* retinotectal projection by antibodies to *Xenopus* N-CAM. *Dev. Biol.* **129,** 217–230.

Friedlander, D. R., Hoffman, S., and Edelman, G. M. (1988). Functional mapping of cytotactin: Proteolytic fragments active in cell–substrate adhesion. *J. Cell Biol.* **107,** 2329–2340.

Friedlander, D. R., Mege, R.-M., Cunningham, B. A., and Edelman, G. M. (1989). Cell sorting-out is modulated by both the specificity and amount of different cell adhesion molecules (CAMs) expressed on cell surfaces. *Proc. Natl. Acad. Sci. U.S.A.* **86,** 7043–7047.

Furley, A. J., Morton, S. B., Manalo, D., Karagogeos, D., Dodd, J., and Jessel, T. M. (1990). The axonal glycoprotein TAG-1 is an immunoglobulin superfamily member with neurite outgrowth-promoting activity. *Cell (Cambridge, Mass.)* **61,** 157–170.

Gennarini, G., Cibelli, G., Rougon, G., Mattei, M.-G., and Goridis, C. (1989). The mouse neuronal cell surface protein F3: A phosphatidylinositol-anchored member of the immunoglobulin superfamily related to chicken contactin. *J. Cell Biol.* **109,** 775–788.

Grumet, M., Hoffman, S., Crossin, K. L., and Edelman, G. M. (1985). Cytotactin, an extracellular matrix protein of neural and non-neural tissues that mediates glia-neuron interaction. *Proc. Natl. Acad. Sci. U.S.A.* **82,** 8075–8079.

Grumet, M., Mauro, V., Burgoon, M. P., Edelman, G. M., and Cunningham, B. A. (1991). Structure of a new nervous system glycoprotein, Nr-CAM, and its relationship to subgroups of neural cell adhesion molecules. *J. Cell Biol.* **113,** 1399–1412.

Harrelson, A. L., and Goodman, C. S. (1988). Growth cone guidance in insects: Fasciclin II is a member of the immunoglobulin superfamily. *Science* **242,** 700–708.

Hirsch, M.-R., Gaugler, L., Deagostini-Bazin, H., Bally-Cuif, L., and Goridis, C. (1990). Identification of positive and negative regulatory elements governing cell-type-specific expression of the neural cell adhesion molecule gene. *Mol. Cell. Biol.* **10,** 1959–1968.

Hoffman, S., and Edelman, G. M. (1983). Kinetics of homophilic binding by E and A forms of the neural cell adhesion molecule. *Proc. Natl. Acad. Sci. U.S.A.* **80,** 5762–5766.

Hoffman, S., and Edelman, G. M. (1987). A proteoglycan with HNK-1 antigenic determinants is a neuron-associated ligand for cytotactin. *Proc. Natl. Acad. Sci. U.S.A.* **84,** 2523–2527.

Hoffman, S., Sorkin, B. C., White, P. C., Brackenbury, R., Mailhammer, R., Rutishauser, U., Cunningham, B. A., and Edelman, G. M. (1982). Chemical characterization of a neural cell adhesion molecule purified from embryonic brain membranes. *J. Biol. Chem.* **257,** 7720–7729.

Hoffman, S., Friedlander, D. R., Chuong, C.-M., Grumet, M., and Edelman, G. M. (1986). Differential contributions of Ng-CAM and N-CAM to cell adhesion in different neural regions. *J. Cell Biol.* **103,** 145–158.

Hoffman, S., Crossin, K. L., and Edelman, G. M. (1988). Molecular forms, binding functions, and developmental expression patterns of cytotactin and cytotactin-binding proteoglycan, an interactive pair of extracellular matrix molecules. *J. Cell Biol.* **106,** 519–532.

Jaffe, S. H., Friedlander, D. R., Matsuzaki, F., Crossin, K. L., Cunningham, B. A., and Edelman, G. M. (1990). Differential effects of the cytoplasmic domains of cell adhesion molecules on cell aggregation and sorting-out. *Proc. Natl. Acad. Sci. U.S.A.* **87**, 3589–3593.

Jhaveri, S., Erzurumlu, R. S., and Crossin, K. (1991). Barrel construction in rodent neocortex: Role of thalamic afferents versus extracellular matrix molecules. *Proc. Natl. Acad. Sci. U.S.A.* **88**, 4489–4493.

Jones, F. S., Burgoon, M. P., Hoffman, S., Crossin, K. L., Cunningham, B. A., and Edelman, G. M. (1988). A cDNA clone for cytotactin contains sequences similar to epidermal growth factor-like repeats and segments of fibronectin and fibrinogen. *Proc. Natl. Acad. Sci. U.S.A.* **85**, 2186–2190.

Jones, F. S., Hoffman, S., Cunningham, B. A., and Edelman, G. M. (1989). A detailed structural model of cytotactin: Protein homologies, alternative RNA splicing, and binding regions. *Proc. Natl. Acad. Sci. U.S.A.* **86**, 1905–1909.

Jones, F. S., Crossin, K. L., Cunningham, B. A., and Edelman, G. M. (1990). Identification and characterization of the promoter for the cytotactin gene. *Proc. Natl. Acad. Sci. U.S.A.* **87**, 6497–6501.

Jones, F. S., Prediger, E. A., Bittner, D. A., DeRobertis, E. M., and Edelman, G. M. (1992a). Cell adhesion molecules as targets for *hox* genes: N-CAM promoter activity is modulated by co-transfection with *Hox 2.5* and *2.4*. *Proc. Natl. Acad. Sci. U.S.A.* **89**, 2086–2090.

Jones, F. S., Chalepakis, G., Gruss, P., and Edelman, G. M. (1992b). Activation of the cytotactin promoter by the homeobox-containing gene, *Evx-1*. *Proc. Natl. Acad. Sci. U.S.A.* **89**, 2091–2095.

Lagenaur, C., and Lemmon, V. (1987). An L1-like molecule, the 8D9 antigen, is a potent substrate for neurite extension. *Proc. Natl. Acad. Sci. U.S.A.* **84**, 7753–7757.

Lemke, G., and Axel, R. (1985). Isolation and sequence of a cDNA encoding the major structural protein of peripheral myelin. *Cell (Cambridge, Mass.)* **40**, 501–508.

Matsuzaki, F., Mege, R.-M., Jaffe, S. H., Friedlander, D. R., Gallin, W. J., Goldberg, J. I., Cunningham, B. A., and Edelman, G. M. (1990). cDNAs of cell adhesion molecules of different specificity induce changes in cell shape and border formation in cultured S180 cells. *J. Cell Biol.* **110**, 1239–1252.

Mayr, E. (1982). "The Growth of Biological Thought: Diversity, Evolution, and Inheritance." Harvard Univ. Press, Cambridge, MA.

Mege, R.-M., Matsuzaki, F., Gallin, W. J., Goldberg, J. I., Cunningham, B. A., and Edelman, G. M. (1988). Construction of epithelioid sheets by transfection of mouse sarcoma cells with cDNAs for chicken cell adhesion molecules. *Proc. Natl. Acad. Sci. U.S.A.* **85**, 7274–7278.

Moos, M., Tacke, R., Scherer, H., Teplow, D., Fruh, K., and Schachner, M. (1988). Neural adhesion molecule L1 is a member of the immunoglobulin superfamily with binding domains similar to fibronectin. *Nature (London)* **334**, 701–703.

Nagafuchi, A., and Takeichi, M. (1988). Cell binding function of E-cadherin is regulated by the cytoplasmic domain. *EMBO J.* **7**, 3679–3694.

Needham, J. (1933). On the dissociability of the fundamental process in ontogenesis. *Biol. Rev. Cambridge Philos. Soc.* **8**, 180–223.

Rakic, P. (1988). Specification of cerebral cortical areas. *Science* **241**, 170–176.

Ranscht, B. (1988). Sequence of contactin, a 130-kD glycoprotein concentrated in areas of interneuronal contact, defines a new member of the immunoglobulin supergene family in the nervous system. *J. Cell Biol.* **107**, 1561–1573.

Ranscht, B., and Dours, M. T. (1989). Selective expression of a novel cadherin in the pathways of developing motor and commissural axons. *Soc. Neurosci. Abstr.* **15**, 959 (abstr.).

Rathjen, F. G., and Schachner, M. (1984). Immunocytological and biochemical characterization of a new neuronal cell surface component (L1 antigen), which is involved in cell adhesion. *EMBO J.* **3**, 1–10.

Reichardt, L. F., and Tomaselli, K. J. (1991). Extracellular matrix molecules and their receptors: Functions in neural development. *Annu. Rev. Neurosci.* **14,** 531–570.

Rieger, F., Grumet, M., and Edelman, G. M. (1985). N-CAM at the vertebrate neuromuscular junction. *J. Cell Biol.* **101,** 285–293.

Rieger, F., Daniloff, J. F., Pinçon-Raymond, M., Crossin, K. L., Grumet, M., and Edelman, G. M. (1986). Neuronal cell adhesion molecules and cytotactin are colocalized at the node of Ranvier. *J. Cell Biol.* **103,** 379–391.

Salzer, J. G., Holmes, W. P., and Colman, D. R. (1987). The amino acid sequences of the myelin-associated glycoproteins: Homology to the immunoglobulin gene superfamily. *J. Cell Biol.* **104,** 957–965.

Sanes, J. R. (1989). Extracellular matrix molecules that influence neural development. *Annu. Rev. Neurosci.* **12,** 491–516.

Schacher, S., Glanzman, D., Barzilai, A., Dash, P., Grant, S. G., Keller, F., Mayford, M., and Kandel, E. R. (1990). Long-term facilitation in *Aplysia:* Persistent phosphorylation and structural changes. *Cold Spring Harbor Symp. Quant. Biol.* **55,** 187–202.

Seeger, M. A., Haffley, L., and Kaufman, T. C. (1988). Characterization of amalgam: A member of the immunoglobulin superfamily from *Drosophila. Cell (Cambridge, Mass.)* **55,** 589–600.

Sperry, R. W. (1963). Chemoaffinity in the orderly growth of nerve fiber patterns and connections. *Proc. Natl. Acad. Sci. U.S.A.* **50,** 703–710.

Spring, J., Beck, K., and Chiquet-Ehrismann, R. (1989). Two contrary functions of tenascin: Dissection of the active sites by recombinant tenascin fragments. *Cell (Cambridge, Mass.)* **59,** 325–334.

Suzuki, S., Sano, K., and Tanihara, H. (1991). Diversity of the cadherin family: Evidence for eight new cadherins in nervous tissue. *Cell Regul.* **2,** 261–270.

Takeichi, M. (1988). The cadherins: Cell-cell adhesion molecules controlling animal morphogenesis. *Development (Cambridge, UK)* **102,** 639–655.

Takeichi, M. (1990). Cadherins: A molecular family important in selective cell–cell adhesion. *Annu. Rev. Biochem.* **59,** 237–252.

Tan, S.-S., Crossin, K. L., Hoffman, S., and Edelman, G. M. (1987). Asymmetric expression in somites of cytotactin and its proteoglycan ligand is correlated with neural crest cell distribution. *Proc. Natl. Acad. Sci. U.S.A.* **84,** 7977–7981.

Thiery, J.-P., Duband, J.-L., Rutishauser, U., and Edelman, G. M. (1982). Cell adhesion molecules in early chick embryogenesis. *Proc. Natl. Acad. Sci. U.S.A.* **79,** 6737–6741.

Thiery, J.-P., Delouvée, A., Grumet, M., and Edelman, G. M. (1985). Initial appearance and regional distribution of the neuron–glia cell adhesion molecule, in the chick embryo. *J. Cell Biol.* **100,** 442–456.

Volk, T., and Geiger, B. (1986). A-CAM—A 135 kD receptor of intercellular adherens junctions. I. Immuno-electron microscopic localization and biochemical studies. *J. Cell Biol.* **103,** 1441–1450.

Walsh, F. S., and Moore, S. E. (1985). Expression of cell-adhesion molecule, N-CAM, in diseases of adult human skeletal-muscle. *Neurosci. Lett.* **59,** 73–78.

Williams, A. F., and Barclay, A. N. (1988). The immunoglobulin superfamily—Domains for cell surface recognition. *Annu. Rev. Immunol.* **6,** 381–405.

Zuellig, R. A., Rader, C., Schroeder, A., Kalousek, M. B., vonBohlenundHalbach, F., Osterwalder, T., Inan, C., Stoeckli, E. T., Affolter, H. U., and Fritz, A. (1992). The axonally secreted cell adhesion molecule, axonin-1: Primary structure, immunoglobulin-like and fibronectin-type-III-like domains and glycosylphosphatidylinositol anchorage. *Eur. J. Biochem.* **204,** 453–463.

EXPLORATION AND SELECTION IN THE EARLY ACQUISITION OF SKILL

Esther Thelen and Daniela Corbetta

Department of Psychology
Indiana University
Bloomington, Indiana 47405

I. Development of Brain and Behavior

The lives of babies seem far removed from the concerns of neuroscientists. In a world measured in microseconds, microliters, micrometers, and microvolts, the endearing but clumsy and whimsical noodlings of infants bear little relevance. What we hope to show in this article, however, is that the behavior of human infants during their first years of life can both inform, and be informed by, contemporary advances in the brain sciences, as reported in many of the other papers in this volume. To do this, we will first describe some research on the perceptual motor development of human infants and its theoretical implications and underpinnings. We will then show how this work is congruent with a selectionist and dynamic theory of brain function. In particular, we will argue that behavioral data from infants are consistent with an epigenetic development, that the driving forces are exploration and selection, that multimodal inputs, and especially movement, are critical, and that new behavior is functionally established and maintained. These behavioral results argue, in turn, for brain function that is distributed and noniconic.

It is axiomatic in the brain and behavioral sciences that the levels of analysis, from the most molecular descriptions of ion channels and neurochemistry to the most macroscopic analysis of individual and social behavior, must ultimately be concordant. Although no one envisions such a complete synthesis in our lifetimes, to deny its possibility leaves us with unacceptable mind–body dualism. Nonetheless, progress toward integrated brain–behavior explanations has been slow in coming, especially in the developmental sciences. Most behavioral theorists and researchers have proceeded without consideration of the biological plausibility of their explanations, or by using very simplistic and, in our view, unsatisfactory accounts of brain–behavior relations. At the same time, developmental behavioral research has not always been well-used by neuroscientists, when it is used at all.

A. Construct of Maturation

To illustrate our point, consider the construct of brain "maturation." This construct is used by neuroscientists and by psychologists who want to invoke a "biological basis" for some developmental change. Here are some examples from the recent developmental literature:

> As the brain matures, it allows for better control of movement with sensory information. The welcome results for the child are major strides in gross and fine motor control. [Edwards, 1992, p. 11]

> The development of improved function in this tract [corticospinal] as a result of myelination is a likely candidate for a neural basis of the maturation of walking. [Konner, 1991, p. 201]

> The finding that synapses develop rather synchronously in all areas of the cerebral cortex raises the possibility that functions mediated in these cortical areas might also emerge in relation to synaptogenesis, that is, concurrently, or nearly so. Specifically, is it possible that cardinal functions of each major cortical area might emerge in at least elementary form in all regions of the cortex simultaneously . . . Perhaps the coincidental timing of a child's first utterance and first step are expressions of concurrent synaptogenesis in the language and motor areas of the cortex. [Goldman-Rakic, 1987, pp. 614–615]

It is incontrovertible that, as we get older, our brains get bigger and more highly differentiated, and that there are changes in myelination, neurotransmitter distribution, conduction speed, and the distribution and density of synapses. The brain "matures." At the same time, we do more things and we do them much better.

Though the effort to relate behavioral changes and their neural underpinnings is laudable, we have not gained much in understanding by invoking brain maturation as a cause of developmental change. Numerous problems arise with this type of explanation: How does one recognize a mature brain structure outside of its functional manifestations? What is a "cardinal" function of a particular brain area? What is a "primitive form" of a cardinal function? What level of correlation is sufficient between structure and function to make a causal link? What behavioral landmarks do we assign as tokens of maturity? As we shall see, these questions are formidable in the light of real neural and behavioral data.

The most serious shortcoming of invoking brain maturation is, however, a disregard for developmental process either at the neural or at the behavioral level. By developmental process we mean the complex, contingent, multiply determined web of interactions that leads the organism from a single cell to a toddler who can climb, sing songs, and tease her baby brother. What developmental research is good for is to uncover this matted web, and to thus put behavioral constraints on neurological explanations and vice versa.

B. Facing Real Developmental Data

The construct of maturation came under question with Thelen's behavioral data on the development of locomotion. Locomotor development has long stood as the "paradigmatic case" (Konner, 1991, p. 199) of a maturational acquisition under genetic control (e.g., McGraw, 1945). One stage in the development of locomotion has been especially intriguing. As is well known, if you hold newborn infants under the armpits, they will produce—reflexively—active stepping movements, often alternating, and always rather surprising in such an otherwise uncoordinated creature. Within a month or two, these movements can no longer be elicited, and infants, when held erect, keep their feet glued to the surface. Stepping movements reappear only 6 or 8 months later, when infants begin to voluntarily step and then walk. In the conventional maturational view, the loss of stepping, as well as its return, was ascribed to improved cortical control over lower, presumably spinal, pathways, first inhibiting the reflex and then facilitating voluntary walking (Forssberg, 1985; McGraw, 1945).

This eminently reasonable explanation began to crumble, however, when Thelen and colleagues looked more closely at newborn stepping and its disappearance. First, it was discovered that at the very same time that 2- and 3-month-old infants refused to step when upright, they continued to make steplike movements when placed supine. These movements were normally called kicking, but because infants were not upright, no one connected kicking to later locomotion. But in terms of the structure of the movements and their underlying muscle patterns, kicking and stepping were identical (Thelen and Fisher, 1982). It was a challenge, therefore, to maturation theory to explain why cortical centers would inhibit movements in one posture and not in another.

Thelen and colleagues proposed a different, and more biomechanical, explanation for the disappearing reflex, namely, that increases in relative body fat during the first postnatal months made the legs difficult to lift in the biomechanically challenging position of upright (Thelen and Fisher, 1982). We confirmed this by a number of experiments varying biomechanical and energetic parameters. In one study, for example, we showed that infants held upright on small treadmills continued to step well throughout the first year, all during the period the brain was supposedly inhibiting the pattern (Thelen and Ulrich, 1991).

The "case of the disappearing reflex" raised two fundamental considerations about locomotor development in particular and about development in general. First, learning to walk was *not* a unitary process directed by increasing cortical control of the legs by the brain. Rather walking, like all skills, involved many subcomponents, some of which, like the ability to step, may be in place early in life, while others emerge later and at different rates (Thelen, 1984; Thelen and Ulrich, 1991). The ultimate performance of the skill required the availability and coordination of all the component parts. And second, that walking development was not strictly a top-down matter, from the brain to the limbs. Nonneural elements clearly influenced whether the motor pattern was performed at all, and indeed determined the configuration of the movement. These included orientation to gravity, muscle mass and body proportion, and energetic constraints, that is, whether the infant was active or quiet (Thelen *et al.*, 1982, 1984). In short, the pattern could not be said to "exist" in some dedicated element in the brain or spinal cord at all, no matter what their state of maturation. The baby stepped or walked only in the immediate context, given his or her total organic status, itself a product of contingent developmental processes. Clearly, the construct of autonomous maturation is an impoverished substitute for process.

II. Dynamic Systems Approach to Development

If not simply brain maturity, how then to conceptualize learning to walk and the acquisition of other skills, in light of the multiple interactions and the shifting and context-dependent nature of performance? Fortunately, about the time of work on the disappearing reflex, there was a growing interest in the works of the movement physiologist Bernstein (1967). Bernstein's insights had profound implications for understanding brain–behavior relations in the control of movement, and for its development as well.

Movements occur, according to Bernstein, because of imbalances in forces caused by changes in muscle tension. Nonetheless, he recognized that there cannot be a one-to-one relationship between the specific patterns of motoneuron firing and the actual movement produced. This is because the limbs and body segments are acting continually in a changing field of forces due to gravity and mechanical actions of the other parts of the body. Thus, a particular muscle contraction has different effects depending on the postural and movement contexts in which it occurs. In addition, muscles and joints have properties of springiness and tension that depend on their degree of stretch and their stiffness, but these relationships are not simple or linear.

To move, then, the devices-be-controlled present the nervous system with a continually changing biodynamic problem. The brain cannot know ahead and store all the possible solutions—all the possible combinations of motor neuron firings needed for the flexible actions of everyday life. Rather, what the brain learns is broad categories of movement—synergies of action—but the details emerge on line, so to speak, in interaction with the periphery. Likewise, Bernstein proposed that these patterns "develop and involute" in relation to the physical demands of the periphery. He showed, for example, that walking involved complex interactions between the movements of the legs, the center of gravity of the body, and the ground. It is these interactions with the periphery that sculpt the patterns of walking, and not some icon of walking living somewhere in the brain.

Bernstein's insights, combined with resurgent interest in the principles and mathematics of complex system dynamics, have inspired new theories of the coordination and control of movement, which, in turn, form the basis of a new way of conceptualizing behavioral development (Kelso *et al.*, 1980; Kugler *et al.*, 1980, 1982). There are two core assumptions to such a dynamic approach to movement control, the first being that patterns of coordination—the trajectories of movement within and among the segments—need not be symbolically "represented" anywhere in the nervous system. Rather, that pattern "self-organizes" in response to information specifying the task, given a particular status of the organism and the physical environment. Self-organization means that given the neural, anatomic, and energetic components of the system (including their history), patterns will arise without their *a priori* specification

(Kugler and Turvey, 1987). (We will illustrate this with infant movement in a later section.) The second core assumption is that these patterns of coordination will obey principles of nonlinear dynamics, in particular, that motor systems will exhibit certain modes, or *attractor states*, where the system prefers to reside, but is not obligated to do so. (For example, walking is the preferred mode for upright locomotion, but people can also hop, skip, jump, or tap dance across the room.) Such attractor states, which are operationally defined, may be more or less stable, but unstable configurations can spontaneously shift into new coordinative modes. Thus, the primary empirical job is to discover the stable attractors in motor patterns and the conditions under which they lose stability and change (Schöner and Kelso, 1988).

Researchers have successfully integrated dynamic theory and data with human cyclic movements such as coordinated finger and arm flexing (Kelso *et al.*, 1981), juggling (Beek, 1989), and skilike whole body movements (Vereijken, 1991). These movements have been well-characterized by models that incorporate features of known physical oscillators such as pendula or springs, but in which the human mover can intentionally vary stiffness, damping, and the timing of energetic spurts by muscular effort. A major concern now in adult movement dynamics is to discover how movers use perceptual information about tasks, environments, and their own movements to match their goals to the dynamics intrinsic to their body.

A. FROM ACTION TO DEVELOPMENT

When we consider human performance as a dynamic system—multiply determined, complex, self-organizing—we shift our focus from static, structural constructs such as motor programs or schema to time-dependent processes. Such a dynamic view also generates a process account of development (Thelen, 1989; Thelen and Ulrich, 1991; Thelen and Smith, 1994). The key here is the assumption that the same general principles that govern the assembly and coordination of behavior in the real time of perception, action, and cognition also apply to changes in developmental time. Specifically, as organisms develop, behavior "soft-assembles," to use Kugler and Turvey's (1987) term, from multiple and coequal elements and components, each of which has its characteristic dynamic, and this assembly represents a preferred state of the organism in a particular environment and task context. Development, then, can be envisioned as a changing landscape of preferred, but not obligatory, behavioral states with varying degrees of stability and instability, rather than as a prescribed series of structurally invariant stages leading to progressive improvement. Although some behavioral preferences are so stable that they take on the quality of a developmental stage, the stability is a function of the organism-in-context, not a set of prior instructions.

That both mental states and the actions they engender are seen as fluid, flexible, task specific, and stochastic means that development proceeds as a series of continual matches between the current dynamics of the individual—the preferred states—and his or her intentions, the demands of the task, and the affordances of the environment. Thus, how individuals solve problems in the real time scale directly affects the solutions that evolve in ontogenetic time. Developmental change is multiply complex, however, because the very architecture of the system is changing through both growth and function. For example, acquiring speech requires a particular anatomical configuration of the speech articulators and a degree of neural control over these structures. As the structures grow, the control processes must be recalibrated. But structural change is also engendered through function—through speaking itself—which molds the peripheral anatomy as well as the central nervous system. Thus, even the set of problems to be solved is dynamic because the state of the system is changing at each succeeding frame of time.

B. USING DYNAMIC PRINCIPLES TO STUDY INFANT DEVELOPMENT

Our central concern, therefore, is to understand development as it happens over these multiple time scales and over multiple levels. This has meant rejecting some of the time-honored experimental designs and analysis techniques of experimental psychology—especially comparing groups of subjects on their performance using analysis of variance. Rather, we began with describing the dynamics of change, of individuals, with dense measurements over long time scales. Because we are interested in stability and change, we consider variability as data—how stable is this pattern?—rather than noise around mean performance. Because dynamic theory has powerful predictions about the behavior of systems during transitions, the idea is to identify these transitions and their component dynamics. Only then will we manipulate the system to try and engender in real time changes seen over developmental time.

In the next section we report on some examples applying a dynamic systems approach to questions of motor skill acquisition in infants. Motor skill is an important window on early mental life, primarily because it is the essential underpinning for all further perception and cognition. But also, motor performance can be measured as a time series, as a continuous readout, so to speak, of how the infant actually explores the space and dynamically solves problems. The task problems involve coordination and control: how the various segments and parts of the body come to cooperate together and how the brain parameterizes or scales movements to fit tasks. From Bernstein, we recognize that coordination and control must be carried out within a physical force environment. Within each following section, we will point out how these behavioral results are consistent with the discoveries at the neural level.

III. Behavioral Dynamics of Learning to Reach

The question of the neural control of the trajectory of arm and hand for reaching is one that is currently generating much interest and controversy among cognitive scientists, neuroscientists, bioengineers, and computer modelers. The debate is unresolved: some claim that the central nervous system (CNS) plans reaches to be smooth and graceful by minimizing irregularities in the path of the hand (Hogan, 1984). Others see the CNS exerting control on the direction of the hand path (Morasso, 1981). Some have offered computational models of the transformation of coordinates from the visual target to the positions of the joints (e.g., Schoechting and Ross, 1984), and still others are looking toward muscle patterns as the invariant level of control (Gottlieb *et al.*, 1989). Finally, a group of models suggests that the CNS is working on the dynamic, biomechanical, characteristics of the controlled limb, its compliance or dynamic stiffness, rather than movement pathway or muscle patterns (e.g., Feldman, 1980; Hogan *et al.*, 1987; Polit and Bizzi, 1978).

The development of reaching has also been of considerable research interest, but the questions have been posed more in terms of the origins of the behavior than its neural control. Here the debate is whether reaching is constructed from disparate perceptual and motor components (Bruner, 1973; Piaget, 1952), if it is innate, that is, configured from birth, and needs only to be refined (Bower *et al.*, 1970; Trevarthen, 1984), or whether reaching comes from maturation of appropriate pathways from the brain (von Hofsten, 1984; Jeannerod, 1988).

Following Bernstein and dynamic theories of movement and development, we have asked the questions of reaching development differently. We believe that this new approach casts light on both the developmental process and the neural control. For us the question of origins can be posed thus: how do infants individually solve the problem of how to get their hands to a desired object given their current developmental status? How do their neural, muscular, perceptual, energetic, and intentional abilities cooperate to perform an action within the physical demands of the task? (We call this preference for certain coordinative solutions the infants' *intrinsic dynamics*.) In other words, how do infants find and assemble a new pattern of coordination within the reaching context?

This approach shifts the emphasis from looking for early prefiguration of reaching (e.g., von Hofsten, 1982) to observing changes in the here-and-now behavior of individual infants as they progress from no reaching to well-coordinated movements. To do this, we observed four infants from when they were 3 weeks old and not even able to lift their heads to when they were 1 year old and reaching for and manipulating objects with considerable skill. Our observations were weekly until 30 weeks and every other week thereafter. A number of features made this study unique. First, we recorded kinematics of the joints of both arms and calculated, using the techniques of inverse dynamics, the distribution and partitioning of forces at the joints. Second, we simultaneously recorded electromyelograms (EMGs) to correlate kinematic and kinetic changes with muscle patterns. These measures allowed us to track the multiple levels of control. Finally, to understand how new forms emerged from ongoing movement, we did not record only the reach, but also the reach embedded in the other arm actions that preceded and followed it. This allowed us to describe infants' intrinsic dynamics and how they modulated these dynamics across development.

A. Transition to Reaching

The most dramatic change during this period was the infants' shift from not being able to reach and touch an object in front of them to a successful attempt. To our surprise, not only did the four infants demonstrate this milestone at different ages, but they solved their task problems in very different ways (Thelen *et al.*, 1993). Here we show how two infants, Gabriel and Hannah, made this transition to reaching.

1. Spontaneous Movements

What was apparent from the start was that Gabriel and Hannah, and the other two infants, faced the task of reaching with very different intrinsic dynamics. That is, from birth, their spontaneous movement patterns were individual and consistent. Gabriel, for example, was a very energetic infant. When we supported him upright in an infant seat, he waved his arms and kicked his legs with great vigor. Hannah, in contrast, was more of a looker than a mover. She was quiet, contemplative, and her movements were small and slow. It is important to remember that before infants first reach at 3, 4, or 5 months, they have spent many waking hours moving their heads and limbs and that the tactile and proprioceptive information generated by those spontaneous movements forms the background dynamics from which intentional reaches must emerge.

Thus, the infants came into the reaching transition having to solve different individual problems. In Figs. 1 and 2, we report kinematic and kinetic variables from the spontaneous movements of Gabriel and Hannah before, during, and after their reaching transition. Notice first the weeks before they learned to reach. Gabriel's movements were fast

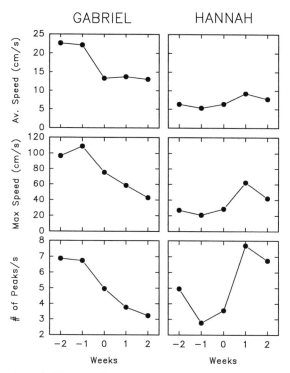

FIG. 1. Hand speed of the overall movement context from which Gabriel's and Hannah's first reaches emerged. Weeks -2 and -1 correspond to the 2 weeks preceding reach onset; reach onset is at week 0, and weeks 1 and 2 correspond to the 2 weeks following reach onset. Top panels: averaged resultant speed across trials and hands by week. Middle panels: averaged maximum resultant speed across trials and hands by week. Bottom panels: averaged number of resultant speed peaks across trials and hands by week.

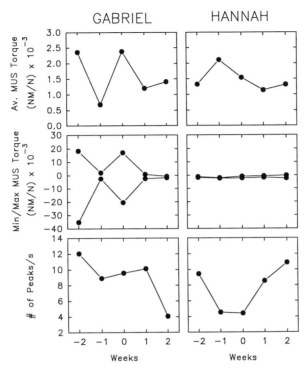

FIG. 2. Shoulder muscle (MUS) torques of the overall movement context from which an infant's first reach emerged. Weeks −2 and −1 correspond to the 2 weeks preceding reach onset; reach onset is at week 0, and weeks 1 and 2 correspond to the 2 weeks following reach onset. Top panels: averaged shoulder MUS torques computed using absolute values. Torques were averaged across trials and arms by week. Middle panels: averaged maximum and minimum shoulder MUS torques across trials and arms by week. Bottom panels: averaged number of MUS torque peaks across trials and arms by week.

and showed many changes of direction. His muscles generated high forces at the shoulder. Hannah's spontaneous movements were much slower, smoother, and were associated with much lower muscle forces. Gabriel's movements were too fast and uncontrolled to contact the toy and Hannah was barely lifting her arm.

2. First Reaches

Gabriel and Hannah fashioned their first reaches by appropriately modulating their spontaneous movements. Gabriel reached first at 15 weeks. To do this, he converted his spontaneous flapping movements by damping down his vigorous forces through changing the compliance characteristics of his arm. This process is illustrated in Figs. 3 and 4.

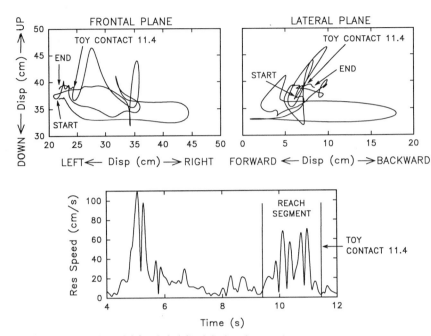

FIG. 3. Exemplar trial for Gabriel's right hand at reach onset showing transition from spontaneous flapping to reaching for toy. Top panels: 8-second hand path in the frontal and lateral planes. Bottom panel: resultant speed for the same segment showing high-velocity flaps at 4–6 seconds and a flap-into-reach at 9.5–11.4 seconds.

Figure 3 shows an example of the continuous hand trajectory of flapping and reach and the high velocity and many changes of direction in the movements before contacting the target. Figure 4 illustrates the patterns of joint angle changes, torques generated at the shoulder, and corresponding EMG for the same flap-into-reach segment. Notice that most of Gabriel's movement was at the shoulder, with the elbow and wrist held stiffly until contact with the toy. This is coincident with the high active and passive torques at the shoulder and more tonic than phasic EMG patterns. These data are also consistent with the stiffness estimates presented in the top panel of Fig. 5. Here, stiffness estimates are plotted for all of Gabriel's first week of reaches as regression lines between the displacement and maximum speed of each unit of acceleration and deceleration [von Hofsten's (1984) "movement units"]. We took into consideration 3 seconds of movement prior to contact and then divided them into 1-second intervals before contact (on the right; 0 seconds). The slope of the regression between displacement and speed estimates stiffness, with a steeper slope indicating a stiffer arm. The important point here is that the slopes remained steep until contact time.

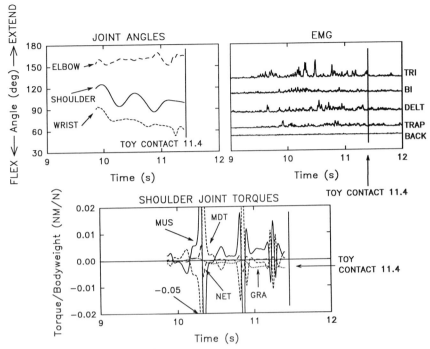

FIG. 4. Top left panel: rotations of the shoulder, elbow, and wrist joints of Gabriel's right hand for the flap-and-reach segment indicated in Fig. 3. Flexion reflects the decreasing joint angles at elbow and wrist, and lifting the arm at the shoulder. Top right panel: EMGs of five muscle groups for the entire 3-second reach segment illustrating tonic coactivation. Bottom panel: torques at the shoulder associated with the same segment. Negative torques work to flex the joints. NET, the sum of all torques rotating the shoulder joint; GRA, torques due to the pull of gravity (note that gravity is the extensor at the shoulder); MDT, shoulder-rotating torques that result from the movement of the other, mechanically linked segments of the arm; MUS, shoulder-rotating torques arising from muscle contraction and tissue deformation.

Hannah's first reaches stand in dramatic contrast. Although she did not reach first until 22 weeks, nearly 2 months later than Gabriel, her first reaches, from a background of quiet movements, were much more controlled and adult-looking. (She was no more accurate or successful, however.) Her trajectories were very smooth and slow, as the exemplar in Fig. 6 shows. Her arm was quite compliant, as illustrated by the differentiated joint movements (Fig. 7) and the very low slopes of stiffness estimates prior to contact (Fig. 8). These patterns resulted from low shoulder torques and very low, tonic muscle activation (Fig. 7).

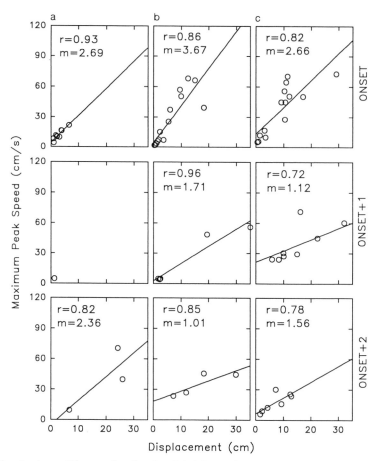

FIG. 5. Arm stiffness estimation for Gabriel's reach segments at (a) 3 to 2, (b) 2 to 1, and (c) 1 to 0 seconds prior to contact during the week of onset and the following 2 weeks. Each point of the scattergram represents hand displacement as a function of the maximum peak speed for a single "movement unit." Regression lines give an estimation of arm stiffness. Steep slopes indicate high stiffness; slopes near 0 indicate a lack of stiffness.

3. Subsequent Modulation

In the 2 weeks following their reach onset, Gabriel and Hannah continued to modify their preferred motor styles individually. Note that Gabriel made his movements more slowly, more smoothly, and with much less force at the shoulder. Hannah's movements got faster and less smooth, but only slightly more forceful overall (Figs. 1 and 2, for all movements). During the reach, however, Hannah increased her estimated stiffness dramatically in the 2 weeks following onset (Fig. 8), whereas Gabriel significantly decreased his estimated stiffness (Fig. 5).

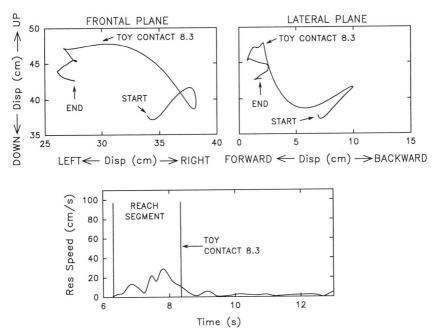

FIG. 6. Exemplar trial for Hannah's right hand at reach onset showing a reach initiated from a quiet starting position. Top panels: 8-second hand path in the frontal and lateral planes. Bottom panel: resultant speed for the same segment showing fewer reversals than for Gabriel.

B. DEVELOPMENTAL IMPLICATIONS OF THE TRANSITION TO REACHING

These data, and those from the other two infants in this study, provide compelling evidence, in our view, of the epigenetic nature of development. By epigenetic we mean that development proceeds in a contingent and historical fashion, whereby new forms arise from ongoing structures and processes, and the end point is not contained in the initial conditions. Gabriel and Hannah faced different here-and-now problems when they wanted to reach out and grab an attractive toy. Gabriel needed to tame his flapping movements, and Hannah needed to generate enough force in her arm to lift it up against gravity and extend it forward. The problems were individual and involved modulating muscle forces over time in relation to a particular task —appropriately scaling arm action to toy location. As Bernstein showed, this coupling between the periphery and the central nervous system can in no way be anticipated by programs or codes installed in the organism, waiting to emerge. What these infants had was a strong intention to grab the toy and to do it using whatever

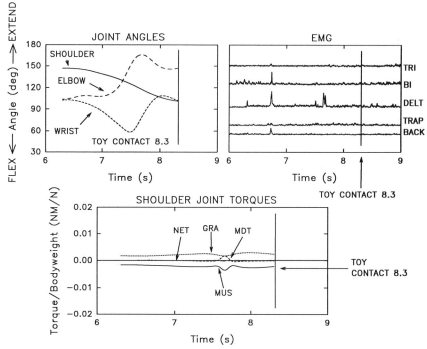

FIG. 7. Top left panel: rotations of the shoulder, elbow, and wrist joints of Hannah's right hand for the reach segment indicated in Fig. 6. Note slow flexion of the shoulder accompanied by smooth changes in the elbow and wrist. Top right panel: EMGs of five muscle groups for the entire 3-second reach segment. Bottom panel: torques at the shoulder associated with the same segment. Negative torques work to flex the joints. NET, the sum of all torques rotating the shoulder joint; GRA, torques due to the pull of gravity (note that gravity is extensor at the shoulder); MDT, shoulder-rotating torques that result from the movement of the other, mechanically linked segments of the arm; MUS, shoulder-rotating torques arising from muscle contraction and tissue deformation.

means they could muster. Indeed, in the early months, we sometimes saw these babies reach toward the toy, not with their arms, but with their heads and open mouths [Rochat's (1989) "oral capture"]. Because the mouth was nearly always the ultimate goal for an object in the hand, when controlling the arm was difficult, the infants tried to simply bypass using the arm and went straight for the object with the mouth.

What we saw both in the matching of individual intrinsic dynamics to the task and in oral capture was the infants' opportunistic marshalling of their available resources, indeed a "soft-assembly" of the components that would do the job. These are real-time discoveries, inspired by a functional goal. The infants were not passive receptacles of instructions

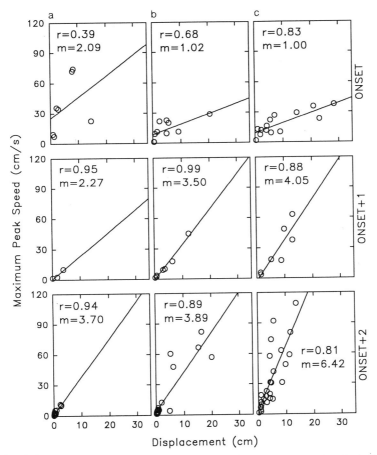

FIG. 8. Arm stiffness estimation for Hannah's reach segments at (a) 3 to 2, (b) 2 to 1, and (c) 1 to 0 seconds prior to contact during the week of onset and the following 2 weeks. Each point of the scattergram represents hand displacement as a function of the maximum peak speed for a single "movement unit." Regression lines between displacement and maximum speed peaks give an estimation of arm stiffness. Steep slopes indicate high stiffness; slopes near 0 indicate a lack of stiffness.

from above, but active explorers of their own force dynamics and active selectors of parameters that did the job.

The theme of this volume and of an exciting new theory of neural ontogeny is that of *selection* in the brain (Edelman, 1987). At the neural level, this means that out of the immensely varied and densely interconnected circuitry, groups of neurons are selected by experience to form a coherent group, the basis of categorization, learning, and memory.

Selection and its copartner exploration must as well be the parallel processes at the behavioral level as the driving forces in both learning and ontogeny (Gibson, 1988; Piaget, 1952). But we understand little about exploration and selection as processes. For instance, in previous studies of reaching, the focus has been on looking for precursors that *look like reaching*. Thus, transient arm extensions toward the direction of the head and gaze in the newborn period (which then disappear) are believed to prefigure intentional reaching that emerges some 4 months later (von Hofsten, 1982, 1984; Trevarthen, 1984). But in the intervening time, infants are not laying still waiting for the reaching icon to pop out again. They are, as we mentioned above, continually moving their heads and limbs, moving while looking, listening, and feeling, getting excited in social interactions and when hungry or in pain, or lying quietly alert, observing the passing scene. They are changing the force parameters of their limbs and feeling the consequences of those scalar changes at the same time that they are taking in the visual, auditory, tactile, and perhaps even chemical sensations that co-occur. Even without consistent successful arm-extended reaches, those 3 or 5 months of continual, coherent, multimodal experience constitute behavioral exploration, exploration with neural consequences. Thus, by the time infants *can* execute a successful reach, they have selected the correct parameters because of months of experience moving and sensing. It is worthy to note, although hardly conclusive, that the two very active infants in our reaching study, Gabriel and Nathan, reached first at 15 and 12 weeks, whereas our two more quiet infants, Hannah and Justin, did not attain this landmark until 22 and 21 weeks. It is certainly worthy of further investigation if the two infants who were constantly in motion simply generated more exploratory movements and thus had an early basis for understanding their arm parameters in relation to the visual task of grabbing the toy.

Additionally, these data point to the primacy of modulations in the stiffness or compliance characteristics of the limbs as the control parameter for early reaches. In these early days, it appeared as though hand path and joint coordination were derived or emergent properties of compliance modulation. The first reaches of these infants were highly variable in kinematics, kinetics, and muscle patterning; the only common element was that their hands eventually got to the toy (Thelen *et al.*, 1993). Yet within this variability, when reaches were slow, the paths were smoother and the joints more individuated. But infants could reach with arms held stiff and movement primarily from the shoulder. In other words, it looked like the infants were working on these force dynamics to get the hand "in the ball park" of the toy, and that further improvements in kinematics were subsequent to this primary parameterization. In the next section, we present some data to substantiate this claim.

C. KINEMATIC IMPROVEMENTS OVER THE FIRST YEAR

After 2 weeks of practice, Gabriel and Hannah were not very accomplished reachers. They sometimes swiped at the toy, often missed, and their reaches were jerky and circuitous. Within a few months, all the infants were consistently reaching and grasping. By the end of the year, they were accomplished reachers functionally, although even then, their reaches were neither as smooth nor as straight as those of adults. The top panels of Figs. 9 and 10 show two measures of "goodness" of reach. The number of velocity peaks indexes the number of increases and decreases in movement speed between the onset of the reach and target. (Adults usually have one or two velocity peaks, depending on the task.) The index of rectilinearity is the ratio between the three-dimensional straight line path from the start of the reach to the target to the actual path of the hand during the reach. A value of 1 means the actual hand path was perfectly straight.

These kinematic measures of the reach segment showed that both Gabriel and Hannah had an initial period of great variability both within and between test sessions. Following about 4 months after onset, both babies seemed to reach a period of much greater stability. Although both infants showed this plateau of improvement in trajectory smoothness and straightness, Hannah was notable in her discovery of a stable and mature-looking reaching pattern by 36 weeks. The bottom panels of Figs. 9 and 10 suggest a reason for these individual differences. This panel depicts the infants' developmental changes in speed of the hand at contact with the toy. Hannah contacted the object more slowly at her first reaches and continued throughout the year. Gabriel's inherently more energetic movements continued to be manifest in his reaching throughout the first year, causing him to hit the toy faster and to have more difficulty producing consistently straight and smooth reaches. Thus, the configuration of the movement trajectory must be considered in relation to the problems of force control, as Bernstein suggested. Gabriel's enthusiastic movements generated high inertial forces, which acted like internal perturbations and affected the control of movement speed at contact. Hannah, in her more deliberate approach, had a slower but smoother reach strategy.

One suggestive interpretation of these overall patterns is that the first 4 months of reaching were a time of intense exploration, with the infants producing movements that varied greatly in speed, smoothness, efficiency, and coordination, leading to a rather sudden selection of reaches that though not adultlike, were "good enough." But we cannot discount that reaching improvement was a function of changes happening in other components of the system, for example, in posture.

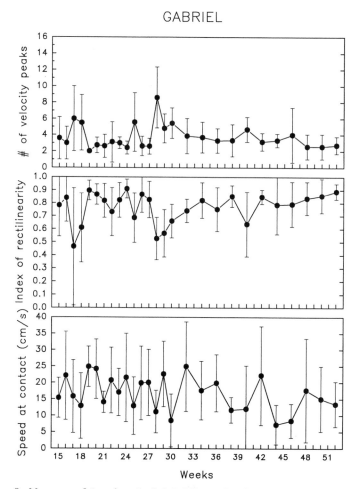

Fig. 9. Measures of "goodness" of Gabriel's reaches from week 15 to week 52. Top panel: number of velocity peaks of the reach averaged across trials by weeks. Middle panel: index of rectilinearity of the path of the hand averaged across trials by weeks. A value of 1 means that the path is perfectly straight. Bottom panel: resultant speed of the hand at contact with the target averaged across trials by weeks.

D. FORCE DYNAMICS AND BIMANUAL COORDINATION

To this point, we have described developmental changes in reaching, considering only the reach of one hand. But our everyday activities require that we coordinate the activities of both arms and hands. For instance, it is common for one hand to stabilize an object, while the other

HANNAH

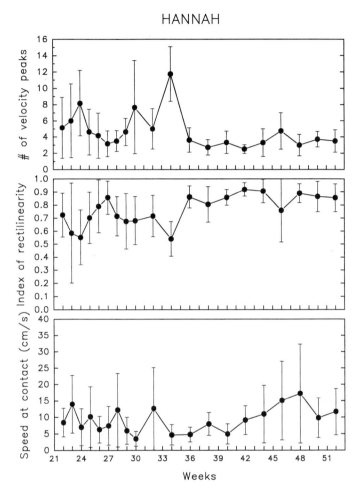

FIG. 10. Measures of "goodness" of Hannah's reaches from week 22 to week 52. Top panel: number of velocity peaks of the reach averaged across trials by weeks. Middle panel: index of rectilinearity of the path of the hand averaged across trials by weeks. A value of 1 means that the path is perfectly straight. Bottom panel: resultant speed of the hand at contact with the target averaged across trials by weeks.

performs a manipulation, such as opening a can of beer. It is an act of deliberate bimanual coordination even when one hand does not move while the other does some functional action such as opening a doorknob.

How do people develop this ability to voluntarily coordinate the arms? The origins of bimanual coordination in infancy have remained obscure. We know that by the end of the first year, infants appropriately reach and grasp small objects with one arm, large objects with two arms, and can use the two hands differentially to stabilize and manipulate (Fagard and Jacquet, 1994; Flament, 1975; Ramsay *et al.*, 1979). But conventional studies of arm and hand use as a function of age in younger infants have led to confusing and conflicting results.

Our longitudinal study of individual infants helps explain why it is difficult to describe a consistent developmental trend in bimanual function and adds further evidence to the importance of learning about force dynamics in early motor control. As we described above, the infants in the study showed strong individual differences in their level of overall motor activity, and we described in detail the reaching development of the most active, Gabriel, and the most quiet, Hannah. Nathan, like Gabriel, was an active mover, and the fourth baby, Justin, was more quiet.

What our analysis of interlimb coordination showed was that Gabriel and Nathan, the two most active infants, began reaching using predominantly two arms simultaneously (Corbetta and Thelen, 1994a,b). That is, when they saw the small toy in front of them, both arms went out and forward, although one hand usually touched the toy first. Most importantly, our analysis of their spontaneous movements—all their movements when they were not actually reaching—revealed that they tended to accelerate and decelerate both arms simultaneously as well. In contrast, the quieter Hannah and Justin did not use as many bimanual reaches when they began to reach, but showed a mixture of one- and two-handed reaches. Moreover, their spontaneous patterns of interlimb coordination did not reveal any predominant tendency to move in synchrony, but rather showed a wide range of desynchronized patterns. Thus, the different styles at reaching onset suggested that coupling was not an obligatory neural pattern but a function of intrinsic, individual energy parameterization of their movements.

These initial intrinsic dynamics were not stable over the first year, however, but sometimes showed developmental shifts. As Hannah speeded up (and stiffened up) her movements in the weeks following onset, she also increased her proportion of two-handed reaches, even though the objects remained small enough to grasp with one hand. Similarly, Justin, who became very active at the end of the first year, reached with two hands at that time. And, Nathan who damped down his initial energetic movements, shifted to more one-handed reaches. Only Gabriel, who remained very active during the entire year, maintained his preference for two-handed reaches.

What these data suggest, then, is that recruitment across the two limbs is part of the same force dynamic parameters as the reaching pattern in one limb. In the early months, coupling is neither hard-wired nor well-matched to the task, but appears to be a function of the infants' overall energetics. When more motoneuron pools are recruited, the activation overflows to both limbs. As in adult movements, asymmetry across the limbs can be maintained only when movements are slow and generated by low forces. As soon as movement speed increases, the asymmetrical patterns become unstable and behavior becomes attracted to symmetrical and synchronized patterns. Desynchronization is difficult or impossible when the system is highly energized (Kelso, 1984; Kelso *et al.*, 1981; Swinnen *et al.*, 1992). The task for infants in bimanual function may be the same as in unimanual reaching, that is, to appropriately parameterize the muscle contractions to allow inhibition of active movements for unimanual reaching and to energize both arms when bimanual reaching is demanded by the task. This hypothesis warrants further experimental test.

IV. Infant Reaching and Neural Dynamics

The lesson from infant reaching is that this new behavior cannot have arisen from a dedicated reaching "device" in the brain, innate or prefigured, and awaiting autonomous, time-dependent processes of "maturation" for its liberation. Following Edelman (1987) and consistent with a dynamic, Bernstein-inspired approach, we suggest that infants begin life with a few simple biases, for example, to look at interesting visual events and to have interesting things in their mouths. They also arrive in the world as perceivers and movers. Because movement always has proprioceptive and haptic consequences, it can also be considered as a perceptual modality. Infants actively move and perceive using whatever capabilities they marshall at the time, and thus they learn from their nondirected as well as their more goal-oriented movements. These early explorations of moving and its perceptual consequences constitute the first postnatal, experience-related neuronal groups—populations of neurons whose activity is strengthened by correlated, multimodal input. Our evidence suggests these early categories may include the relative compliances of the limbs or other articulators. If getting something into the mouth is desirable, then infants would rapidly learn to contract muscles of the arm so as not to slam into their faces with their fists, or to adjust sucking movements to the flow of the milk from the breast. These explorations build the basic repertoire of a body sense, of knowing where the limbs are and the parameters of muscles needed to change the limbs and posture (Thelen and Smith, 1994).

As the earliest arm movements are rarely coordinated with vision, but are more self-directed, the earliest coherent neural maps may well be of proprioception and tactile inputs—presumably of correlated force levels detected by joint and muscle proprioceptors along with pressure and skin deformation. As muscles and bones strengthen and limbs and torso grow, and as vision and its control also improve, the visual correlates of posture and movement increasingly become associated as movements are carried out within the visual field. The initial role of vision in reaching, however, may be to convince the infant that there is something interesting out there to put in the mouth and to roughly specify its location, that is, to provide a concept of an object. Recent work by Clifton and associates supports the primacy of proprioception in getting the hand to the object. They found that normal infants, provided with either the sight or the sound of a toy, initially reached equally well in the light and in the dark, that is, with without the sight of their hands (Clifton *et al.*, 1993). Thus, as we also suggested, babies are unlikely to construct a reach initially from a visual comparison between hand and object. Of course, these early reaches are not very accurate, and vision may become increasingly important for an accurate reach and grasp.

The question naturally arises about blind children. Infants who are blind from birth are significantly delayed in reaching for objects outside of their close personal space. This is because without vision they lack the motivation to reach forward and grasp things; they appear not to have the concept of an object to reach for. Indeed, only after extended manual and auditory exploration of objects do these babies reach for a sounding toy away from their bodies, and they are also delayed in searching for a sounding toy that is displaced from an original location (Bigelow, 1992). Blind infants are also delayed in the onset of forward locomotion, although their motor systems are intact. The problem is similar; they appear to lack a visually specified goal for moving forward. Interestingly, only after blind infants master reaching do they learn to walk (Bigelow, 1992). That is, once they discover manually that there are objects in extrapersonal space—goals that sighted infants have recognized soon after birth—they are motivated to discover a motor solution of how to obtain a distant goal.

These results on normal and blind infants point again to the epigenetic and "problem-solving" nature of development, consistent with a process of exploration and selection. There are many pathways to adaptive behavior not rigidly specified by a maturational timetable. Just as Gabriel and Hannah had to find their own solutions, so blind babies must discover an object concept by alternative perceptual means.

When early behavioral development is thus conceptualized as dynamic, emergent, continuous, and selected, it is not useful to ask what part of the brain must "mature" in order for some milestone to appear. We believe that brain–behavior questions need to be reformulated to better reflect both the behavioral realities and contemporary trends in the neurosciences. The behavioral realities are that performance does not "reside" in any privileged form, but is assembled from multiple components, which will have asynchronous developmental courses. Some components may act as rate limiters, that is, be necessary but not sufficient contributors to developmental change, but that does not mean these components "house" the behaviors in question. Such a view of behavior is consistent with the growing emphasis on the dynamic, distributed, and population nature of complex brain function (e.g., Damasio, 1989; Singer, 1990; Georgopoulos, 1991). Evidence is rapidly accumulating that central nervous system function is an emergent property of widely distributed, densely interconnected networks, and at all levels from sensory processing, motor control, memory, and higher cognitive functions. The brain–behavior question thus shifts to understanding the contribution of these multiple influences and their separate and multiple paths of mutual influence.

Especially important, in our view, is a new understanding of the mutual influences of brain and behavior, rather than assuming the conventional brain-to-behavior path of causality. An important example comes from the elegant studies of Diamond (e.g., 1990) on the role of the dorsolateral prefrontal cortex in a class of tasks used to measure spatial remembering of hidden objects. A wealth of data on humans and monkeys point to the involvement of this brain area in successful solution of the Piagetian "A-not-B error" and various other delayed-response tasks. Diamond concluded that maturation of the dorsolateral prefrontal cortex enables infants to solve this class of tasks. Other research, however, shows that the structure-to-function chain is not the simple developmental pathway. Indeed, research by Acredolo (1988) and others demonstrated that it is experience that is directly correlated with solving these tasks, and not experience practicing the task. Rather, it is locomotor experience—independent crawling—that correlates with the hidden object task. Infants, who through their own self-generated movement, have explored a spatial landscape, learn and remember the location of objects when they or the objects are displaced.

Thus, the traditional question must be reformulated to ask, how is behavior changing the brain? Again, this view is entirely consistent with the growing and exciting demonstrations of amazing plasticity in the brain, even in the brains of adult animals (see, for example, Kaas, 1991; Merzenich et al., 1990). That function is sculpting brain must now be considered as a primary postnatal developmental mechanism (see Thelen and Smith, 1994, for extended discussion and models). And that the function may not prefigure the behavior in question speaks dramatically to the distributed and noniconic nature of brain processes.

Acknowledgments

This work was supported by the National Institutes of Health, Grant RO1 HD22830, and by a Research Career Development Award (KO2 MH00718) from the National Institute of Mental Health to Esther Thelen.

References

Acredolo, L. P. (1988). Infant mobility and spatial development. *In* "Spatial Cognition: Brain Bases and Development" (J. Stiles-Davis, M. Kritchevsky, and U. Bellugi, eds.), pp. 156–166. Erlbaum, Hillsdale, NJ.

Beek, P. J. (1989). "Juggling Dynamics." Free Univ. Press, Amsterdam.

Bernstein, N. (1967). "The Co-ordination and Regulation of Movements." Pergamon, New York.

Bigelow, A. E. (1992). Locomotion and search behavior in blind infants. *Infant Behav. Dev.* **15**, 179–189.

Bower, T. G. R., Broughton, J., and Moore, M. (1970). The coordination of vision and touch in infancy. *Percept. Psychophys.* **8**, 51–53.

Bruner, J. S. (1973). Organization of early skilled action. *Child Dev.* **44**, 1–11.

Clifton, R. K., Muir, D. W., Ashmead, D. H., and Clarkson, M. G. (1993). Is visually guided reaching in early infancy a myth? *Child Dev.* **64**, 1099–1110.

Corbetta, D., and Thelen, E. (1994a). Interlimb coordination in the development of reaching. *In* "Motor Development: Aspects of Normal and Delayed Development" J. H. A. van Rossum and J. L. Laszlo, eds.), pp. 11–24. VU Univ. Press, Amsterdam.

Corbetta, D., and Thelen, E. (1994b). Shifting patterns of interlimb coordination in infants' reaching: A case study. *In* "Interlimb Coordination: Neural, Dynamical and Cognitive Constraints" (S. P. Swinnen, H. Heuer, J. Massion, and P. Casaer, eds.), pp. 413–438. Academic Press, San Diego.

Damasio, A. R. (1989). Time-locked multiregional retroactivation: A systems-level proposal for the neural substrates of recall and recognition. *Cognition* **33**, 25–62.

Diamond, A. (1990). The development and neural bases of memory functions as indexed by the A-not-B and delayed response tasks in human infants and infant monkeys. *Ann. N. Y. Acad. Sci.* **608**, 267–398.

Edelman, G. M. (1987). "Neural Darwinism: The Theory of Neuronal Group Selection." Basic Books, New York.

Edwards, C. T. (1992). Motor development in the preschool years. *In* "Assessing and Screening Preschoolers: Psychological and Educational Dimensions" (E. V. Nuttall, I. Romero, and J. Kalesnik, eds.), pp. 9–22. Allyn & Bacon, Boston.

Fagard, J., and Jacquet, A. Y. (1994). Changes in reaching and grasping objects of different sizes between 7 and 13 months of age. Unpublished.

Feldman, A. G. (1980). Superposition of motor programs. I. Rhythmic forearm movements in man. *J. Neurosci.* **5**, 81–90.

Flament, F. (1975). "Coordination et prévalence manuelle chex le nourrisson." Editions du CNRS, Paris.

Forssberg, H. (1985). Ontogeny of human locomotor control. I. Infant stepping, supported locomotion, and transition to independent locomotion. *Exp. Brain Res.* **57**, 480–493.

Georgopoulos, A. P. (1991). Higher order motor control. *Annu. Rev. Neurosci.* **14**, 361–377.

Gibson, E. J. (1988). Exploratory behavior in the development of perceiving, acting and the acquiring of knowledge. *Annu. Rev. Psychol.* **39**, 1–41.

Goldman-Rakic, P. S. (1987). Development of control circuitry and cognitive function. *Child Dev.* **58**, 601–622.

Gottlieb, G. L., Corcos, D. M., and Agarwal, G. C. (1989). Strategies for the control of voluntary movements with one degree of freedom. *Behav. Brain Sci.* **12**, 189–250.

Hogan, N. (1984). An organizing principle for a class of voluntary movements. *J. Neurosci.* **4**, 2745–2754.

Hogan, N., Bizzi, E., Mussa-Ivaldi, F. A., and Flash, T. (1987). Controlling multijoint motor behavior. *Exercise Sport Sci. Rev.* **15**, 153–190.

Jeannerod, M. (1988). "The Neural and Behavioural Organization of Goal-Directed Movements." Clarendon Press, Oxford.

Kaas, J. H. (1991). Plasticity of sensory and motor maps in adult mammals. *Annu. Rev. Neurosci.* **14**, 137–167.

Kelso, J. A. S. (1984). Phase transitions and critical behavior in human bimanual coordination. *Am. J. Physiol.* **246**, R1000–R1004.

Kelso, J. A. S., Holt, K. G., Kugler, P. N., and Turvey, M. T. (1980). On the concept of coordinative structures as dissipative structures. II. Empirical lines of convergence. *In* "Tutorials in Motor Behavior" (G. E. Stelmach and J. Requin, eds.), pp. 49–70. North-Holland Publ., New York.

Kelso, J. A. S., Holt, K. G., Rubin, P., and Kugler, P. N. (1981). Patterns of human interlimb coordination emerge from the properties of non-linear limit cycle oscillatory processes: Theory and data. *J. Mot. Behav.* **13**, 226–261.

Konner, M. (1991). Universals of behavioral development in relation to brain myelination. *In* "Brain Maturation and Cognitive Development: Comparative and Cross-Cultural Perspectives" (K. R. Gibson and A. C. Petersen, eds.), pp. 181–223. de Gruyter, New York.

Kugler, P. N., and Turvey, M. T. (1987). "Information, Natural Law, and the Self-Assembly of Rhythmic Movement." Erlbaum, Hillsdale, NJ.

Kugler, P. N., Kelso, J. A. S., and Turvey, M. T. (1980). On the concept of coordinative structures as dissipative structures. I. Theoretical lines of convergence. *In* "Tutorials in Motor Behavior" (G. E. Stelmach and J. Requin, eds.), pp. 3–47. North-Holland Publ., New York.

Kugler, P. N., Kelso, J. A. S., and Turvey, M. T. (1982). On the control and coordination of naturally developing systems. *In* "The Development of Movement Control and Coordination" (J. A. S. Kelso and J. E. Clark, eds.), pp. 5–78. Wiley, New York.

McGraw, M. B. (1945). "The Neuromuscular Maturation of the Human Infant." Columbia Univ. Press, New York.

Merzenich, M. M., Allard, T. T., and Jenkins, W. M. (1990). Neural ontogeny of higher brain function: Implications of some recent neurophysiological findings. *In* "Information Processing in the Somatosensory System" (O. Franz and P. Westman, eds.), pp. 293–311. Macmillan, London.

Morasso, P. (1981). Spatial control of arm movements. *Exp. Brain Res.* **42**, 223–227.

Piaget, J. (1952). "The Origins of Intelligence in Children." International Universities Press, New York.

Polit, A., and Bizzi, E. (1978). Processes controlling arm movements in monkeys. *Science* **201**, 1235–1237.

Ramsay, D. S., Campos, J. J., and Fenson, L. (1979). Onset of bimanual handedness in infants. *Infant Behav. Dev.* **2**, 69–76.

Rochat, P. (1989). Object manipulation and exploration in 2- to 5-month old infants. *Dev. Psychol.* **25**, 871–884.

Schöner, G., and Kelso, J. A. S. (1988). Dynamic pattern generation in behavioral and neural systems. *Science* **239**, 1513–1520.

Singer, W. (1990). The formation of cooperative cell assemblies in the visual cortex. *J. Exp. Biol.* **153**, 177–197.

Soechting, J. F., and Ross, B. (1984). Psychophysical determination of coordinate representation of human arm orientation. *Neuroscience* **13**, 595–604.

Swinnen, S. P., Walter, C. B., Serrien, D. J., and Vandendriessche, C. (1992). The effect of movement speed on upper-limb coupling strength. *Hum. Movement Sci.* **11**, 615–636.

Thelen, E. (1984). Learning to walk: Ecological demands and phylogenetic constraints. *Adv. Infancy Res.* **3**, 213–150.

Thelen, E. (1989). Self-organization in developmental processes: Can systems approaches work? *In* "Minnesota Symposia in Child Psychology" (M. Gunnar and E. Thelen, eds.), Vol. 22, pp. 77–117. Erlbaum, Hillsdale, NJ.

Thelen, E., and Fisher, D. M. (1982). Newborn stepping: An explanation for a "disappearing reflex." *Dev. Psychol.* **18**, 760–775.

Thelen, E., and Smith, L. B. (1994). "A Dynamic Systems Approach to the Development of Cognition and Action." MIT Press, Cambridge, MA.

Thelen, E., and Ulrich, B. D. (1991). Hidden skills: A dynamic systems analysis of treadmill stepping during the first year. *Monogr. Soc. Res. Child Dev.* 223, **56**(1, Ser. No. 223).

Thelen, E., Fisher, D. M., Ridley-Johnson, R., and Griffin, N. (1982). The effects of body build and arousal on newborn infant stepping. *Dev. Psychobiol.* **15**, 447–453.

Thelen, E., Fisher, D. M., and Ridley-Johnson, R. (1984). The relationship between physical growth and a newborn reflex. *Infant Behav. Dev.* **7**, 479–493.

Thelen, E., Corbetta, D., Kamm, K., Spencer, J. C., Schneider, K., and Zernicke, R. F. (1993). The transition to reaching: Mapping intention and intrinsic dynamics. *Child Dev.* **64**, 1058–1098.

Trevarthen, C. (1984). How control of movement develops. *In* "Human Motor Actions: Bernstein Reassessed" (H. T. A. Whiting, ed.), pp. 223–261. North-Holland Publ., Amsterdam.

Vereijken, B. (1991). "The Dynamics of Skill Acquisition." Krips Repo, Meppel, The Netherlands.

von Hofsten, C. (1982). Eye–hand coordination in the newborn. *Dev. Psychol.* **18**, 450–461.

von Hofsten, C. (1984). Developmental changes in the organization of prereaching movements. *Dev. Psychol.* **20**, 378–388.

POPULATION ACTIVITY IN THE CONTROL OF MOVEMENT

Apostolos P. Georgopoulos

Veterans Affairs Medical Center
Minneapolis, Minnesota 55417

This review summarizes key observations and concepts concerning the role of neuronal populations in specification and control of the direction of movement and isometric force. Large populations of neurons in the motor cortex are engaged with reaching movements. This engagement is fairly early, starting approximately 60 msec following target onset. Single cells are directionally broadly tuned, but the neuronal population carries an unambiguous directional signal. The outcome of this population code can be visualized as a vector that points in the direction of the upcoming movement during the reaction time, during an instructed delay period, and during a memorized delay period. Moreover, when a mental transformation is required for the generation of a reaching movement in a different direction from a reference direction, the population vector provides a direct insight into the nature of the cognitive process by which the required transformation is achieved.

The problem we are investigating concerns the neural mechanisms of spatially directed motor output, including reaching movements and isometric forces exerted by the arm. For this purpose, we have trained rhesus monkeys to operate three devices to produce motor outputs in various directions in space. The first device allows movements in two-dimensional space (Fig. 1); the monkey moves an articulated manipulandum from one point to another on a planar working surface (Georgopoulos et al., 1981, 1982). The second device allows reaching movements in three-dimensional space (Fig. 2); the monkey pushes buttons placed at various points in three-dimensional space (Georgopoulos et al., 1986; Schwartz et al., 1988). Finally, an isometric force device allows exertion of two-dimensional isometric forces on a rigid handle (Georgopoulos et al., 1992). In all three paradigms, we focused on the neural coding of the direction of the motor output, be it movement or isometric force. The salient finding of these studies has been that the activity of single cells in the motor cortex is broadly tuned with respect to the direction of the motor output (Georgopoulos et al., 1982, 1992; Schwartz et al., 1988). In general, the intensity of cell discharge varied as a cosine function of this direction (Figs. 3 and 4). The peak of this function is the direction for which the cell activity is most intense; this is the cell's

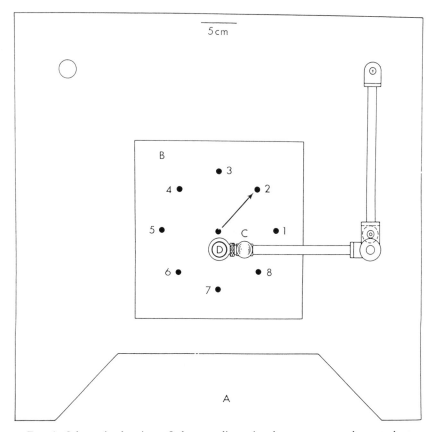

FIG. 1. Schematic drawing of the two-dimensional apparatus used to study two-dimensional movements of monkeys. The monkey sat at A, in front of the working surface, B. The numbered light-emitting diodes (LEDs) were placed on a circle of 8 cm radius. The monkey held the articulated manipulandum at its distal end (C) and captured a lighted LED within a transparent plexiglass circle (D). The arrow indicates the direction of one movement. The x–y motion of the center of that circle was monitored every 10 msec with a resolution of 0.125 mm. (Modified from Georgopoulos *et al.*, 1981; reproduced with permission.)

preferred direction. The preferred directions ranged throughout the directional continuum without any particular tendency to cluster (Fig. 5). The similarity of the directional tuning in two- and three-dimensional movements, and in two-dimensional isometric forces, provides a common background on the problem of how motor direction could be specified in a unique fashion within the neuronal population, as follows.

The broad directional tuning indicates that a given cell participates

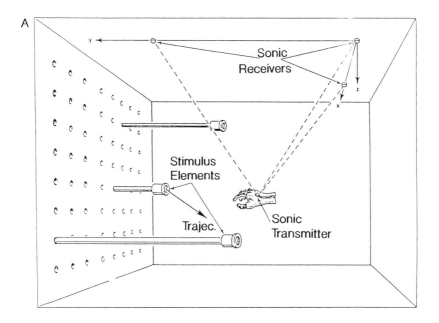

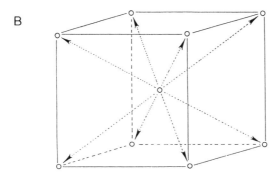

FIG. 2. Schematic drawing of the apparatus used to study free reaching movements in three-dimensional space. (A) The monkey reached toward and pushed lighted buttons mounted at the end of metal rods threaded through a heavy metal plate. The movement trajectory was monitored using an ultrasonic system. (B) Schematic diagram of the location of the nine buttons used. Dotted lines indicate directions of movements. (From Schwartz *et al.*, 1988; reproduced with permission. Copyright by Society for Neuroscience.)

in movements of various directions, and that a movement in a particular direction will involve the activation of a whole population of cells. Given that single cells are directionally tuned, we proposed a vectorial neuronal population code for the direction of reaching (Georgopoulos *et al.*, 1983, 1986, 1988, 1992): (1) a particular cell vector represents the contribution

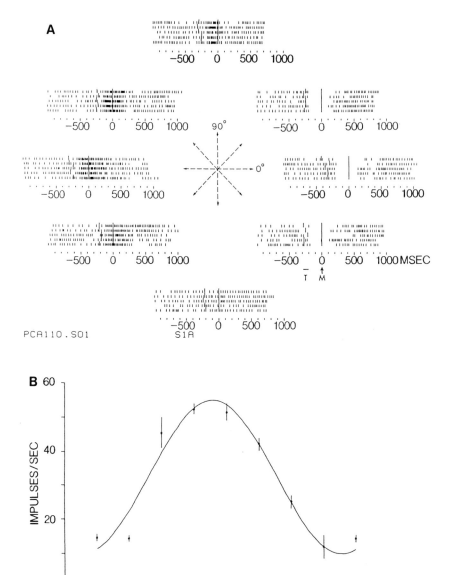

FIG. 3. Broad directional tuning in two-dimensional space of a cell recorded in the arm area of the motor cortex. (A) Impulse activity during five trials with movements in the directions indicated in the drawing at the center. Short vertical bars indicate the occurrence of an action potential. Rasters are aligned to the onset of movement (M). Longer vertical bars preceding the onset of movement indicate the onset of the target (T). (B) Average frequency of discharge (±SEM) from the onset of the stimulus until the entry to the target window are plotted against the direction of movement. Continuous curve is a cosine function fitted to the data using multiple regression analysis. (From Georgopoulos *et al.*, 1982; reproduced with permission. Copyright by Society for Neuroscience.)

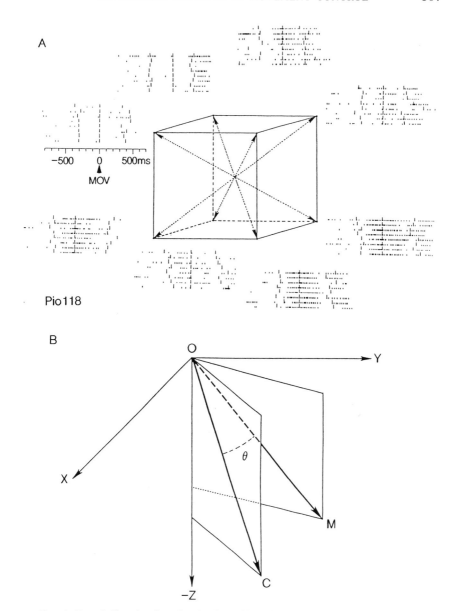

FIG. 4. Broad directional tuning in three-dimensional space of a motor cortical cell. (A) Impulse activity is shown in raster form for eight trials in eight movement directions indicated in the drawing at center. MOV, Onset of movement. (B) Principle of directional tuning: C is the preferred direction of the cell whose rasters are shown in A; M is the direction of a movement; θ is the angle between C and M. The cell activity varies in a linear fashion with $\cos(\theta)$. (Adapted from Georgopoulos *et al.*, 1986; reproduced with permission. Copyright by AAAS, 1986.)

of a directionally tuned cell and points in the cell's preferred direction; (2) cell vectors are weighted by the change in cell activity during a particular movement; and (3) the sum of these vectors (i.e., the population vector) provides the unique outcome of the ensemble coding operation. We found that the population vector points in the direction of movement for two-dimensional movements (Fig. 6; Georgopoulos *et al.*, 1983), and three-dimensional movements (Fig. 7; Georgopoulos *et al.*, 1986, 1988), and in the direction of net force for two-dimensional isometric forces (Georgopoulos *et al.*, 1992).

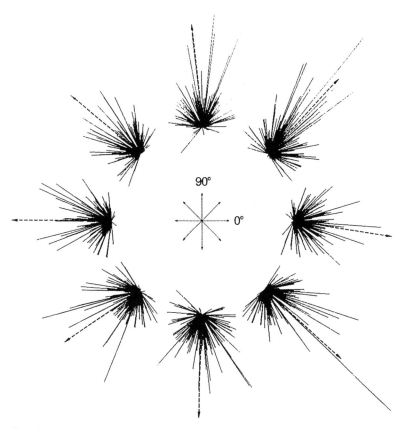

FIG. 6. Neuronal population coding of the direction of two-dimensional reaching movements. Vectorial contributions of single cells (continuous lines, $N = 241$) add to yield the population vector (interrupted line). Each cluster represents the same population; the movement directions are shown in the diagram at the center. The population vector points in or near the direction of the movement. (From Georgopoulos *et al.*, 1983; reproduced with permission.)

What do we gain and lose with this coding scheme? First, we gain a unique spatial measure. It is remarkable that we start with purely *temporal* spike trains, and through their tuning and the interpretation of this tuning in a vectorial fashion, we end up with a unique *spatial* outcome that is isomorphic in space with the direction of the movement. Second, we gain a continuous coding of directions by the same ensemble without depending on specific cells to code uniquely for specific directions. And third, this kind of coding is resistant to cell loss (Georgopoulos *et al.*, 1988). The main drawback of this coding scheme is that it is energetically inefficient, because the whole ensemble is engaged for any particular movement. We could have devised another scheme by which only a small number of cells, very specific for a particular direction, would be activated, and this would have been energetically inexpensive. Be that as it may, our code is a distributed one and involves the whole population.

The next step in our investigation was to find out whether we could get useful information *in time*, that is, whether we can use the population vector to acquire information during the reaction time about the upcoming movement direction. And indeed, this was the case (Georgopoulos *et al.*, 1984, 1988). Figure 8 illustrates two examples in which the movement was instructed to be in two different directions. We calculated the population of vector every 20 msec during the reaction time. It can be

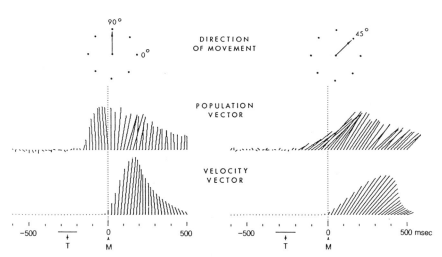

FIG. 8. Population vectors computed every 20 msec for movements in two different directions. Instantaneous velocity vectors are also shown. Notice that the population vector lengthens well before the movement begins and points in the approximate direction of the upcoming movement. M, Onset of movement; T, target. (From Georgopoulos *et al.*, 1984; reproduced with permission.)

seen that after the stimulus was given and approximately 180 msec before the onset of the movement, the population vector lengthens and points in the direction of the upcoming movement. The same also held for three-dimensional movements (Georgopoulos *et al.*, 1988) and isometric forces (Georgopoulos *et al.*, 1992).

These findings provided us with the tools for probing time-varying, directional processes involved in cognitive function. The diagram in Fig. 9 is from Edelman's book (Edelman, 1992). The connection between neuroscience and psychology is a crucial one, and it was on this connection that we focused our research during the past several years. Our strategy to attack this problem is shown in Table I. First, we have to select a cognitive process for study. Second, we need a variable on which this process will operate. Third, we need to understand the neural coding of the variable outside the process. Finally, we design an experiment and look at the neural representation of the process, having understood the coding for the variable on which the process operates.

The variable of interest in our case is the direction of the motor output, and the population vector provides the neural coding of that variable. The next question is how can we use the population vector as a *probe* to decipher brain events underlying a cognitive process. If we formulate a problem properly and devise an appropriate task, we can then record the activity of cells during a task, and use the population

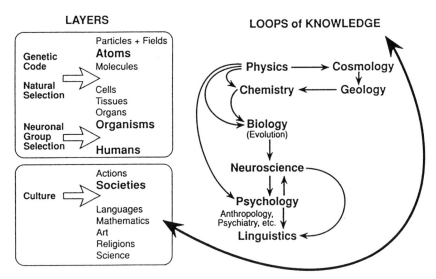

FIG. 9. Layers of biological organization and loops of knowledge. (From Figure 14-1 from "Bright Air, Brilliant Fire" by Gerald Edelman. Copyright © 1992 by Basic Books, Inc. Reprinted by permission of Basic Books, a division of Harper Collins Publishers, Inc.)

TABLE I
Steps in Deciphering Brain Mechanisms of Cognitive Processes

1. Select a variable of interest
2. Find the neural coding of the variable outside the cognitive process
3. Select a cognitive process operating on the variable of interest
4. Record brain activity during cognitive processing and infer how the variable is operated on

vector as a probe to elucidate how the motor cortex deals with a cognitive directional process.

As a first step in that direction, we investigated the changes in cell activity in the motor cortex during two delay tasks that involved either an instructed delay, during which the target was continuously present, or a memorized delay, during which information about the direction of movement had to be kept in mind before a go signal was given. In the latter task, the target light was presented for 300 msec and was turned off, and, after a memorized delay, the *go* signal was given for the monkey to move its arm in the direction of the target that disappeared (Smyrnis *et al.*, 1992). Making the correct movement depended on keeping in mind the position of that target. In contrast, in the nonmemorized delay task, the target came on and stayed on until the *go* signal was given. During this delay period there was information available all the time about the direction of the upcoming movement.

Tanji and Evarts (1976) had shown previously that motor cortical cells can be activated during imposed delays, in the absence of an immediate motor output. We confirmed that approximately one-half of the cells in the motor cortex changed activity during the delay periods in our tasks (Georgopoulos *et al.*, 1989; Smyrnis *et al.*, 1992). However, the simple knowledge that cells change activity during a task does not provide the crucial information concerning the *content* of the process in which a cell participates. We gained valuable insight in this problem by the population vector analysis. The population vector during the nonmemorized (Georgopoulos *et al.*, 1989) or the memorized (Fig. 10; Smyrnis *et al.*, 1992) delay period pointed in the direction of the upcoming movement. Therefore, the directional information carried by the population vector in these tasks identified the content of the process in a direct fashion.

Another interesting point concerns the strength of the signal. Figure 11 plots the length of the population vector over time in the memorized and nonmemorized delay tasks. There are two phases in this time course. First, the population vector increases shortly after the cue onset, and

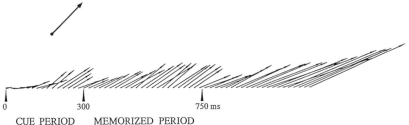

0   300   750 ms

CUE PERIOD   MEMORIZED PERIOD

FIG. 10. Population vectors in the memorized delay task for the direction indicated are plotted every 20 msec. The arrow on top indicates the direction of the cue signal present during the first 300 msec of the delay period. (From Smyrnis *et al.*, 1992; reproduced with permission.)

then decreases at the end of the cue period. This phase is almost the same in both tasks. However, during the memorized delay period, there is a sustained, longer population vector in the memorized compared to the nonmemorized delay task (Fig. 11; stippled area). It is intriguing that there is a stronger signal in the absence of the target stimulus, which may reflect the higher demand for keeping information in mind. This brings us to a peculiar hypothesis about the motor cortex; namely, that this structure may be more active when there is lack of external information and the information has to be constructed from memory, rather than when everything is given for a particular movement.

We now move to the third and central part of this psychology–neuro-

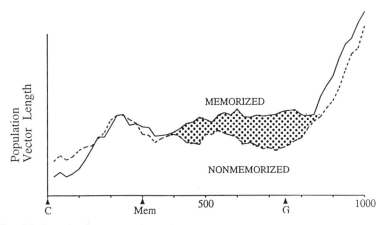

FIG. 11. Length of mean resultant of the population vector is plotted against time for the two delay tasks. C, Cue onset; G, minimum time of onset of the *go* signal. (From Smyrnis *et al.*, 1992; reproduced with permission.)

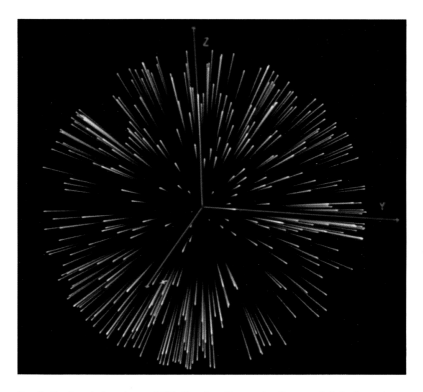

Fig. 5. Preferred directions of 475 directionally tuned cells recorded during a three-dimensional reaching task. Lines are vectors of unit length. (From Schwartz et al., 1988; reproduced with permission. Copyright by the Society for Neuroscience.)

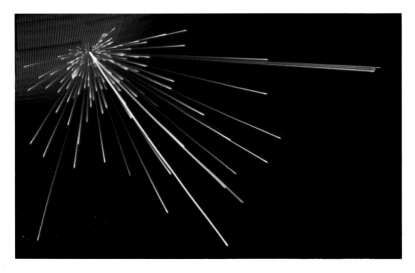

FIG. 7. Neuronal population coding of the direction of three-dimensional reaching movements. Vectorial contributions of single cells (light blue lines) add to the yield of the population vector (orange), the direction of which is close to the direction of the movement (yellow). (From Georgopoulos et al., 1988; reproduced with permission. Copyright by the Society for Neuroscience.)

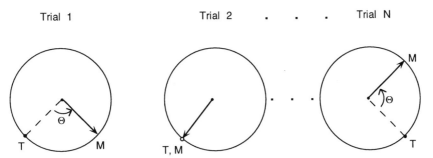

FIG. 12. Schematic directional transformation experiment. Three typical trials are shown. T, Stimulus; M, movement. Open and filled circles indicate trials of direct and transformation tasks, respectively.

science interplay. We first studied human subjects, to learn how they perform and solve a particular problem. From the results of these studies we formulated hypotheses about the psychological process(es) underlying the solution of the problem. Then, we trained monkeys to solve the same

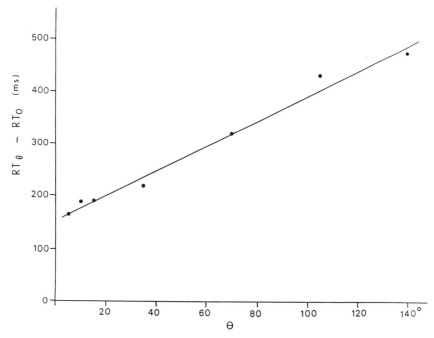

FIG. 13. Increase of reaction time with instructed transformation angle (see text). (From Georgopoulos and Massey, 1987; reproduced with permission.)

problem and recorded the activity of cells in the motor cortex, trying to interpret the results of the psychological experiments on the basis of the results of the neurophysiological studies.

The problem we studied is illustrated in Fig. 12. Subjects were trained to start from the center of the plane in the two-dimensional device. But when the target shifted to a peripheral location, the light would be either dim or bright. The brightness level gave the subject the clue to either move the handle in the direction of the light (*direct* task) or away from the light at an instructed angle, clockwise or counterclockwise (*transformation* task). These trials were randomized in terms of the stimulus position and the condition of brightness. This task is quite difficult. The problem can be solved in different ways (Georgopoulos and Massey, 1987), which makes the studies interesting. For example, subjects can form a lookup table in their mind to associate specific stimuli with specific movements, given the particular instructions: they look at their table to determine which is which. But for any given trial, and however the subjects solve the problem, they have to derive the direction of their movements on the basis of the stimulus direction. The basic finding from the human studies is shown in Fig. 13: it takes more time to generate movements when the subject is instructed to move away from the target for a given angle, and the increasing reaction time is a linear function of the angle that the subject is instructed to move away from the stimulus direction.

This finding cannot be explained by the above hypothesis involving a lookup table, because in that case we would have to suppose that it takes more time to search for one angle than for another; and there is no *a priori* reason for that supposition. We might expect longer reaction times but not a dependence of the increase of the reaction time on the angle. The most parsimonious explanation for these findings is shown

Task   Reaction time

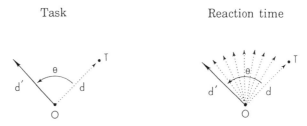

FIG. 14. O, Movement origin; T, stimulus location; d, stimulus direction; d', movement direction; θ, transformation angle. Dotted lines indicate hypothesized rotation of imagined movement direction.

in Fig. 14. If the task is to move away from a stimulus direction at a given angle, then our results would be explained by the idea that the subject rotates a representation of the motor intention from the stimulus direction toward the movement direction. If the instruction is for a short angle, then the process would take less time. However, more time would be needed for a larger angle because the subject has to go through the intermediate directions. This idea is very similar to the mental rotation hypothesis advanced by Shepard and Cooper (1982) to explain the monotonic increase of the reaction time with orientation angle, when a judgment has to be made whether a visual image is normal or mirror image. In both cases a mental rotation is postulated. We thought that we could identify the neural representation of the motor intention by the population vector, and we were curious to see if the population vector would rotate in this task. The null hypothesis was that the motor cortex is involved only in the generation of movement and therefore the population vector would just point in the direction of the upcoming movement.

To our surprise, we found that the population vector rotated over time. In these experiments, the animals were trained to move, in the transformation trials, at 90° counterclockwise from the stimulus direction. An example is shown in Fig. 15. The movement was the same as for the above experiment, but was made in the direct task (left panel) or the transformation task (right panel). In the latter, the movement had to be 90° counterclockwise from the stimulus direction. It can be seen that in the direct task the population vector points in the direction of the upcoming movement, whereas in the transformation task it rotates counterclockwise from the stimulus direction to the movement direction. An interesting question is whether one would see a moving wave across the cortex during the rotation period. We believe that we would not, because the cells are distributed within the arm area of the motor cortex and the cells' latencies are very similar within that area. Therefore we would not expect to see a spatial movement of the population but we cannot test this idea at the moment.

It could be argued that the population vector rotation does not necessarily imply a rotation per se. For example, there could be two subsets of neurons, one pointing in the stimulus direction and the other in the movement direction. If their intensity changes accordingly, their vector sum would seem to be rotating without a "true" rotation, that is, without involving cells with a preferred direction intermediate between the stimulus and movement directions. This idea is a strong prediction of a "true rotation," namely, during the reaction time, there is a preferential recruit-

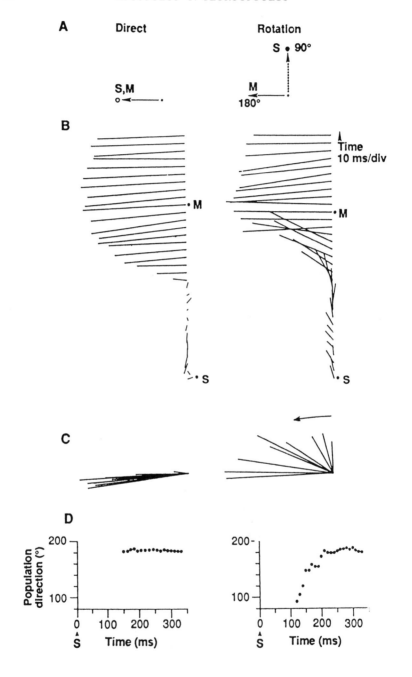

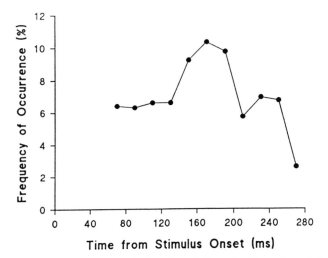

FIG. 16. Percentage of cells recruited at times indicated with preferred directions at or near the intermediate direction. Data points are centered on the middle of 20-msec bins. See text for explanation. (N = 94, 119, 150, 91, 185, 203, 104, 122, 71, 90, and 78 for the 20-msec time bins used, from 60–80 to 260–280 msec.) (From Lurito *et al.*, 1991; reproduced with permission.)

ment of cells with preferred directions intermediate between those of the stimulus and those of the movement. Figure 16 shows that cells of preferred directions within 20° in the intermediate direction (between

---

FIG. 15. Results from direct and rotation movements. (A) Task. Open and filled circles indicate dim and bright light, respectively. Interrupted and continuous lines with arrowheads indicate stimulus (S) and movement (M) direction, respectively. (B) Neuronal population vectors calculated every 10 msec from the onset of the stimulus, S, at positions shown in A until after the onset of the movement (M). When the population vector lengthens, for the direct case (left) it points in the direction of the movement, whereas for the rotation case (right) it points initially in the direction of the stimulus and then rotates counterclockwise (from 12 o'clock to 9 o'clock) and points in the direction of the movement. (C) Ten successive population vectors from B are shown in a spatial plot, starting from the first population vector that increased significantly in length. Notice the counterclockwise rotation of the population vector (right panel). (D) Scatter plots of the direction of the population vector as a function of time, starting from the first population vector that increased significantly in length following stimulus onset (S). For the direct case (left), the direction of the population vector is in the direction of the movement (~180°); for the rotation case (right) the direction of the population vector rotates counterclockwise from the direction of the stimulus (~90°) to the direction of the movement (~180°). (From Georgopoulos *et al.*, 1989; reproduced with permission. Copyright by AAAS, 1989.)

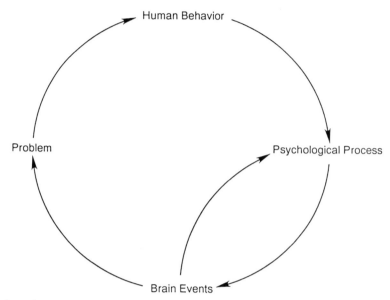

FIG. 17. Cognitive neuroscience conceptual loop. Links between studies probing the relation between psychology and neuroscience.

stimulus and movement) were preferentially engaged during the middle of the reaction time, as predicted by the rotation hypothesis. Therefore, we are dealing with a dynamic cognitive process evolving in time (Freyd, 1987). Interestingly, the mean rotation rate (about 400°/second (Lurito *et al.*, 1991) and the range of rates observed for different stimulus directions were very similar to those obtained in the human studies.

And these studies, in a way, close the circle (Fig. 17). We started with the problem of spatial transformation, and obtained the linear increase of the reaction time with the angle. On the basis of these findings, we hypothesized the rotation of an internal representation of the directional motor intention and then, with the same task, we directly visualized the hypothesized rotation in the rotation of the population vector. And so we closed the loop in the circle.

Acknowledgment

This work was supported by USPHS Grants NS17413 and PSMH48185.

References

Edelman, G. M. (1992). "Bright Air, Brilliant Fire: On the Matter of the Mind." Basic Books, New York.

Freyd, J. J. (1987). Dynamic mental representations. *Psychol. Rev.* **94,** 427–438.

Georgopoulos, A. P., and Massey, J. T. (1987). Cognitive spatial–motor processes 1. The making of movements at various angles from a stimulus direction. *Exp. Brain Res.* **65,** 361–370.

Georgopoulos, A. P., Kalaska, J. F., and Massey, J. T. (1981). Spatial trajectories and reaction times of aimed movements: Effects of practice, uncertainty, and change in target location. *J. Neurophysiol.* **46,** 725–743.

Georgopoulos, A. P., Kalaska, J. F., Caminiti, R., and Massey, J. T. (1982). On the relations between the direction of two-dimensional arm movements and cell discharge in primate motor cortex. *J. Neurosci.* **2,** 1527–1537.

Georgopoulos, A. P., Caminiti, R., Kalaska, J. F., and Massey, J. T. (1983). Spatial coding of movement: A hypothesis concerning the coding of movement direction by motor cortical populations. *Exp. Brain Res., Suppl.* **7,** 327–336.

Georgopoulos, A. P., Kalaska, J. F., Crutcher, M. D., Caminiti, R., and Massey, J. T. (1984). The representation of movement direction in the motor cortex: Single cell and population studies. *In* "Dynamic Aspects of Neocortical Function" (G. M. Edelman, W. E. Gall, and W. M. Cowan, eds.), pp. 501–524. Wiley, New York.

Georgopoulos, A. P., Schwartz, A. B., and Kettner, R. E. (1986). Neuronal population coding of movement direction. *Science* **233,** 1416–1419.

Georgopoulos, A. P., Kettner, R. E., and Schwartz, A. B. (1988). Primate motor cortex and free arm movements to visual targets in three-dimensional space. II. Coding of the direction of movement by a neuronal population. *J. Neurosci.* **8,** 2928–2937.

Georgopoulos, A. P., Crutcher, M. D., and Schwartz, A. B. (1989). Cognitive spatial-motor processes. 3. motor cortical predication of movement direction during an instructed delay period. *Exp. Brain Res.* **75,** 183–194.

Georgopoulos, A. P., Ashe, J., Smyrnis, N., and Taira, M. (1992). Motor cortex and the coding of force. *Science* **256,** 1692–1695.

Lurito, J. L., Georgakopoulos, T., and Georgopoulos, A. P. (1991). Cognitive spatial–motor processes. 7. The making of movements at an angle from a stimulus direction: Studies of motor cortical activity at the single cell and population levels. *Exp. Brain Res.* **87,** 562–580.

Schwartz, A. B., Kettner, R. E., and Georgopoulos, A. P. (1988). Primate motor cortex and free arm movements to visual targets in three-dimensional space. I. Relations between single cell discharge and direction of movement. *J. Neurosci.* **8,** 2913–2927.

Shepard, R. N., and Cooper, L. A. (1982). "Mental Images and Their Transformations." MIT Press, Cambridge, MA.

Smyrnis, N., Taira, M., Ashe, J., and Georgopoulos, A. P. (1992). Motor cortical activity in a memorized delay task. *Exp. Brain Res.* **92,** 139–151.

Tanji, J., and Evarts, E. V. (1976). Anticipatory activity of motor cortex neurons in relation to direction of an intended movement. *J. Neurophysiol.* **39,** 1062–1068.

SECTION II
DISCUSSION

The uniting theme of the contributions in this section is the issue of *variability*. The evidence for the existence of variability in biological structures, particularly the nervous system, is overwhelming. There is variability at the level of the structure and morphology of neuronal circuits, as well as in the dynamics of neuronal populations and in behavioral performance. What makes variability an important issue is that selection cannot occur without it; the absence of variability (except that present as "noise") is a hallmark of an instructive system or of a selective system in which previously occurring selective events have ceased. Though selective systems share a set of principles (outlined in great detail in the Section I), the origin of variability differs for each biological case. In natural selection a major source of variability is provided by randomly occurring genetic mutations. In the immune system "shuffling" of the genetic material coding for parts of antibody molecules leads to expression of diverse molecules varying with respect to the domains binding to antigens. Perhaps the most complicated case of all is presented by the nervous system: variability exists at multiple levels of organization (neurons, neuronal populations, neuronal maps, etc.) and it involves biochemistry, cell morphology, and dynamics.

Much of this variability originates during embryonic development, resulting in a primary repertoire of variant circuits that is ready to respond differentially to events in the environment surrounding the organism. Partly concurrent with morphogenesis is an extended phase of sensorimotor development, during which the nervous system and musculoskeletal apparatus engage in behavioral performance that varies significantly even for identical external stimuli. This represents an example of *dynamic* variability, partly a result of underlying structural variations at the level of circuitry. Structural variability translates into dynamic variability, yielding a primary repertoire of exploratory movements constantly refined and shaped by selection.

To a large degree, both morphological and dynamic development are due to *epigenetic processes* that act in addition to more direct genetic control. Epigenetic processes have a highly adaptive and regulatory character. This becomes especially evident when looking at Crossin's diagram illustrating the action of morphoregulatory loops. The networklike appearance of molecular interactions and the multilevel nature of morphoregulatory events (involving genes, molecules, cells, and cell collectives) are reminiscent of similar multilevel characteristics of neuronal networks. A view of development that emphasizes epigenetic interactions and

121

morphoregulation contrasts sharply with other proposals exclusively based on strict genetic control. Given the evidence, the view that all that is required for the appropriate formation of neuronal connectivity is the presence on the surface of neurons of unique molecular tags (serving as instructional cues) must be rejected.

With respect to the significance of selectional processes there is *continuity* between development and adaptation (plasticity) during mature function. Embryonic development leads to the formation of the three-dimensional structure of the embryo with its microscopic variations. This developmental stage continues, once initial connectivity is set up, with the activity-dependent formation of specific circuitry (for example, in the cerebral cortex). Starting from an exuberance of connections only those that link neurons that are coactive within a critical time window are maintained; others are lost. In this case, variant connectivity, under the influence of self-generated and externally triggered neural activity, is subject to differential stabilization or destabilization, a process under selectional control. Subsequently, the resultant connectivity can support selective processes at the next higher level, for example, involving the selection of neuronal groups in various tasks and contexts. Evidently, selectional events in the brain occur at different times as well as at different organizational levels. The main point is that developmental processes do not come to an abrupt half at the end of embryogenesis; rather, they manifest themselves as neuronal plasticity and reorganization in the adult organism.

Furthermore, as the discussion of motor development by Thelen and Corbetta shows, the consideration of selectional processes removes to some extent the old antagonism between *nature and nurture*. In view of the evidence it is unlikely that preformed "motor programs" exist anywhere in the brain; by the same token the brain is not a "tabula rasa." Instead, spontaneous exploration by the organism within the constraints provided by its body structure, workspace, and neurological setup leads to the adaptive formation of movement categories or "synergies." Thus, a selectionist theoretical framework unites nativist and empiricist approaches to an understanding of motor development by placing dual emphasis on preexisting constraints and ongoing exploration and selection.

There are several commonalities between morphogenesis and motor development. We have already commented on the fact that neither appears to be controlled by rigidly defined sets of rules. Also, common to both morphogenesis and motor development is that they require the action of large *populations* of cells. In general, the developmental fate or the activity of a single neuron will have little impact on overall function.

The population aspects of both processes are evident; the formation of cell collectives during development parallels the action of cell collectives as neuronal populations during adult neuronal function. Given the cooperative nature of most primary developmental processes, it is perhaps not surprising to find that neuronal populations such as those described by Georgopoulos form the basic functional units in the adult brain. But the analysis of neuronal population activity needs an underlying theoretical framework of how these populations are structured. One such scheme (discussed in more detail in Section III) is that tightly coupled local neuronal groups interact through intraareal and interareal connections. This arrangement includes elements of a local as well as a more global nature and could be useful in guiding future explorations of cortical population activity. It remains to be seen whether Georgopoulos' analysis of motor cortical populations can be understood within the framework of this model.

SECTION III

FUNCTIONAL SEGREGATION AND INTEGRATION IN THE BRAIN

This section addresses a question that has been central to neuroscience since its very beginnings: How does the activity of functionally segregated populations of neurons give rise to a unified perceptual scene and to an integrated behavior?

This problem of integration in the context of the visual system is introduced in the chapter by Giulio Tononi and addressed theoretically with the help of large-scale computer simulations. It is proposed that integration in the brain is achieved in large part through the process of reentry, the recurrent parallel exchange of neural signals between neuronal groups taking place at many different levels of organization: locally within populations of neurons, within a single brain area, and across different areas. A first computer model demonstrates that the cooperative dynamics within a neuronal group can give rise to temporally coherent activity. A second model shows how the brain may solve the problem of perceptual grouping and figure–ground segregation, and demonstrates how some of the Gestalt laws may emerge naturally from the anatomy and physiology of a primary visual area. Finally, a large-scale model of the visual system illustrates a solution to the problem of "binding" the activity of functionally segregated brain areas dealing with different attributes of an object, such as form, color, and location. The model makes specific suggestions as to the neural basis of certain classes of psychological phenomena, paradigmatic examples of which are form-from-motion and motion capture.

In the following chapter, Wolf Singer summarizes his work and other studies suggesting that stimulus properties are signaled in the brain not only by the activity levels of neurons, but also by their temporal correlations. He reviews the evidence that spatially segregated neurons in the visual cortex exhibit synchronized responses for a few hundreds of milliseconds if activated by coherent stimuli, both within a single area and between different areas. Such synchronization can change dynamically depending on the stimulus configuration, and allows for the coexistence of more than one synchronous "assembly" of neuronal groups. He also discusses the mechanisms underlying such stimulus-dependent synchronization. Much emphasis is given in this context to the network of reciprocal cortico-cortical connections that link different groups and areas. Singer points out that such connections are subject to a selective process of differential amplification. Such process leads to preferential connections among groups of neurons with similar stimulus specificities that reflect some of the regularities in the world. The selective nature of such processes is nicely demonstrated by the plasticity of these connectivity patterns and by the ensuing patterns of synchronization revealed in Singer's studies on strabismic cats.

Whereas the first two chapters suggest that synchronous activity may mediate the integration of the activity of distributed neuronal groups and areas, Ernst Pöppel's chapter is concerned mainly with the range of the temporal aspects of integration. In this context, two time intervals, 30 msec and 3 seconds, are especially relevant. Pöppel reviews several experiments indicating that the nervous system can organize a response to stimuli requiring multimodal integration only at intervals that are multiples of 30 msec. Pöppel's view is that this is characteristic of a relaxation oscillator that has an intrinsic periodicity of 30 msec but that can be reset almost instantaneously by the stimulus. This would be consistent with the oscillatory activity in the 40-Hz range reported by Singer and by other investigators using different approaches. Pöppel then discusses several examples, ranging from psychology to poetry and to music, indicating that the brain can integrate into a coherent conscious scene events spanning at most 3 seconds, but not more.

REENTRY AND THE PROBLEM OF CORTICAL INTEGRATION

Giulio Tononi

The Neurosciences Institute
La Jolla, California 92037

I. The Problem of Integration

Though much is known about the properties of single nerve cells and the function of specific brain areas in isolation, the integrative aspect of brain function has remained more elusive. Modern anatomical studies of the visual cortex have revealed a mosaic of functionally segregated areas that deal individually with different attributes of visual objects, such as form, color, and motion, and that are linked by an intricate system of cortico-cortical connections (Zeki and Shipp, 1988; Felleman and Van Essen, 1991). Evidence for the segregation of function in the visual cortex has also been provided by the identification of multiple parallel processing streams, such as the magnocellular and parvocellular systems (Livingstone and Hubel, 1987), as well as by the distinction between a set of occipitoparietal visual areas responding specifically to spatial attributes (such as object location) and of another set of occipito-temporal visual areas responding to characteristic features of objects (Mishkin *et al.*, 1983; Desimone *et al.*, 1984; Maunsell and Newsome, 1987). Functional segregation is a consequence of neural development and of the responsivity of neuronal groups to correlations in their input. A system based on many locally specialized elements (or neuronal groups)

Copyright © 1994 by Academic Press, Inc.
All rights of reproduction in any form reserved.

has several advantages. For instance, locally specialized elements deal with restricted aspects of the stimulus domain, but can do so in considerable detail. In addition, such a system is economical in terms of the number and the length of the connections required for proper functioning. However, the brain does not work just as a collection of specialized groups of neurons. For instance, different visual attributes, such as form, color, and motion, are perceived in register and are referred to the corresponding objects. More generally, a visual scene is perceived as unitary and coherent, and this makes possible a coherent behavioral output.

How the integration of functionally segregated areas may occur in the brain is the theme of the present contribution (see Table I). After briefly examining different approaches to the problem, we will propose the process of reentry as a solution to the problem of integration, and we will illustrate it using several computer simulations. We will also present a measure, called neural complexity, that captures the interplay of functional segregation and integration in the brain.

II. Reentry as a Solution to Integration in the Brain

Any system composed of several functionally segregated modules is capable of some degree of integration if the modules can produce a

TABLE I
SOME REQUIREMENTS FOR INTEGRATION IN THE BRAIN

Integration occurs among heterogeneous and functionally specialized elements

The mechanisms of integration must be consistent with anatomy and physiology

Integration must obey strict temporal constraints

Integration takes place at several different levels of organization:

    Locally within groups of neurons

    Within an area (linking)

    Among different areas (binding)

    Among different regions

Integration must allow for some degree of differentiation (multiple objects)

Integration implies effectiveness as a whole (cooperativity): units must interact cooperatively in such a way that the effects they produce are different from those they would produce independently

An integrated system should provide a powerful substrate for selection simultaneously at several places and levels coherent behavior by virtue of acting together in the environment. Simple animals (or artifacts) can rely on such "behavioral" integration for relatively simple tasks (cf., e.g., Brooks, 1989). It is apparent, however, that more sophisticated behaviors require integration to take place within the nervous system. An important distinction is that between a strictly hierarchical and a reentrant model of integration. Most earlier attempts of explaining neural integration have been based on the notion that the brain is organized hierarchically with a progressive increase in the specificity of its neurons from the sensory periphery to more central areas. According to one version of this model, perceptual integration is achieved by the confluence of diverse processing streams at a very high hierarchical level, or "master area" (for a related theory of perception, see Barlow, 1972). Although feedforward convergence is an important anatomical feature of the cortex, as demonstrated by multimodal areas and by neurons with complex response properties (e.g., "face" cells), a master area, the activity of which represents entire perceptual or mental states, has not been found. In any case, such a possibility is conceptually unlikely, given the combinatorial explosion required by convergence in a single place.

A neurally based theory of spatiotemporal integration that does not require a master area was proposed by Edelman (1978) within the framework of the theory of neuronal group selection (TNGS), and has since been considerably extended and refined (Edelman, 1987, 1989; Finkel and Edelman, 1989; Sporns et al., 1989, 1991b; Tononi et al., 1992a,b). Two of the main tenets of this theory are that neurons act together in local collectives called *neuronal groups* and that they communicate with each other and correlate their activity by a process called *reentry*. Reentry can be defined as the "ongoing parallel signaling between separate [neuronal groups in] maps along ordered anatomical connections" (Edelman, 1989, p. 49), and it occurs in both directions simultaneously and recursively. Reentry is a dynamic process; its anatomic substrates are reciprocal cortico-cortical and cortico-thalamic connections, and it is governed both by the statistics of neuronal discharges and by the topology of the connection patterns. Because reentry is inherently parallel and it takes place simultaneously between vast numbers of neurons in virtually all cortical maps, it is not to be confused with the notion of feedback. As a consequence of its reciprocal and recursive features, reentry can resolve conflicts between the responses of different areas as well as construct new neuronal response properties. We call this its *constructive* function. Another fundamental consequence of reentry is the emergence of temporal correlations in the activity of neuronal groups within a cortical area as well as between different areas (its *correlative* function).

III. Evidence for Reentry in the Brain

Examples of the anatomical substrates of reentrant systems abound in the cerebral cortex. A recent detailed survey of 32 different areas of the monkey visual system and of their interconnections (Felleman and Van Essen, 1991) revealed that 242 out of a total of 305 pathways (i.e., 80%) are reciprocal; only 5 pathways have clearly been identified as unidirectional. Reentrant connections exist between visual areas at the same or different hierarchical levels and can occur in a variety of geometrical patterns (diffuse, registered, convergent–divergent, etc.; see Edelman, 1989). Though, in some cases, return projections may be anatomically diffuse and largely modulatory in character (Zeki and Shipp, 1988), they can in other cases directly drive neurons in lower areas (Mignard and Malpeli, 1991).

Recent experiments have provided evidence for the existence of neuronal groups in the cerebral cortex and for cooperative interactions within groups that lead to coherent firing (see the contributions by Singer and by Pöppel in the present volume). Orientation-selective neurons in the cat primary visual cortex show stimulus-dependent oscillatory discharges at around 40 Hz when presented with a stimulus of optimal orientation (Gray and Singer, 1989). These oscillations can be observed in single cells, but are most clearly visible in local populations of cells (recorded as a multiunit activity or a local field potential). As a result of local cooperative processes, neurons within such neuronal groups tend to discharge in a synchronous fashion.

Further experiments indicate that reentry along reciprocal anatomical connections may play a role in the generation of temporal correlations among groups. When a single long light bar is moved across the receptive fields of spatially separated neurons with similar orientation specificity, cross-correlations reveal that their oscillatory responses are synchronized (Eckhorn et al., 1988; Gray et al., 1989; Engel et al., 1990). The synchronization becomes weaker if a gap is inserted into the stimulus contour and it disappears completely if two parts of the contour are moved separately and in opposite directions. Synchrony is established rapidly, often within 100 msec, and single episodes of coherency last for 50–500 msec. Frequency and phase of the oscillations change continuously and stochastically but stay within the range of 40–60 Hz and ±3 msec, respectively (Gray et al., 1992). Synchronization of oscillatory activity was observed between cortical areas V1 and V2 (Eckhorn et al., 1988), between the two cortical hemispheres (Engel et al., 1991a), and between striate and extrastriate cortical areas (Engel et al., 1991b).

One of the best demonstrations so far of the importance of reentry in establishing temporal correlations comes from a recent experiment by Engel *et al.* (1991a). The experiment shows stimulus-dependent correlations between neurons located in the two hemispheres of cat visual cortex in response to two simultaneously presented stimuli, one on each side of the visual midline. The correlations disappear when the corpus callosum is cut, a direct indication that reentrant signaling along reciprocal cortico-cortical connections is responsible for their generation. It is important to note that, after the cut, both hemispheres continue to show neuronal activity at normal levels, so that their mean activity levels remain unchanged. This experiment strongly corroborates the view that mean activity rates alone are an insufficient indicator of neural integration, and that the temporal characteristics of neuronal firing are indeed essential in this process. The fact that perceptual processes in the two cortical hemispheres of human split brain patients appear to be disconnected (Gazzaniga, 1987) strongly suggests that also the unitary nature of consciousness depends on reentrant signaling (Edelman, 1989), in this case across the corpus callosum.

IV. Computer Simulations

The interpretation of the experimental evidence for reentry can be significantly complemented by large-scale simulations that serve to illustrate and test its role in the integration of brain function. These simulations are an example of synthetic neural modeling, an approach that stresses the importance of analyzing complex interactions across multiple levels of organization and of linking neural function to behavioral output (see Reeke, this volume, and Reeke *et al.*, 1990). Models help to make intuition more precise, illustrate theoretical assumptions, test their self-consistency, illuminate experimental results, and make predictions amenable to experimental investigation. In some cases, models can substitute for experiments that would be too difficult or unethical to perform.

Here we will briefly summarize some of our work that reflects the different levels of integration in the brain, namely, intragroup, intraareal, and interareal. We will then reexamine some criteria for cortical integration in view of the performance of these models. Finally, we will discuss the importance of the integration of functionally segregated areas at a still larger scale, and its relevance to conscious perception.

A. NEURONAL GROUPS: GENERATION OF COHERENT ACTIVITY

Within the few hundreds of milliseconds necessary for perceptual as well as behavioral integration, a single cell in the cortex will generally produce only a few, apparently stochastic spikes. As a consequence, the behavior of a single cell is not reliable enough for the establishment of significant temporal correlations within this short period of time. Moreover, it appears that the effect of the discharge of a single cell on any given target cell is negligible. Only when a few dozens of cells happen to fire together does their target change its probability of firing (cf. Abeles, 1991). These and other findings (e.g., Eckhorn *et al.*, 1988; Gray and Singer, 1989; Gray *et al.*, 1989) suggest that the relevant units of cortical function are neuronal groups rather than single cells, as predicted by the TNGS. Correlated activity in a population, recorded as a multiunit activity or a local field potential, is statistically more reliable and allows the establishment of significant correlations with other groups. Moreover, because cells in a group tend to share their anatomical projections, as suggested by the "patchy" nature of cortico-cortical connections (see, e.g., Amir *et al.*, 1993), their correlated discharge will generally be effective in modifying the probability of firing of target neurons and often of a whole target group.

In several computer simulations (Sporns *et al.*, 1989, 1991a,b), we modeled neuronal groups as collections of 40 to 160 excitatory cells and 20 to 80 inhibitory cells. In all simulations, the activity function of each cell is such that inputs arriving within a time period of a few milliseconds (the time constant of the cell) are summed and thus have a cooperative effect; inputs separated by longer time intervals act independently and noncooperatively. The interactions between excitatory and inhibitory cells within a group are responsible for the generation of oscillatory activity and, together with the local cooperative interactions among excitatory cells, they lead to the emergence of correlated activity within the group (Fig. 1). As in the experimental data, the activity of a single cell often does not seem to be periodic over a short time period, whereas the activity of the group as a whole does. Our simulations show that such coherent oscillatory behavior based on sparsely connected local populations of neurons is an inherently rich and variable phenomenon, a result that is in full accord with experiment (Gray *et al.*, 1992). Thus, the coherent activity of neuronal groups overcomes the intrinsic unreliability of single cells and represents a first, elementary step for establishing functionally significant correlations.

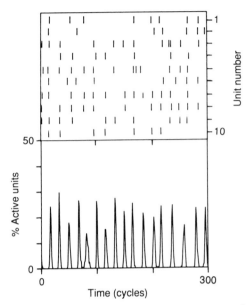

FIG. 1. Single unit activity (top) and population activity (bottom) of orientation-selective units responding to a simulated light bar in preferred orientation moving through the unit's receptive field. Ten different orientation-selective units within the same neuronal group are recorded simultaneously (top) and their activity is compared to the population activity of that group (bottom). Only a few single units appear to discharge at regular intervals, making identification of oscillatory behavior without the use of statistical techniques difficult. The instantaneous frequency of the neuronal groups shifts significantly around 40 Hz. A varying proportion of the group's constituent units participates in each oscillation cycle. (From Sporns *et al.*, 1989; reproduced with permission.)

B. Intraareal Reentry: Modeling Perceptual Grouping, Figure–Ground Segregation, and Gestalt Laws

An early instance of the problem of integration at the level of a single cortical area is represented by a classical problem in visual perception, that of perceptual grouping and figure–ground segregation. These two processes, both of fundamental importance in perceptual organization, refer to the ability to group together elementary features into discrete objects and to segregate these objects from each other and from the background. Gestalt psychologists have extensively investigated the factors influencing grouping and the distinction between figure and ground, and have described a number of laws, such as those of similarity, continuity, proximity, and common motion (Wertheimer, 1923; Koffka, 1935;

Köhler, 1947). However, their attempts to identify the underlying neural mechanisms, such as postulating the existence of isomorphic brain fields, have failed.

We have addressed the problem of perceptual grouping and segmentation in vision in a model illustrating the effects of intraareal reentry (Sporns *et al.*, 1991b). The model consists of an input array, four sets of elementary feature detectors, and four repertoires of orientation- and direction-selective neuronal groups representing a primary cortical area. Each neuronal group is explicitly modeled as a local population of excitatory and inhibitory neurons, as described above. On external stimulation, local recurrent network interactions give rise to oscillatory activity. Intraareal reentrant connections link adjacent groups of the same stimulus specificity. Groups of different specificities are connected only if they have overlapping receptive fields, whereas groups of similar specificities have more extended lateral connections, which fall off with distance. These assumptions (see Table II) are justified by anatomical and physiological observations in the visual cortex (Gilbert and Wiesel, 1989; Luhmann *et al.*, 1990). An important feature incorporated into this extended model consists of rapid and reversible changes in synaptic efficacies, depending on correlations between presynaptic activity and postsynaptic depolarization. These can change on a very short time scale (in the range of tens of milliseconds, if a single iteration is taken to correspond to 1 msec). The increased efficacy of reentrant connections among correlated groups rapidly amplifies and stabilizes correlations. Evidence for voltage-dependent interactions among orientation columns linked by horizontal connections has been provided (Hirsch and Gilbert, 1991).

Previous models (Sporns *et al.*, 1989, 1991a) had already shown that reentrant interactions within a single cortical area can give rise to temporal correlations between neighboring as well as distant groups with a

TABLE II

SOME ANATOMICAL AND PHYSIOLOGICAL CONSTRAINTS INCORPORATED IN THE MODEL OF
PERCEPTUAL GROUPING AND FIGURE–GROUND SEGREGATION

Neurons with specific response properties (orientation, direction) and topographic organization

Strong local interactions among excitatory and inhibitory neurons (neuronal groups)

Preferential connections among neuronal groups with similar orientation and direction selectivity

Connection density falls off with distance

Many connections are voltage dependent

near zero phase lag. In accord with experiments (Gray *et al.*, 1989; Engel *et al.*, 1990), correlations are found between units in groups that have nonoverlapping receptive fields if a long, continuous moving bar is presented. These distant correlations disappear if two collinear short bars (separated by a gap) are moved separately with the same velocity. In an extension of these results, the model was presented with an extended pattern composed of several bars moving coherently, embedded in a background of vertical and horizontal bars moving right, left, up, and down at random (Fig. 2). The groups responding to the bars that move in the same direction are rapidly linked by coherent oscillations (within 60–100 msec after stimulus onset), even though the lateral spread of the connections from each group is much less than the size of the object. The ability to establish specific linking (grouping) is directly related to the ability to achieve segmentation. Accordingly, there is no coherency

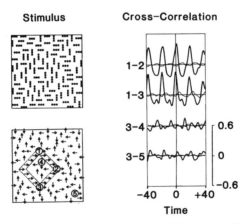

FIG. 2. An example of grouping and segmentation in the model of Sporns *et al.* (1991b). Left: Stimulus presented to the model, consisting of 100 vertically and horizontally oriented light bars moving right, left, up, and down. In the top panel the light bars are shown at their starting positions; the bottom panel shows their corresponding directions of movement indicated by arrows. Encircled numbers with arrows in the bottom panel refer to the locations of recorded neuronal activity; corresponding cross-correlations are displayed on the right. Electrodes 1–3 recorded from neurons responding to the figure; electrodes 4 and 5 recorded from neurons responding to the background. Right: Cross-correlograms of neuronal responses to the stimulus shown on the left. Cross-correlograms are computed over a 100-msec sample period and are subsequently averaged over 10 trials. Numbers refer to the locations of neuronal groups within the direction-selective repertoires (see left). Four correlograms are shown (figure–figure; 1–2, 1–3; figure–ground: 3–4, 3–5), computed between msec 201 and 300 after stimulus onset. The correlograms are scaled and shift predictors (thin lines, averaged over nine shifts) are displayed for comparison. (From Sporns *et al.*, 1991b; reproduced with permission.)

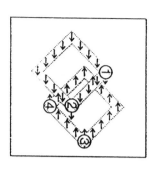

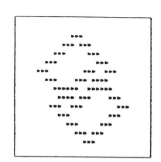

Stimulus

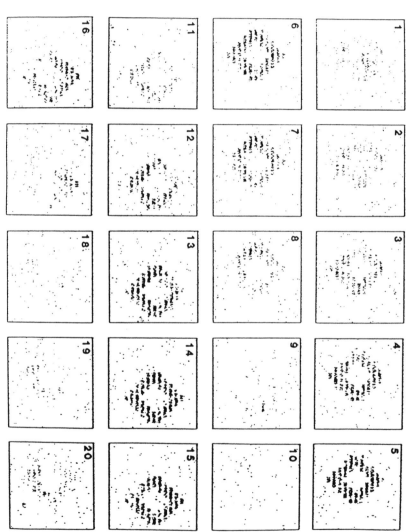

among groups responding to elements of the figure and those responding to elements of the background; the latter include elements moving in the same direction as the figure, but placed some distance away. The model is also able to segregate a figure from a coherent background of identical texture moving in a different direction or from another, overlapping figure (Fig. 3). All these results are strongly dependent on the presence of rapid changes in synaptic efficacy.

This computer model may serve as an example of *linking*, the establishment of correlations among features belonging to the same feature domain (in this case, orientation and direction of motion). It shows that, at least in principle, the neural basis for the integration and segregation of elementary features into objects and background might be the pattern of temporal correlations among neuronal groups. In addition, because the resulting grouping and segregation are consistent with the Gestalt laws of continuity, proximity, similarity, common orientation, and common motion, it suggests that the neural basis for these laws is to be found implicitly in the specific pattern of connectivity incorporated into the architecture as well as in the ensuing dynamics of short-term correlations.

C. INTERAREAL REENTRY: SOLVING THE BINDING PROBLEM

In a recent model (Tononi *et al.*, 1992b), we generalized the previous results to multiple areas of the visual system, and we coupled these areas to a simple behavioral output. This eliminates the problem of the homunculus, i.e., the need to deduce potential outputs through interpretation of specific patterns of neural activity and correlations from

---

FIG. 3. Frames taken from a movie (right) showing the responses of direction-selective groups in the model of figure–ground segregation (Sporns *et al.*, 1991b) to a stimulus (left) containing two identical and overlapping, but differently moving, figures. The frames show a continuous period of 20 msec (20 iterations) recorded about 150 msec after stimulus onset. Each frame displays the entire array of neuronal groups (16 × 16) selective for motion to the right and to the left, and arranged in an interleaved fashion (this accounts for the striped pattern). Each small dot within the array is an active neuron. For the first 10 msec (frames 1–10), mostly groups responding to the figure moving right are active; subsequently these groups are silent and groups responsive to the other figure become active (frames 11–20). The array of groups has been segregated into two cohorts oscillating independently from each other (in this movie segment they happen to be 180° out of phase). Notice that neuronal activity is strongly correlated both locally (in neighborhoods corresponding to groups) as well as over the entire extent of the figure. (Left: modified from Sporns *et al.*, 1991b; reproduced with permission; right: from Tononi *et al.*, 1992a; reproduced with permission.)

the point of view of a privileged observer. We introduced a new computational scheme to deal explicitly and efficiently with short-term temporal correlations among large numbers of units. The model received input from a color video camera and contained nine functionally segregated areas divided into three parallel anatomical streams for form, color, and motion; the areas were connected by reciprocal pathways. Altogether, 10,000 units were linked by about 1,000,000 connections between areas at different levels (*forward* and *backward*), areas at the same level (*lateral*),

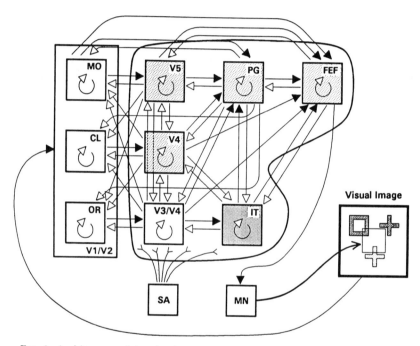

FIG. 4. Architecture of the visual cortex model. Segregated visual maps are depicted as boxes; pathways (composed of many thousands of individual connections) are indicated by arrows. The model comprises three parallel streams involved in the analysis of visual motion (MO; top row), color (CL; middle row), and form (OR, bottom row). Areas are finely (no shading) or coarsely (light shading) topographic, or nontopographic (heavy shading). The visual image (sampled by a color camera) is indicated at the extreme right. The output of the system (simulated foveation movements under the control of eye motoneurons MN) is indicated at the bottom. Filled arrowheads indicate voltage-independent pathways; open arrowheads indicate voltage-dependent pathways. Curved arrows within boxes indicate intraareal connections. The box labeled SA refers to the diffusely projecting saliency system used in the behavioral paradigm; the general area of projection is outlined. The complete system contains a total of about 10,000 neuronal units and of about 1,000,000 connections. (From Tononi *et al.*, 1992b; reproduced with permission.)

TABLE III
SOME ORGANIZATIONAL PRINCIPLES INCORPORATED IN
THE VISUAL SYSTEM MODEL

Functional specialization

Parallel organization

Hierarchical organization

Selective intraareal connections

Forward, backward, and lateral interareal connections

Topographic and nontopographic mapping

Forward connections increase functional specialization

Backward connections terminate more diffusely

Many connections are voltage dependent

Most pathways are reciprocal

Modulatory diffuse projection systems

Behavioral output

---

and within an area (*intrinsic*) (Fig. 4). Table III lists some organizational principles in the visual system model.

The various areas can be grouped into three streams for form, color, and motion (cf. Livingstone and Hubel, 1987), or into two systems, an "occipitotemporal" one related to the identity ("what"), and an "occipito-parietal" one related to the location of an object ("where"; cf. Mishkin *et al.*, 1983; Maunsell and Newsome, 1987).

There is a progressive increase in receptive field size from "lower" to "higher" areas, and units acquire more complex response properties. For instance, units in V1/V2 OR respond to oriented line segments, units in V3/V4 respond to corners, and units in IT respond to entire objects such as crosses or squares in a position-invariant way (cf. Desimone *et al.*, 1984). Units in V1/V2 CL respond to wavelength, whereas those in V4 display some degree of color constancy (cf. Zeki, 1983a,b). Units in V1/V2 MO are responsive to local motion, and those in V5 are responsive to pattern motion (cf. Movshon *et al.*, 1985).

All areas have systems of horizontal connections that locally and preferentially connect units with similar feature specificity, e.g., similar orientation preference (cf. Gilbert and Wiesel, 1989). Forward connections are generally organized in such a way that a small region of a "higher" area receives input from a larger region of a "lower" area. This is responsible for the increased size of the receptive fields at "higher" levels.

Furthermore, forward connections tend to preserve or enhance functional specificity, as seen in the separate projections from the three subdivisions of V1/V2 to V3, V4, and V5, and in the increasingly complex response properties of, e.g., IT. Backward connections are more divergent: for example, each of V3/V4, V4 and V5 project back to all three subsystems of V1/V2, although they receive from only one of them (cf. Zeki and Shipp, 1988). Lateral connections have mixed characteristics. In agreement with the experimental literature (see Felleman and Van Essen, 1991), all intraareal and most interareal pathways in the simulations are reciprocal.

The model includes an output stage consisting of area FEF and a set of oculomotor neurons driving a simulated foveation response, which can be used for operant conditioning. Reward for foveating objects characterized by a particular conjunction of attributes (e.g., a red cross in a particular position) is mediated by the activation of a *saliency* or *value system*. Such a system incorporates the following characteristics: it responds to salient events, either evolutionarily or experientially selected; it is activated phasically by such events, signaling a change in expectation; it projects diffusely to many brain areas, thus allowing a global signal simultaneously to control many local interactions; it releases modulatory substances that can influence local activity and plasticity changes, thus providing a substrate for selection (for a discussion of value systems in the context of selection, see the general discussion at the end of Section I of this volume). The saliency system reflects some aspects of those brain nuclei (e.g., the noradrenergic locus coeruleus and the cholinergic nucleus basalis) that project diffusely to wide areas of the cortex (Amaral and Sinnamon, 1977; Mesulam *et al.*, 1983). Among the many postulated functions of these nuclei are the signaling of salient environmental events and the gating of synaptic plasticity (Foote *et al.*, 1983; Richardson and DeLong, 1990; Barnes and Pompeiano, 1991; Napier *et al.*, 1991; cf. Friston *et al.*, 1994a).

The model's performance is summarized in Table IV. Consistent with functional segregation, areas within each of the separate streams (motion, form, and color) have specialized characteristics similar to corresponding areas in the cortex. Reentrant interactions between the streams provide possible neural bases for two psychophysical effects, the construction of *form-from-motion* boundaries and *motion capture*. Form-from-motion illustrates the *constructive* aspect of reentry: reentrant signals from a hierarchically "higher" area (V5) interact with signals coming from the periphery to construct responses consistent with form from motion in area V1/V2 OR, which disappear when reentrant inputs are cut. We

TABLE IV
FUNCTIONS OF THE VISUAL SYSTEM MODEL

Streams	Modeled functions
Motion	Perceptual grouping and figure–ground segregation (Gestalt laws); pattern motion
Form	Position-invariant recognition; generalization
Color	Simultaneous color contrast; color constancy
Motion plus form	Structure from motion
Motion plus form plus color	Motion capture
Complete system	Linking and binding of attributes of one or multiple objects within and among multiple areas; conditioning using distributed synaptic changes; effectiveness of short-term correlations; object discrimination simultaneously based on position, form, and color

suggest that several other classes of perceptual phenomena involving cooperative interactions of different submodalities or modalities will be found to be associated with the activation of specific populations of neurons through reentrant interactions among different areas or subdivisions of an area. A simulation of motion capture illustrates the *correlative* properties of reentry: in this case, rather than radically altering the response properties of neuronal units, reentry leads to the emergence of short-term correlations between units in the motion and color streams. We propose that such short-term correlations lie at the basis of this and similar perceptual capture phenomena.

Reentrant interactions within and between the multiple areas of the complete system give rise to temporal correlations between units responding to different visual attributes across multiple pathways and between topographic as well as nontopographic areas. At the same time, the model is able unambiguously to differentiate between two or more objects present in the same visual scene and thus it solves the so-called *binding problem*. The model produces a behavior (simulated foveation) that can be conditioned using diffusely projecting units to signal saliency and thereby influence the modification of cortico-cortical connections. Specific patterns of activity and correlations result in a foveation response that simultaneously depends on color, form, and location, thus achieving integration without the need for a hierarchically superordinate area.

D. The Models and Some Requirements for Cortical Integration

Although we cannot present here a detailed analysis of the performance of the previous models (the reader is referred to the original papers), we will briefly discuss how the simulations satisfy several requirements that are needed for a satisfactory solution to the problem of cortical integration (Table I).

As we have seen, the brain is characterized by the interplay of integration with functional segregation. Thus, cortical integration must occur among neuronal groups and areas that are *functionally segregated* and that are characterized by heterogeneous and rather specialized properties. For example, in the simulation illustrated in the visual system model, the behavioral response depends on the integration of form-, color-, and location-related signals, each represented by functionally specialized areas (IT, V4, and PG, respectively). In the model, lesions *within* areas such as IT, V4, or PG impair the ability to discriminate visual form, color, or location, respectively. On the other hand, lesioning the reentrant pathways *between* these areas prevents the integration of these signals.

The models described here are strictly *based on anatomical and physiological criteria*, as indicated in Tables II and III. Our model of the visual system achieves integration of functionally segregated areas through their reentrant interactions and does not require any master area, consistent with the fact that no single area receives projections from all functionally segregated areas responding to the various visual submodalities (Zeki and Shipp, 1988). The model avoids the problem of combinatorial explosion, in that it can respond in a specific way even to unfamiliar objects for which prior representations (such as specialized "detectors") do not exist (cf. Treisman *et al.*, 1990).

Furthermore, integration takes place at many *different levels of organization* (Sporns *et al.*, 1991a). We propose that such different levels of integration are mediated by reentry over intragroup, intraareal, interareal, and interregional connections (e.g., between the cortex and the thalamus, the basal ganglia, the claustrum). In the model of perceptual grouping, we demonstrated the interplay between intragroup and intraareal interactions. Most of the results obtained with the visual system model are instead based on the interplay between intraareal and interareal reentry. It is likely that the contribution to integration of interregional reentry is similarly important, although we have not yet explored this issue extensively in computer simulations.

There is evidence that perceptual and behavioral integration is accomplished in many cases in as little as 50 to 500 msec (Blumenthal, 1977;

Biederman, *et al.*, 1982). On the other hand, there is also evidence that for most purposes integration over time does not extend beyond a few seconds (Pöppel, 1985, 1988; Pöppel *et al.*, 1991). These data pose strong *temporal constraints* on any mechanism proposed for perceptual and behavioral integration. In agreement with such strict temporal constraints, all the effects obtained in the simulations require very few iterations. Even the establishment of a globally coherent pattern over all areas of the simulated visual system, and a subsequent discriminatory foveation response, can take as few as 8 iterations in the computer. If one assigns realistic values for the modeled variables and parameters, 8–10 iterations can be taken to correspond in this case to 200–300 msec of real time.

Neurons can show correlated activity at several time scales (cf. Nelson, *et al.*, 1992a,b). Thus, when responding to the presence of several different objects in a single visual scene, many neurons will increase their mean firing rate together, resulting in significant correlations on a time scale of hundreds of milliseconds. These correlations indicate that those objects and features are simultaneously present in a coherent visual scene. On the other hand, correlations over shorter time scales, i.e., milliseconds, allow neurons with an increased mean firing rate to group and segregate differentially, e.g., to bind selectively various attributes of different objects. Thus, both the simultaneous presence and the relationships between the elements are preserved in the pattern of correlations between neuronal groups. In the present models, the ability to "differentiate" between two or more objects presented simultaneously in the visual field was demonstrated in figure–ground segregation and in the discriminatory response to more than one object. The capacity of the models to carry out such differentiation is nevertheless limited; consistent with experimental studies (Treisman and Schmidt, 1982; see also Keele *et al.*, 1988), in the presence of several simultaneously presented objects there is an increase in erroneous responses (illusory conjunctions).

It is important to realize that the concept of integration is meaningful only if it is strictly tied to effectiveness, in this case *effectiveness as a whole*, a notion that can be related to that of *cooperativity* which, in physics and chemistry (cf. Haken, 1973) indicates the emergence of a state that depends on multiple nonlinear interactions among several elements. In the present models, integration is achieved when different areas, or groups of neurons within an area, cooperate to produce a global state of the system, reflected in specific patterns of activity and correlations. In the visual system model, the discrimination behavior depends on the emergence of such patterns. Eliminating the reentrant connections within and between the various areas does not abolish their separate responses but prevents the emergence of such specific patterns and, as a result, impairs the discrimination behavior (Tononi et al., 1992b). The fact that the elements of the model exert different effects depending on the presence or absence of reentrant connections illustrates the requirement that integration must be effective. This model also shows that, if the units are sensitive to temporal coincidences, short-term correlations can be effective by themselves, and should not be considered an epiphenomenon.

A highly integrated system often appears to be a nightmare when seen from an engineer's or instructionist point of view. The assignment of credit or of fault to specific elements or connections becomes almost impossible. From a selectionist point of view, however, an integrated system is a powerful substrate. In fact, *selection can act at all places and levels simultaneously.* In other words, whatever cooperative interactions among several elements and across several levels lead to a positive outcome can be selected. Another consequence is that synaptic changes contributing to learning can be widely distributed. In the visual system model, because saliency-related diffuse projections affect virtually the entire cortical mantle, entire cortical states and all of the cooperative interactions that lead to their establishment can be selected during reinforcement. This results in synaptic changes in many different pathways, including some whose involvement in the task at hand may not be immediately obvious. In a task that requires several specialized areas, the system can allocate a large number of connections in different pathways. Thus, this model reconciles distributed synaptic changes in learning with functional segregation while avoiding the error of "equipotentiality" (Lashley, 1950).

V. Complexity: Functional Segregation and Integration Reconciled

Recently, we have considered the relationship between functional segregation and integration in the brain from a more general theoretical perspective (Tononi et al., 1994). By making certain simplifying assumptions, we have shown that these two organizational aspects can be formulated within a unified framework. In such a framework, functional segregation and integration are characterized in terms of deviations from statistical independence among the components of a neural system, measured using the concepts of statistical entropy and mutual information (Papoulis, 1991). For instance, consider a bipartition of a neural system

X into a jth subset X_j^k composed of k components (which can be taken to represent neuronal groups) and its complement $X - X_j^k$. The deviation from statistical independence between X_j^k and $X - X_j^k$ is measured by their mutual information MI:

$$\text{MI}(X_j^k; X - X_j^k) = H(X_j^k) + H(X - X_j^k) - H(X)$$

where $H(X_j^k)$ and $H(X - X_j^k)$ are the entropies of X_j^k and $X - X_j^k$ considered independently, and $H(X)$ is the entropy of the system considered as a whole. MI $= 0$ if X_j^k and $X - X_j^k$ are statistically independent and MI > 0 otherwise.

The integration I(X) of a neural system is then defined as the total deviation from independence among all its n components and can be measured through a single measure that is a generalization of the notion of mutual information. I(X) is defined as the difference between the sum of the entropies of all individual components $\{x_i\}$ considered independently and the entropy of X considered as a whole:

$$\text{I}(X) = \sum_{i=1}^{n} H(x_i) - H(X)$$

If the n components of the system are completely independent, as when neuronal groups are completely desynchronized, integration is zero. If, on the other hand, such groups show strong deviations from independence, as when they are fully synchronized, integration is high.

Measuring integration in terms of deviation from statistical independence allows us simultaneously to characterize functional segregation and integration within a neural system, by considering the average integration for subsets of increasing size. Functional segregation is expressed by the relative statistical independence of the activity of individual neuronal groups if these groups are considered in small subsets, i.e., a few at a time (low average integration for small subsets). Conversely, functional integration is expressed by a high degree of statistical dependence when neuronal groups are considered in large subsets, i.e., many at a time (high average integration for large subsets).

This leads to the formulation of a measure, called *neural complexity* (C_N), which reflects the interplay between functional segregation and integration within a neural system, and which is defined as follows:

$$C_N(X) = \sum_{k=1}^{n} \left[(k/n)\text{I}(X) - \langle \text{I}(X_j^k) \rangle \right]$$

where we consider all subsets X^k composed of k out of n components of the system ($1 \leq k \leq n$) and the average integration for subsets of size k is denoted as $\langle \text{I}(X_j^k) \rangle$ {the index j indicates that the average is taken over all $n!/[k! \, (n - k)!]$ combinations of k components}. In essence, C_N measures how much the increase of average integration with increasing subset size deviates from linearity, i.e., roughly speaking, how much the whole is more integrated than its parts (Fig. 5A). C_N can be shown to

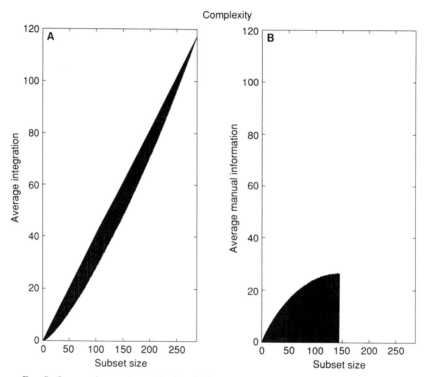

Fig. 5. Integration and complexity obtained from simulations of a primary visual area as in the model of Sporns *et al.* (1991b). The simulated cortical area contains 512 neuronal groups in two arrays (16 by 16) and modeled as collections of 40 excitatory and 20 inhibitory neurons that are mutually interconnected, as summarized in Table II (details in Sporns *et al.*, 1991b). No external input is provided to the network; neuronal group activity is triggered by intrinsic gaussian noise, as in Tononi *et al.* (1994), but with different parameters for the average noise. The groups tend to discharge in an oscillatory fashion. To compute complexity, we sampled the mean activity traces of groups forming the central 12-by-12 portion of the two arrays (one for each orientation preference) for 8000 time steps and derived the covariance matrix. (A) Complexity computed and expressed as the difference between a linear increase of integration and the observed average integration for increasing subset size. (B) Complexity computed and expressed as the sum, over increasing subset size, of the average mutual information between subsets of neuronal groups and the rest of the system. Complexity corresponds to the shaded area in both A and B and its numerical value, in both cases, is 2640.3

be equivalent to the mutual information between each part of a neural system and the rest, summed over all possible bipartitions:

$$C_N(X) = \sum_{k=1}^{n/2} \langle MI(X_j^k; X - X_j^k) \rangle$$

Thus, for complexity to be high, the average mutual information between each component and the rest of the brain must be high, indicating that the system is very integrated. At the same time, the average mutual information must be higher the larger the subset one is considering. This indicates that each component has a rather specialized function, in that considering more components provides additional mutual information (Fig. 5B). Thus, consistent with intuitive notions and with current attempts in physics and biology to conceptualize complex systems, C_N is high for systems such as the vertebrate brain that conjoin local specialization with global integration. On the other hand, C_N is low for systems that are composed either of completely independent parts or of parts that show completely homogeneous behavior.

As an illustration, we calculated the complexity associated with the primary visual area used in our model of perceptual grouping and figure–ground segregation (Sporns *et al.*, 1991b). Neuronal activity was triggered by uncorrelated gaussian noise rather than by patterned external input. We observed that certain structural characteristics of cortical connectivity, as incorporated in the model, are associated with high values of C_N. These characteristics include a high density of connections, strong local connectivity helping to organize cells into neuronal groups, patchiness in the connectivity among neuronal groups, and a large number of short reentrant circuits. A broader exploration of this new arena of theoretical neuroanatomy will require the successful extension of the present analysis to other important characteristics, for example, the diffuse terminations of back-projections and the distribution of inhibitory connections. We hope that, together with the demonstrations offered by computer simulations, the introduction of a general measure of complexity that encompasses both functional segregation and integration should resolve many issues raised by conflicting views on local versus global functions.

VI. Conclusion: Functional Segregation, Integration, and Consciousness

The previous discussion shows that computer simulations can help to define the problem of integration in more precise terms, to clarify integration as a concept, to illustrate a process, reentry, that can serve as a mechanism to achieve the integration, and finally to make experimental predictions. Examples of such predictions are the proposed neuronal basis for psychophysical phenomena, such as form from motion, motion capture, and some of the Gestalt laws; the claim that short-term correlations will be found across different cortical areas; the important role attributed to backward and lateral connections and to voltage-dependent mechanisms; and the conclusion that synaptic changes during conditioning will be widely distributed.

Perhaps most important, such large-scale models indicate that it should be possible to start addressing even higher levels of integration on a firm structural basis. As was suggested before, the problem of integration, which is first encountered in considering linking and binding, culminates with the integration or unity of consciousness. According to William James, being "an integral thing not made of parts" (James, 1890, p. 177) is indeed an important property of consciousness. On the other hand, every conscious state requires the integration of a very large amount of specific elements and relations to acquire its full meaning. "Consciousness . . . is of a teeming multiplicity of objects and relations, and what we call simple sensations are results of discriminative attention, pushed often to a very high degree" (James, 1890, p. 224).

A detailed, biologically based analysis of what brain structures and processes are involved in the emergence of consciousness is contained in Edelman (1989). This analysis concludes that even the most basic or primary form of consciousness presupposes complex brain systems dealing with perceptual categorization, memory, learning, biological self–nonself distinction, conceptual categorization, a memory of past value-category associations, and a reentrant pathway by which this memory can discriminate current perceptual categorizations (Edelman, 1989). To attain the degree of integration required by such structures and processes, reentry must take place simultaneously across several brain regions in arrangements that have been called *global mappings* (Edelman, 1987). Structures such as the thalamus, the basal ganglia, the claustrum, and the hippocampus may be particularly important in linking parts of global mappings despite the long distances among brain areas. Due to their strategic position, they may facilitate the fast interaction among remote brain regions by establishing more direct synaptic routes among them, and allow the locking-in of distributed brain systems involved in the emergence of consciousness. In this respect, the experimental results that show how the activity of distant neuronal groups can lock in with near zero phase lag should be considered as an important indication of the presence and the effects of reentry.

Thus, in contrast to simplistic proposals that refer consciousness to a place in the brain, to a special class of neurons, or to a special kind of neuronal activity, we argue that consciousness results from the integration of many specialized perceptual and cognitive processes that are carried out in parallel in different parts of our brain. We also propose that, in order to give rise to conscious experience, such integration should be fast, taking place on a time scale extending from a few tens of milliseconds up to perhaps a few seconds, and that reentry is a key process through which integration is obtained. Thus, correlates of conscious experience should be sought in sets of relationships among functionally specialized neuronal groups which interact tightly and rapidly among themselves, forming within the thalamocortical system a large, but ever-changing, "core" of elements that are strongly integrated over hundreds of milliseconds. Finally, we suggest that it should be possible to actually measure the extent of the interplay of functional segregation and integration in the working brain by means of the notion of neural complexity. Some preliminary results using complexity measures on data obtained from functional neuroimaging are pointing in this direction (Friston, *et al.*, 1994b).

References

Abeles, M. (1991). "Corticonics." Cambridge Univ. Press, Cambridge, UK.

Amaral, D. G., and Sinnamon, H. M. (1977). The locus coeruleus: Neurobiology of a central noradrenergic nucleus. *Prog. Neurobiol.* **9**, 147–196.

Amir, Y., Harel, M., and Malach, R. (1993). Cortical hierarchy reflected in the organization of intrinsic connections in macaque monkey visual cortex. *J. Comp. Neurol.* **334**, 19–46.

Marlow, H. B. (1972). Single units and sensation: A neuron doctrine for perceptual psychology? *Perception* **1**, 371–394.

Barnes, C. D., and Pompeiano, O. (1991). Neurobiology of the locus coeruleus. *Prog. Brain Res.* **88**.

Biederman, I., Mezzanotte, R. J., and Rabinowitz, J. C. (1982). Scene perception: Detecting and judging objects undergoing relational violations. *Cognit. Psychol.* **14**, 143–177.

Blumenthal, A. L. (1977). "The Process of Cognition." Prentice-Hall, Englewood Cliffs, NJ.

Brooks, R. A. (1989). A robot that walks; emergent behaviors from a carefully evolved network. *Neural Comput.* **1**, 253–262.

Desimone, R., Albright, T. D., Gross, C. G., and Bruce, C. (1984). Stimulus selective properties of inferior temporal neurons in the macaque. *J. Neurosci.* **4**, 2051–2062.

Eckhorn, R., Bauer, R., Jordan, W., Brosch, M., Kruse, W., Munk, M., and Retiboeck, H. J. (1988). Coherent oscillations: A mechanism of feature linking in the visual cortex? Multiple electrode and correlation analyses in the cat. *Biol. Cybernet.* **60**, 121–130.

Edelman, G. M. (1978). Group selection and phasic re-entrant signalling: A theory of higher brain function. *In* "The Mindful Brain" (G. M. Edelman and V. B. Mountcastle, eds.), pp. 51–100. MIT Press, Cambridge, MA.

Edelman, G. M. (1987). "Neural Darwinism: The Theory of Neuronal Group Selection." Basic Books, New York.

Edelman, G. M. (1989). "The Remembered Present: A Biological Theory of Consciousness." Basic Books, New York.

Engel, A. K., König, P., Gray, C. M., and Singer, W. (1990). Stimulus-dependent neuronal oscillations in cat visual cortex. II. Inter-columnar interaction as determined by cross-correlation analysis. *Eur. J. Neurosci.* **2**, 588–606.

Engel, A. K., König, P., Kreiter, A. K., and Singer, W. (1991a). Interhemispheric synchronization of oscillatory neuronal responses in cat visual cortex. *Science* **252**, 1177–1179.

Engel, A. K., Kreiter, A. K., König, P., and Singer, W. (1991b). Synchronization of oscillatory neuronal responses between striate and extrastriate visual cortical areas of the cat. *Proc. Natl. Acad. Sci. U.S.A.* **88**, 6048–6052.

Felleman, D. J., and Van Essen, D. C. (1991): Distributed hierarchical processing in the primate cerebral cortex. *Cereb. Cortex* **1**, 1–47.

Finkel, L. H., and Edelman, G. M. (1989). The integration of distributed cortical systems by reentry: A computer simulation of interactive functionally segregated visual areas. *J. Neurosci.* **9**, 3188–3208.

Foote, S. L., Bloom, F. E., and Aston-Jones, G. (1983). Nucleus locus coeruleus: New evidence of anatomical and physiological specificity. *Physiol. Rev.* **63**, 844–914.

Friston, K. J., Tononi, G., Reeke, G. N., Sporns, O., and Edelman, G. M. (1994a). Value-dependent selection in the brain: Simulation in a synthetic neural model. *Neuroscience* **59**, 229–243.

Friston, K. J., Tononi, G., Sporns, O., and Edelman, G. M. (1994b). Submitted.

Gazzaniga, M. S. (1987). Perceptual and attentional processes following callosal section in humans. *Neuropsychologia* **25**, 119–133.

Gilbert, C. D., ,and Wiesel, T. N. (1989). Columnar specificity of intrinsic horizontal and corticocortical connections in cat visual cortex. *J. Neurosci.* **9**, 2432–2442.

Gray, C. M., and Singer, W. (1989). Stimulus-specific neuronal oscillations in orientation columns of cat visual cortex. *Proc. Natl. Acad. Sci. U.S.A.* **86**, 1698–1702.

Gray, C. M., König, P., Engel, A. K., and Singer, W. (1989). Oscillatory responses in cat visual cortex exhibit inter-columnar synchronization which reflects global stimulus properties. *Nature (London)* **338**, 334–337.

Gray, C. M., Engel, A. K., König, P., and Singer, W. (1992). Synchronization of oscillatory neuronal responses in cat striate cortex: Temporal properties. *Visual Neurosci.* **8**, 337–347.

Haken, H. (1973). "Synergetics: Cooperative Phenomena in Multi-Component Systems." Teubner, Stuttgart.

Hirsch, J. A., and Gilbert, C. D. (1991). Synaptic physiology of horizontal connections in the cat's visual cortex. *J. Neurosci.* **11**, 1800–1809.

James, W. (1890). "The Principles of Psychology." Holt, New York.

Keele, S. W., Cohen, A., Ivry, R., Liotti, M., and Yee, P. (1988). Tests of a temporal theory of attentional binding. *J. Exp. Psychol.* **14**, 444–452.

Koffka, K. (1935). "Principles of Gestalt Psychology." Harcourt, New York.

Köhler, W. (1947). "Gestalt Psychology." Liveright, New York.

Lashley, K. S. (1950). In search of the engram. *Symp. Soc. Exp. Biol.* **4**, 454–482.

Livingstone, M. S., and Hubel, D. H. (1987). Psychophysical evidence for separate channels for the perception of form, color, movement and depth. *J. Neurosci.* **7**, 3416–3468.

Luhmann, H. J., Greuel, J. M., and Singer, W. (1990). Horizontal interactions in cat striate cortex. I. Anatomical substrate and postnatal development. *Eur. J. Neurosci.* **2**, 344–357.

Maunsell, J. H. R., and Newsome, W. T. (1987). Visual processing in monkey extrastriate cortex. *Annu. Rev. Neurosci.* **10**, 363–401.

Mesulam, M., Mufson, E. J., Levey, A. I., and Wainer, B. H. (1983). Cholinergic innervation of cortex by the basal forebrain: Cytochemistry and cortical connections of the septal area, diagonal band nuclei, nucleus basalis (substantia innominata), and hypothalamus in the rhesus monkey. *J. Comp. Neurol.* **214**, 170–197.

Mignard, M., and Malpeli, J. G. (1991). Paths of information flow through visual cortex. *Science* **251**, 1249–1251.

Mishkin, M., Ungerleider, L. G., and Macko, K. A. (1983). Object vision and spatial vision: Two cortical pathways. *Trends Neurosci.* **6**, 414–417.

Movshon, J. A., Adelson, E. H., Gizzi, M. S., and Newsome, W. T. (1985). The analysis of moving visual patterns. *In* "Pattern Recognition Mechanisms" (C. Chagas, R. Gattass, and C. Gross, eds.), pp. 117–152. Springer-Verlag, Berlin.

Napier, T. C., Kalivas, P. W., and Hanin, I. (1991). The basal forebrain: Anatomy to function. *Adv. Exp. Med. Biol.* **295**, 1.

Nelson, J. I., Salin, P. A., Munk, M. H. J., Arzi, M., and Bullier, J. (1992a). Spatial and temporal coherence in cortico-cortical connections: A cross-correlation study in areas 17 and 18 in the cat. *Visual Neurosci.* **9**, 21–38.

Nelson, J. I., Novak, L. G., Couvet, G., Munk, M. H. J., and Bullier, J. (1992b). Synchronization between cortical neurons depends on activity in remote areas. *Soc. Neurosci. Abstr.* **11**, 8.

Papoulis, A. (1991). "Probability, Random Variables, and Stochastic Processes." McGraw-Hill, New York.

Pöppel, E. (1985). "Grenzen des Bewusstseins. Über Wirklichkeit und Welterfahrung." Deutsche Verlags Anstalt, Stuttgart.

Pöppel, E. (1988). "Mindworks. Time and Conscious Experience" (Engl. ed.). Academic Press, Orlando, FL.

Pöppel, E., Chen, L., Glünder, H., Mitzdorf, U., Ruhnau, E., Schill, K., and von Steinbüchel, N. (1991). Temporal and spatial constraints for mental modelling. *In* "Frontiers in Knowledge-Based Computing" (V. P. Bhatkar and K. M. Rege, eds.), pp. 57–67. Narosa, New Delhi.

Reeke, G., Jr., Finkel, L. H., Sporns, O., and Edelman, G. M. (1990). Synthetic neural modeling: A multilevel approach to the analysis of brain complexity. *In* "Signal and Sense: Local and Global Order in Perceptual Maps" (G. M. Edelman, W. E. Gall, and W. M. Cowan, eds.), pp. 607–707. Wiley, New York.

Richardson, R. T., and DeLong, M. R. (1990). Context-dependent responses of primate nucleus basalis neurons in a go/no-go task. *J. Neurosci.* **10**, 2528–2540.

Sherrington, C. (1947). "The Integrative Action of the Nervous System," 2nd ed. Yale Univ. Press, New Haven, CT.

Sporns, O., Gally, J. A., Reeke, G. N., Jr., and Edelman, G. M. (1989). Reentrant signaling among simulated neuronal groups leads to coherency in their oscillatory activity. *Proc. Natl. Acad. Sci. U.S.A.* **86**, 7265–7269.

Sporns, O., Tononi, G., and Edelman, G. M. (1991a). Dynamic interactions of neuronal groups and cortical integration. *In* "Nonlinear Dynamics of Neural Networks" (H. G. Schuster, ed.), pp. 205–240. VCH, Weinheim.

Sporns, O., Tononi, G., and Edelman, G. M. (1991b). Modeling perceptual grouping and figure–ground segregation by means of active reentrant connections. *Proc. Natl. Acad. Sci. U.S.A.* **88**, 129–133.

Tononi, G., Sporns, O., and Edelman, G. M. (1992a). The problem of neural integration: Induced rhythms and short-term correlations. *In* "Induced Rhythms in the Brain" (E. Basar and T. Bullock, eds.), pp. 365–393. Birkhäuser, Boston, MA.

Tononi, G., Sporns, O., and Edelman, G. M. (1992b). Reentry and the problem of integrating nultiple cortical areas: Simulation of dynamic integration in the visual system. *Cereb. Cortex* **2**, 310–335.

Tononi, G., Sporns, O., and Edelman, G. M. (1994). A measure for brain complexity: Relating functional segregation and integration in the nervous system. *Proc. Natl. Acad. Sci. U.S.A.* **91**, 5033–5037.

Treisman, A., and Schmidt, H. (1982). Illusory conjunctions in the perception of objects. *Cognit. Psychol.* **14,** 107–141.

Treisman, A., Cavanagh, P., Fischer, B., Ramachandran, V. S., and von der Heydt, R. (1990). Form perception and attention. *In* "Visual Perception: The Neurophysiological Foundations (L. Spillman and J. Werner, eds.), pp. 273–316. Academic Press, San Diego.

Wertheimer, M. (1923). Untersuchungen zur Lehre von der Gestalt II. *Psychol. Forsch.* **4,** 301–350.

Zeki, S. M. (1983a). Color coding in the cerebral cortex: the reaction of cells in monkey visual cortex to wavelengths and colors. *Neuroscience* **9,** 741–765.

Zeki, S. M. (1983b). Color coding in the cerebral cortex: The responses of wavelength-selective and colour-coded cells in monkey visual cortex to changes in wavelength composition. *Neuroscience* **9,** 767–781.

Zeki, S. M., and Shipp, S. (1988). The functional logic of cortical connections. *Nature* (*London*) **335,** 311–317.

COHERENCE AS AN ORGANIZING PRINCIPLE OF CORTICAL FUNCTIONS

Wolf Singer

Max Planck Institut für Hirnforschung
D-60528 Frankfurt, Germany

I. Introduction

The preceding papers, in particular the one by Tononi, provide an excellent conceptual framework for the present contribution. Therefore, I shall not spend too much time on the discussion of current hypotheses of cortical processing. Rather, I shall concentrate on the review of recent experimental results on the dynamics of neuronal interactions in the neocortex and on mechanisms of use-dependent synaptic plasticity of neocortical connections. Because the experiments that I shall be describing have been designed to test a set of precise predictions, it is indispensable to briefly recapitulate the arguments that led to the formulation of these predictions. This will cause some redundancy, but, on the other hand, it will make it more explicit where and to what extent there is agreement or disagreement between theories, simulated network models, and experimental data.

The ability to record the activity of individual nerve cells *in situ* and in awake behaving animals has revealed a very rich repertoire of neurons

153

with highly specialized response properties. This evidence has been taken as support of the hypothesis that the activation of individual neurons can represent a code for highly complex and integrated functions, a notion that is commonly addressed as the "single-neuron doctrine" (Barlow, 1972). However, as already mentioned by Tononi, there have always also been proposals that additional and rather different coding principles might be realized in the nervous system of higher vertebrates and mammals. Most of these proposals are extensions of Donald Hebb's postulate that neuronal representations of sensory or motor patterns should consist of assemblies of cooperatively interacting neurons rather than of individual cells. This coding principle implies that information is contained not only in the activation level of individual neurons, but also, and actually to a crucial extent, in the relations between the activities of distributed neurons. If true, a complete description of a particular neuronal state would have to take into account not only the rate and the specificity of individual neuronal responses, but also the relations between discharges of distributed neurons.

Over the past decade, the assembly hypothesis has received more and more support both from experimental results and from theoretical considerations. A strong prediction of the single-neuron doctrine is that there ought to be neurons that respond with very high selectivity to only a small set of perceptual objects and *in extremis* to only one object. By extrapolation of this coding strategy to motor systems, one is led to postulate the existence of command neurons whose activation should lead in a highly selective way to the execution of specific motor acts. However, search for individual neurons responding with the required selectivity to individual perceptual objects was only partly successful and has so far revealed specificity only for faces and for a limited set of objects with which the animal had been previously extensively familiarized (Gross *et al.*, 1972; Baylis *et al.*, 1985; Desimone *et al.*, 1984, 1985; Perrett *et al.*, 1987; Rolls, 1991; Miyashita, 1988; Sakai and Miyashita, 1991). And even in these cases it is likely that a particular face or object evokes responses in a very large number of neurons. Recordings from motor centers such as the deep layers of the tectum and areas of the motor cortex provided no evidence for command neurons that exist in simple nervous systems and code for specific motor patterns. Rather, these latter studies provided strong support for a population code, because the trajectory of a particular movement could be predicted correctly only if the relative contributions of a large number of neurons were considered (Georgopoulos, 1990; Mussa-Ivaldi *et al.*, 1990; Sparks *et al.*, 1990). Arguments favoring the possibility of relational codes have also been derived from the concept of coarse coding. There are numerous examples that behaviorally determined discrimination between stimulus features can be superior to the discriminating abilities of individual sensory neurons (for review, see Lehky and Sejnowski, 1990). It has been proposed, therefore, that the information about the precise location of a stimulus and about specific features is not contained solely in the responses of the few neurons that are optimally activated, but is encoded in the graded responses of the ensemble of neurons that respond to a particular stimulus. Further indications for the putative significance of relational codes are provided by theoretical studies that attempted to simulate certain aspects of pattern recognition and motor control in artificial neuronal networks. Single-cell codes were found appropriate for the representation of a limited set of well-defined patterns, but the number of required representational elements scaled very unfavorably with the number of representable patterns. Moreover, severe difficulties were encountered with functions such as scene segmentation and figure–ground distinction because single-cell codes turned out to be too rigid and inflexible, again leading to a combinatorial explosion of the required representational units.

By implementing population or relational codes, some of these problems can be alleviated (Abeles, 1991; Braitenberg, 1978; Crick, 1984; Edelman, 1987, 1989; Edelman and Mountcastle, 1978; Grossberg, 1980; Hebb, 1949; Palm, 1982, 1990; Singer, 1985, 1990; Sporns et al., 1989, 1991; von der Malsburg, 1985). The essential feature of assembly coding is that individual cells can participate at different times in the representation of different sensory or motor patterns. The assumption is that just as a particular feature can be present in many different patterns, a neuron coding for this feature can be shared by many different representations. This reduces substantially the number of cells required for the representation of different patterns and allows for considerably more flexibility in the generation of new representations.

II. Binding Problems

Population or assembly codes provide viable solutions for a multiplicity of representational problems, but they also introduce new constraints. For the evaluation of population codes it is indispensable that responses that participate in the representation of a particular content can be identified unambiguously as belonging together; they need to be bound together. In the case of coarse coding of individual stimulus features, responses representing the same feature need to be associated selectively and hence have to be distinguished from responses to other features. Similar distinctions are required if, at higher levels of processing, whole perceptual objects are represented by cell assemblies. Again, responses of cells participating in the representation of the same object need to be identified and segregated from responses to other objects. If only a single feature is present, binding problems do not arise because in that case all responses can be associated with each other indiscriminately. But the environment of the organism is usually crowded with different perceptual objects and features. Hence, a large number of neurons will be active simultaneously and because of broad tuning many of them will be coactivated by different features that may even belong to different perceptual objects. For a successful association of responses coding for the same feature, for the selective association of features belonging to the same object, and for the segregation of different objects from one another and from background, it is therefore indispensable to have a mechanism that permits to select, from the many simultaneous responses, those responses that can be related to one another in a "meaningful" way and that avoids false conjunctions.

One way to achieve such unambiguous binding is grouping by convergence, a strategy that retransforms population codes into single-cell codes. In the case of coarse coding this would require selective convergence of the outputs of cells participating in the coding of a particular feature onto higher order cells. If the thresholds of these higher order cells are adjusted so that they respond only to a particular constellation of input activities, these higher cells could signal with high precision the presence and location of a particular feature. A similar strategy could be applied at higher processing levels for the selective association of cells that respond to the component features of perceptual objects. The set of feature-selective neurons that respond to the component features of a particular object would have to be connected selectively to a higher order neuron, and the thresholds of this higher order neuron would have to be adjusted so that this cell responds only to one particular activation pattern of the connected feature detectors. The response of this higher order neuron would then provide an unambiguous description of the relations between the component features and hence would be equivalent to the representation of a particular pattern or perceptual object. In this scheme the features of the object are bound together by convergence of fixed connections that link neurons representing component features with neurons representing the whole pattern. The relations between features are encoded by the specific architecture of these convergent connections.

The hypothesis of "binding by convergence" makes several predictions on neuronal response properties. First, if the responses constituting the coarse code of a particular feature are bound by convergence onto higher order cells, neurons should exist at higher levels of processing that are more sharply tuned for stimulus features than cells at more peripheral levels. Available data suggest that this is usually not the case. Second, if responses representing the component features of perceptual objects are bound by convergence onto higher order cells, one expects to find higher order cells with object-specific responses. However, though it is true that cells occupying higher levels in the processing hierarchy tend to be selective for more complex constellations of features than cells at lower levels, many continue to respond to rather simple geometrical patterns (Gallant et al., 1993; Tanaka et al., 1991). The difficulties with the experimental identification of object-specific cells have already been mentioned. Moreover, no single area in the visual processing stream has yet been identified that could serve as the ultimate site of convergence and that would be large enough to accommodate the vast number of neurons that are required if all distinguishable objects, including their many different views, were represented by individual neurons. Finally, the point has been made that "binding by convergence" may not be flexible enough to account for the rapid formation of representations of new patterns. Alternative proposals for the solution of the binding problem have therefore been proposed.

The proposal most pertinent to the experimental data reviewed in this article is that the population responses that need to be bound together are distinguished by a temporal code (von der Malsburg, 1985; von der Malsburg and Schneider, 1986). A similar suggestion, although formulated less explicitly, had been made previously by Milner (1974). Both hypotheses assume that the responses of neurons participating in the encoding of related contents get organized in time through reciprocal interactions, with the effect that they eventually come to discharge in synchrony. Thus, neurons having joined into an assembly coding for the same feature or at higher levels, for the same perceptual object, would be identifiable as members of the assembly because their responses would contain episodes during which their discharges are synchronous. If the temporal window for the evaluation of coincident firing is kept in the millisecond range, relations between the activities of spatially distributed neurons can be defined very selectively (von der Malsburg, 1985; Shimizu et al., 1986; Abeles, 1991; Softky and Koch, 1993). Hence, if such temporal patterning is combined with population coding, the number of different features or patterns that can be represented by a given set of neurons is substantially larger than if binding is achieved by convergence.

III. Predictions

If an assembly of cells coding for a common feature or a common perceptual object or a particular motor act is distinguished by the temporal coherence of the responses of the constituting neurons, precise and experimentally testable predictions can be derived.

1. Spatially segregated neurons should exhibit synchronized response episodes if activated by a single stimulus or by stimuli that can be grouped together into a single perceptual object.

2. Synchronization should be frequent among neurons within a particular cortical area, but it should also occur between cells distributed across different cortical areas if these cells respond to a common feature or perceptual object.

3. The probability that neurons synchronize their responses both within a particular area and across areas should reflect some of the Gestalt criteria used for perceptual grouping.

4. Individual cells must be able to change rapidly the partners with which they synchronize their responses if stimulus configurations change and require new associations.

5. If more than one object is present in a scene, several distinct assemblies should form. Cells belonging to the same assembly should exhibit synchronous response episodes whereas no consistent temporal relations should exist between the discharges of neurons belonging to different assemblies.

6. Synchronization should occur as the result of a self-organizing process that is based on mutual and parallel interactions between distributed cortical cells.

7. The connections determining synchronization probabilities should be highly specific because the criteria according to which distributed responses are bound together reside in the functional architecture of these connections.

8. The synchronizing connections should allow for interactions at levels of processing where responses of neurons express already some feature selectivity, in order to permit feature-specific associations. This predicts that cortico-cortical connections contribute to synchronization.

9. The synchronizing connections should be endowed with adaptive synapses allowing for use-dependent long-term modifications of synaptic gain in order to permit the acquisition of new grouping criteria when new object representations are to be installed during perceptual learning.

10. These use-dependent synaptic modifications should follow a correlation rule whereby synaptic connection should strengthen if pre- and

postsynaptic activity is often correlated, and they should weaken in case there is no correlation. This is required to enhance grouping of cells that code for features that often occur in consistent relations, as is the case for features constituting a particular object.

11. These grouping operations should occur over multiple processing stages because search for "meaningful" groupings has to be performed at different spatial scales and according to different feature domains. This could be achieved by distributing the grouping operations over different cortical areas in which different neighborhood relations are realized with respect to the representation of retinal location and of feature domains by remapping of inputs.

In order to test these predictions it is necessary to record simultaneously from spatially distributed neurons in the brain, to search for systematic temporal correlations among their responses, and to investigate stimulus-dependent variations of synchronization probabilities. It is not sufficient to analyze the probability of correlations in spontaneous activity, because this reveals only the architecture and coupling strength of connections (Gerstein and Perkel, 1972) but not the dynamic properties of the network, which emerge solely on stimulation. Therefore, and because of restrictions of space, the numerous studies using correlation techniques for the analysis of anatomical connectivity are not included herein. They have been reviewed in detail elsewhere (Singer, 1993).

IV. Experimental Testing of Predictions

Systematic search for the predicted stimulus-dependent synchronization phenomena between spatially distributed cortical neurons had been initiated by the observation that adjacent neurons in the cat visual cortex can engage in highly synchronous discharges when presented with their preferred stimulus (Gray and Singer, 1987). Neurons recorded simultaneously with a single electrode were found to engage transiently in synchronous discharges. In these multiunit recordings the synchronous discharges appear as clusters of spikes that often follow one another at rather regular intervals of 15 to 30 msec. These sequences of synchronous rhythmic firing usually last no more than a few hundred milliseconds and may occur several times during a single passage of moving stimuli (Fig. 1). Accordingly, autocorrelograms computed from such response epochs often exhibit a periodic modulation (Gray and Singer, 1987, 1989; Eckhorn et al., 1988; Gray et al., 1990; Schwarz and Bolz, 1991;

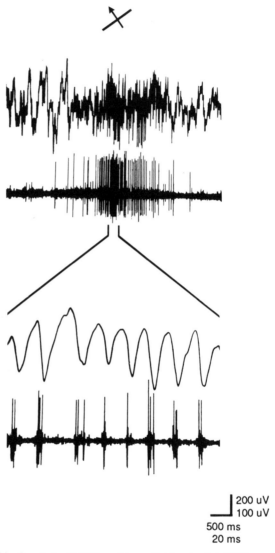

200 uV
100 uV
500 ms
20 ms

FIG. 1. Multiunit activity (MUA) and large field potential (LFP) responses, recorded from area 17 in an adult cat, to the presentation of an optimally oriented light bar moving across the receptive field. Oscilloscope records of a single trial showing the response to the preferred direction of movement. In the upper two traces, at a slow time scale, the onset of the neuronal response is associated with an increase in high-frequency activity in the LFP. The lower two traces display the activity at the peak of the response at an expanded time scale. Note the presence of rhythmic oscillations in the LFP and MUA (35–45 Hz) that are correlated in phase with the peak negativity of the LFP. Upper and lower voltage scales are for the LFP and MUA, respectively (adapted from Gray and Singer, 1989).

Livingstone, 1991). During such episodes of synchronous firing a large oscillatory field potential is recorded by the same electrode, the negative deflections being coincident with the cells' discharges. The occurrence of such a large field response indicates that, in the vicinity of the electrode, many more cells than those actually picked up by the electrode must have synchronized their discharges (Gray and Singer, 1989).

Neither the time of occurrence of these synchronized response episodes nor the phase of the oscillations is related to the position of the stimulus within the neuron's receptive field. When cross-correlation functions are computed between responses to subsequently presented identical stimuli, these "shift predictors" reveal no relation between the temporal patterning of successive responses (Gray and Singer, 1989; Gray *et al.*, 1990). The synchronization of the responses is thus not caused by some common spatial structure of the receptive fields of the simultaneously recorded cortical neurons.

This phenomenon of local response synchronization has been observed with multiunit and field potential recordings in several independent studies in different areas of the visual cortex of anesthetized cats [areas 17, 18, 19, and posterior medio-lateral suprasylvian cortex (PMLS)] (Eckhorn *et al.*, 1988, 1992; Gray and Singer, 1989; Gray *et al.*, 1990; Engel *et al.*, 1991a), in area 17 of awake cats (Raether *et al.*, 1989; Gray and Viana di Prisco, 1993), in the optic tectum of awake pigeons (Neuenschwander and Varela, 1990), and in the visual cortex of anesthetized (Livingstone, 1991) and awake behaving monkeys (Kreiter and Singer, 1992; Eckhorn *et al.*, 1993). Similar synchronization phenomena have been observed in a variety of nonvisual structures (for review, see Singer, 1993).

Subsequently, it has been shown with multielectrode recordings in anesthetized and awake cats (Engel *et al.*, 1990; Gray *et al.*, 1989; Gray and Viana di Prisco, 1993; Raether *et al.*, 1989) and anesthetized and awake monkeys (Kreiter and Singer, 1992; Kreiter *et al.*, 1992; Eckhorn *et al.*, 1993) that similar response synchronization can occur also between spatially segregated cell groups within the same visual area. Interestingly, the synchronization of responses over larger distances also occurs with zero phase lag. Hence, if the cross-correlograms show any interaction at all, they typically have a peak centered around zero delay. The half-width at half-height of this peak is in the order of 2–3 msec, indicating that most of the action potentials that showed some consistent temporal relation had occurred nearly simultaneously. This peak is often flanked on either side by troughs, which result from pauses between the synchronous bursts. When the duration of these pauses is sufficiently constant throughout the episode of synchronization, the cross-correlograms show in addition a periodic modulation with further side peaks and troughs. But such regularity is not a necessary requirement for synchronization to occur. There are numerous examples from anesthetized cats (see, e.g., Engel *et al.*, 1991c; Nelson *et al.*, 1992a) and especially from awake monkeys (Kreiter and Singer, 1992) that responses of spatially distributed neurons can become synchronized and lead to cross-correlograms with significant center peaks without engaging in rhythmic activity that is sufficiently regular to produce a periodical modulation of averaged auto- and cross-correlograms.

V. Dependence of Response Synchronization on Stimulus Configuration

As outlined above, the hypothesis of temporally coded assemblies requires that the probabilities with which distributed cells synchronize their responses should reflect some of the Gestalt criteria applied in perceptual grouping. Another and related prediction is that individual cells must be able to change the partners with which they synchronize, whereby the selection of partners should occur as a function of the patterns used to activate the cells. In this section experiments are reviewed that were designed to address these predictions. Detailed studies on anesthetized cats and anesthetized and awake monkeys have revealed that the synchronization probability for remote groups of cells is determined both by factors within the brain as well as by the configuration of the stimuli (Engel *et al.*, 1990, 1991a,b,c; Gray *et al.*, 1989; Kreiter *et al.*, 1992; König *et al.*, 1993). In general, synchronization probability within a particular cortical area decreases with increasing distance between the cells. If cells are so closely spaced that their receptive fields overlap, the probability is high that their responses will exhibit synchronous epochs if evoked with a single stimulus. The latter condition requires that the orientation and direction preferences of the cell pairs are sufficiently similar or that their tuning is sufficiently broad to allow for coactivation by a single stimulus. As recording distance increases, synchronization probability becomes more and more dependent on the similarity between the orientation preferences of the neurons (Ts'o *et al.*, 1986; Engel *et al.*, 1990).

Concerning the dependence of synchronization probability on stimulus configuration, single linearly moving contours have so far been found to be most efficient. Gray *et al.* (1989) recorded multiunit activity from two locations in cat area 17 separated by 7 mm. The receptive fields of the cells were nonoverlapping, had nearly identical orientation preferences, and were spatially displaced along the axis of preferred orientation. This enabled stimulation of the cells with bars of the same orientation under three different conditions: two bars moving in opposite directions, two bars moving in the same direction, and one long bar moving across both fields coherently. No significant correlation was found when the cells were stimulated by oppositely moving bars. A weak correlation was present for the coherently moving bars. But the long bar stimulus resulted in a robust synchronization of the activity at the two sites (Fig. 2). This effect occurred in spite of the fact that the overall number of spikes produced by the two cells and the oscillatory patterning of the responses were similar in the three conditions.

In related experiments Engel et al. (1991a,b) demonstrated in the cat that the synchronization of activity between cells in areas 17 and area PMLS and between areas 17 in the two hemispheres exhibits a similar dependence on the properties of the visual stimulus (Fig. 3). These findings indicate that the global properties of visual stimuli can influence the magnitude of synchronization between widely separated cells located within and between different cortical areas. Single contours but also spatially separate contours that move coherently and therefore appear as parts of a single figure are more efficient in inducing synchrony among the responding cell groups than are incoherently moving contours, which appear as parts of independent figures.

These results indicate clearly that synchronization probability depends not only on the spatial segregation of cells and on their feature preferences, the latter being related to the cells' position within the columnar architecture of the cortex, but also, and to a crucial extent, on the configuration of the stimuli. So far, synchronization probability appears to reflect rather well some of the Gestalt criteria for perceptual grouping. The high synchronization probability of nearby cells corresponds to the binding criterion of "vicinity," the dependence on receptive field similarities agrees with the criterion of "similarity," the strong synchronization observed in response to continuous stimuli obeys the criterion of "continuity," and the lack of synchrony in responses to stimuli moving in opposite directions relates to the criterion of "common fate."

Experiments have also been performed in order to test the prediction that simultaneously presented but different contours should lead to the organization of two independently synchronized assemblies of cells (Engel et al., 1991c; Kreiter et al., 1992). If groups of cells with overlapping receptive fields but different orientation preferences are activated with a single moving light bar, they synchronize their responses (Engel et al., 1990, 1991c). Usually, synchrony is established between all responding

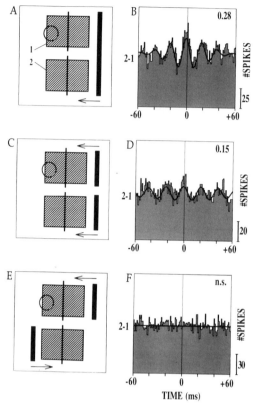

F<small>IG</small>. 2. Long-range synchronization is influenced by stimulus coherence. Multiunit activity was recorded from two sites in area 17 of cat visual cortex that were separated by 7 mm. The two cell groups preferred vertical orientations. (A, C, E) Plots of the receptive fields. The collinear arrangement of the fields allowed the comparison of three different stimulus paradigms: a long, continuous light bar moving across both fields (A), two independent light bars moving in the same direction (C), and the same two bars moving in opposite directions (E). The circle represents the center of the visual field, and the thick line drawn across each receptive field indicates the preferred orientation. (B, D, F) The respective cross-correlograms obtained with each stimulus paradigm. Using the long light bar, the two oscillatory responses were synchronized, as indicated by the strong modulation of the cross-correlogram with alternating peaks and troughs (B). If the continuity of the stimulus was interrupted, the synchronization became weaker (D), and it totally disappeared if the motion of the stimuli was incoherent (F). This change of the stimulus configuration affected neither the strength nor the oscillatory nature of the two responses (not shown). The graph superimposed on each of the correlograms represents a Gabor function that was fitted to the data to assess the strength of the modulation (Engel *et al.*, 1990). The number in the upper right corner indicates the "relative modulation amplitude," a measure of correlation strength that was determined by computing the ratio of the amplitude of the Gabor function to its offset. ns, Not significant; scale bars indicate the number of spikes (from Engel *et al.*, 1992).

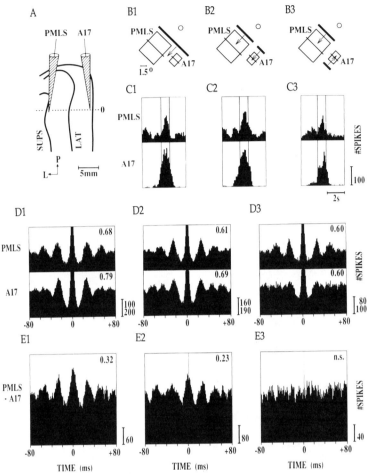

FIG. 3. Interareal synchronization is sensitive to global stimulus features. (A) Position of the recording electrodes. A17, area 17; LAT, lateral sulcus; SUPS, suprasylvian sulcus; P, posterior; L, lateral. (B1–B3) Plots of the receptive fields of the PMLS and area 17 recording. The diagrams depict the three stimulus conditions tested. The circle indicates the visual field center. (C1–C3) Peristimulus time histograms for the three stimulus conditions. The vertical lines indicate 1-second windows for which autocorrelograms and cross-correlograms were computed. (D1–D3) Comparison of the autocorrelograms computed for the three stimulus paradigms. Note that the modulation amplitude of the correlograms is similar in all three cases (indicated by the number in the upper right corner). (E1–E3) Cross-correlograms computed for the three stimulus conditions. The number in the upper right corner represents the relative modulation amplitude of each correlogram. Note that the strongest correlogram modulation is obtained with the continuous stimulus. The cross-correlogram is less regular and has a lower modulation amplitude when two light bars are used as stimuli, and there is no significant (n.s.) modulation with two light bars moving in opposite direction (from Engel *et al.,* 1991a).

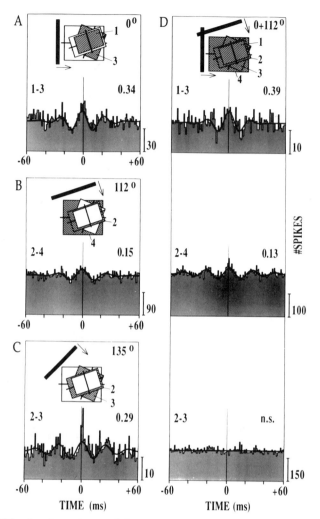

Fig. 4. Stimulus dependence of short-range interactions. Multiunit activity was recorded from four different orientation columns of area 17 of cat visual cortex separated by 0.4 mm. The four cell groups had overlapping receptive fields and orientation preferences of 22° (group 1), 112° (group 2), 157° (group 3), and 90° (group 4), as indicated by the thick line drawn across each receptive field in A–D. The figure shows a comparison of responses to stimulation with single moving light bars of varying orientation (left) and with the combined presentation of two superimposed light bars (right). For each stimulus condition, the shading of the receptive fields indicates the responding cell groups. Stimulation with a single light bar yielded a synchronization between all cells activated by the respective orientation. Thus, groups 1 and 3 responded synchronously to a vertically orientated (0°) light bar (A), groups 2 and 4 to a light bar at an orientation of 112° (B), and cell groups 2 and 3 to a light bar of intermediate orientation. (C) Simultaneous presentation of two stimuli with orientations of 0° and 112°, respectively, activated all four groups (D). However, in this case the groups segregated into two distinct assemblies, depending on which stimulus was closer to the preferred orientation of each group. Thus,

neurons, including those that are activated only suboptimally. This agrees with the postulate derived from the hypothesis of coarse coding that all responses of cells participating in the representation of a stimulus ought to be bound together. However, if such a set of groups is stimulated with two independent spatially overlapping stimuli that move in different directions, the activated cells split into two independently synchronized assemblies. Cells whose feature preferences match better with stimulus 1 form one synchronously active assembly, and those matching better with stimulus 2, the other (Fig. 4). Thus, although the two stimuli now evoke graded responses in all of the recorded groups, cells representing the same stimulus remain distinguishable because their responses exhibit synchronized response epochs while showing no consistent correlations with responses of cells activated by different stimuli. To extract this information requires a read-out mechanism that is capable of evaluating coincident firing at a millisecond time scale. A recent analysis of the integrative properties of cortical pyramidal cells suggests that, in these cells, the window for effective temporal summation may indeed be as short as a few milliseconds (Softky and Koch, 1993). If the extent of coactivation of the simultaneously recorded cells is assessed only on a coarse time scale (tens to hundreds of milliseconds), any read-out mechanism would have difficulty in deciding whether the cells had been activated by one composite figure whose features satisfy the preferences of the active cells or by two independent figures that excite the same set of cells. This would render it difficult to utilize coarse codes for the representation of stimulus features and it would in addition compromise the process of scene segmentation.

Another important issue of these experiments is the demonstration that individual cells can actually change the partners with which they synchronize when stimulus configurations change. Cell groups that engaged in synchronous response episodes when activated with a single

responses were synchronized between groups 1 and 3, which preferred the vertical stimulus, and between 2 and 4, which preferred the stimulus oriented at 112°. The two assemblies were desynchronized with respect to each other, and so there was no significant synchronization between groups 2 and 3. The cross-correlograms between groups 1 and 2, 1 and 4, and 3 and 4 were also flat (not shown). Note that the segregation cannot be explained by preferential anatomical wiring of cells with similar orientation preference (Ts'o et al., 1986) because cell groups can readily be synchronized in all possible pair combinations in response to a single light bar. The correlograms are shown superimposed with their Gabor function. The number in the upper right of each correlogram indicates the relative modulation amplitude. ns, Not significant; scale bars indicate the number of spikes (from Engel et al., 1991c).

stimulus no longer did so when activated with two stimuli, but then synchronized with other groups. This agrees with the prediction of the assembly hypothesis that interactions between distributed cell groups should be variable and influenced by the constellation of features in the visual stimulus.

VI. Synchronization between Areas

Experiments have also been designed to test the prediction that cells distributed across different cortical areas should be able to synchronize their responses if they respond to the same contour. This prediction applies not only for interactions between cells distributed within different visual areas in the same hemisphere, but also for cells in different hemispheres. The reason is that because of the partial decussation of the optic nerves, neurons responding to a figure extending across the vertical meridian are distributed across both hemispheres. Because the responses of these cells have to be related to one another in the same way as those of cells located within the same hemisphere, response synchronization should occur also across hemispheres and depend on stimulus configurations in the same way as intrahemispheric synchronization. In the cat, interareal synchronization of unit responses has been observed between cells in areas 17 and 18 (Eckhorn *et al.*, 1988, 1992; Nelson *et al.*, 1992a), between cells in areas 17 and 19 and 18 and 19 (Eckhorn *et al.*, 1992), between cells in area 17 and area PMLS, an area specialized for motion processing (Fig. 3) (Engel *et al.*, 1991a; Nelson *et al.*, 1992b), and even between neurons in A17 of the two hemispheres (Engel *et al.*, 1991b; Eckhorn *et al.*, 1992; Munk *et al.*, 1992). In the macaque monkey synchronous firing has been observed between neurons in areas V1 and V2 (Bullier *et al.*, 1992; Roe and Ts'o, 1992). Whenever tested, interareal and intraareal synchronization depended in a similar way on receptive field constellations and stimulus configurations (Engel *et al.*, 1991a,b).

VII. Synchronizing Connections

It is commonly assumed in interpretations of cross-correlation data that synchronization of neuronal responses with zero phase lag is indicative of common input (Gerstein and Perkel, 1972). Because response synchronization occurred often in association with oscillatory activity in the β- and γ-range, it has been proposed that the observed synchronization phenomena in the visual cortex are due to common oscillatory input from subcortical centers (Llinas and Ribary, 1993), where such oscillatory patterning of responses has also been observed (Steriade *et al.*, 1991, 1993; Ghose and Freeman, 1992; Pinault and Deschênes, 1992a,b; for a more extensive discussion of this issue, see Singer, 1993, 1994).

If the synchronization phenomena observed at the cortical level were solely a reflection of common subcortical input, this would be incompatible with the postulated role of synchronization in perceptual grouping. The hypothesis requires that synchronization probability depends to a substantial extent on interactions between the neurons whose responses actually represent the features that need to be bound together. Because cells in subcortical centers possess only very limited feature selectivity, one is led to postulate that cortico-cortical connections should also contribute to the synchronization process. This postulate is supported by the finding that synchronization between cells located in different hemispheres is abolished when the corpus callosum is cut (Engel *et al.*, 1991b; Munk *et al.*, 1992). This is direct proof (1) that cortico-cortical connections contribute to response synchronization and (2) that synchronization with zero phase lag can be brought about by reciprocal interactions between spatially distributed neurons despite considerable conduction delays in the coupling connections. Thus, synchrony is not necessarily an indication of common input but may also be the result of a dynamic organization process that establishes coherent firing by reciprocal interactions.

Simulation studies are now available to confirm that synchrony can be established without phase lag by reciprocal connections, even if these have slow and variable conduction velocities (König and Schillen, 1991; Schillen and König, 1990; Schuster and Wagner, 1990a,b). Use-dependent developmental selection of cortico-cortical connections could further contribute to the generation of architectures that favor synchrony. During early postnatal development, cortico-cortical connections are susceptible to use-dependent modifications and are selected according to a correlation rule (Löwel and Singer, 1992; see below). This should favor consolidation of connections whose activity is often in synchrony with the activity of their respective target cells. Hence, it is to be expected that connections are selected not only according to their feature-specific responses but also as a function of conduction velocities that allow for a maximum of synchrony.

However, the possibility to achieve synchrony through reciprocal cortical connections does not exclude a contribution of common input to the establishment of cortical synchronization. Especially if temporal patterns of responses need to be coordinated across distant cortical areas, bifurcating cortico-cortical projections, or divergent cortico-petal projections from subcortical structures such as the "nonspecific" thalamic nuclei, the basal ganglia and the nuclei of the basal forebrain could play an important role. By modulating in synchrony the excitability of selected cortical areas they could influence very effectively the probability with which neurons distributed across these selected areas engage in synchronous firing. This would be a mechanism by which attentional mechanisms could establish links between distributed cortical activity (see, e.g., Crick and Koch, 1990; Ribary *et al.*, 1991). A contribution of diverging cortical back-projections to long-range synchronization is suggested by the observation that unilateral focal inactivation of a prestriate cortical area reduces intraareal and interhemispheric synchrony in area 17 (Nelson *et al.*, 1992b). A contribution of thalamic mechanisms to the establishment of cortical synchrony has yet to be demonstrated.

VIII. Experience-Dependent Modifications of Cortico-cortical Connections and Synchronization Probabilities

The theory of assembly coding implies that the criteria according to which particular features are grouped together, rather than others, reside in the functional architecture of the assembly forming coupling connections. It is of particular interest, therefore, to study the development of the synchronizing connections, to identify the rules according to which they are selected, to establish correlations between their architecture and synchronization probabilities, and, if possible, to relate these neuronal properties to perceptual functions.

In mammals cortico-cortical connections develop mainly postnatally (Callaway and Katz, 1990; Innocenti, 1981; Luhmann *et al.*, 1986; Price and Blakemore, 1985a) and attain their final specificity through an activity-dependent selection process (Callaway and Katz, 1991; Innocenti and Frost, 1979; Luhmann *et al.*, 1990; Price and Blakemore, 1985b). It has been found that strabismus, when induced in 3-week-old kittens, leads to a profound rearrangement of cortico-cortical connections. Normally, these connections link cortical territories irrespective of whether these are dominated by the same or by different eyes. In the strabismics, by contrast, the tangential intracortical connections come to link with high selectivity only territories served by the same eye. The functional correlate of these changes in the architecture of cortico-cortical connections is a modification of synchronization probabilities. In strabismics response synchronization no longer occurs between cell groups connected to different eyes, whereas it is normal between cell groups connected to the same eye (König *et al.*, 1990, 1993).

These results have several implications. First, they are compatible with the notion that tangential intracortical connections contribute to response synchronization (see above). However, as strabismus also abolishes convergence of projections from the two eyes onto common cortical target cells, this result is also compatible with the view that synchrony is caused by common input. Second, these results agree with the postulates of the assembly hypothesis that the assembly-forming connections should be susceptible to use-dependent modifications and be selected according to a correlation rule. Third, the modifications of intracortical connections and synchronization probabilites add to the list of substrate changes that may be related to the specific perceptual deficits associated with early-onset squint. Strabismic subjects usually develop normal monocular vision in both eyes but they become unable to fuse signals conveyed by different eyes into coherent percepts even if these signals are made retinotopically contiguous by optical compensation of the squint angle (von Noorden, 1990). Thus, in strabismics, binding mechanisms appear to be abnormal or missing between cells driven from different eyes. The lack of cortico-cortical connections and the lack of response synchronization could be one of the reasons for this deficit in addition to the loss of binocular neurons.

These correlations are, for the least, compatible with the view that the architecture of cortico-cortical connections, by determining the probability of response synchronization, could set the criteria for perceptual grouping. Because this architecture is shaped by experience, this opens up the possibility that some of the binding and segmentation criteria are acquired or modified by experience.

Interestingly, the synapses of these cortico-cortical connections remain adaptive in the adult. Whereas in the mature cortex activity no longer induces modifications of the architecture of connections, experiments in slices indicate clearly that synapses in the mature visual cortex can undergo long-term potentiation (LTP) (Artola and Singer, 1987) and long-term depression (LTD) (Artola *et al.*, 1990). LTP and LTD have also been described in numerous other cortical areas, suggesting that these forms of synaptic plasticity are constitutive for neocortical processing (for review, see Artola and Singer, 1993). Both LTP and LTD have associative properties. LTP leads to selective strengthening of connections that have a high probability of being active in temporal contiguity with the respective postsynaptic neuron; LTD causes selective weakening of connections that are either totally inactive while other excitatory inputs to the same cell are very active, or whose activity is less well correlated with that of the postsynaptic target, i.e., with other excitatory inputs. A detailed description of these synaptic modification rules is contained in a review by Artola and Singer (1993) and is not repeated here. The conclusion is that these modification rules closely resemble those governing experience-dependent selection of circuits during early development, and because the latter have the effect to strengthen excitatory interactions between cells that are often active in synchrony [for review of the developmental constraints, see Singer (1990)]. It follows that sensory experience can continue to modify effectively the coupling between cortical neurons even after the end of developmental processes [for a review of these adaptive phenomena, see Garraghty and Kaas (1992)]. Because strengthened connections in turn increase the probability that neurons synchronize their responses, it is conceivable that these use-dependent modifications of synaptic coupling serve to modify existing assemblies and to generate new assemblies. In the context of the assembly hypothesis such experience-dependent changes of binding probabilities are equivalent with genuine learning processes, because they serve to modify grouping criteria and hence the relation between sensory patterns and corresponding cell assemblies.

IX. Correlation between Perceptual Deficits and Response Synchronization in Strabismic Amblyopia

Rather direct indications for a relation between experience-dependent modifications of synchronization probabilities and perceptual functions have come from a study of strabismic cats who had developed amblyopia. Strabismus, when induced early in life, not only abolishes binocular fusion and stereopsis but may also lead to amblyopia of one eye (von Noorden, 1990). This condition develops when the subjects solve the problem of double vision not by alternating use of the two eyes but by constantly suppressing the signals coming from the deviated eye. The amblyopic deficit usually consists of reduced spatial resolution and distorted and blurred perception of patterns. A particularly characteristic phenomenon in amblyopia is crowding, the drastic impairment of the ability to discriminate and recognize figures if these are surrounded with other contours. The identification of neuronal correlates of these deficits in animal models of amblyopia has remained inconclusive because the contrast sensitivity and the spatial resolution capacity of neurons in the retina and the lateral geniculate nucleus were found normal. In the visual cortex, identification of neurons with reduced spatial resolution or otherwise abnormal receptive field properties remained controversial (for a discussion, see Crewther and Crewther, 1990; Blakemore and Vital Durand, 1992). However, multielectrode recordings from striate cortex of cats exhibiting behaviorally verified amblyopia have revealed highly significant differences in the synchronization behavior of cells driven by the normal and the amblyopic eye, respectively. The responses to single moving bars that were recorded simultaneously from spatially segregated neurons connected to the amblyopic eye were much less well synchronized with one another than were the responses recorded from neuron pairs driven through the normal eye (Roelfsema et al., 1994). This difference was even more pronounced for responses elicited by gratings of different spatial frequency. For responses of cell pairs activated through the normal eye the strength of synchronization tended to increase with increasing spatial frequency, whereas it tended to decrease further for cell pairs activated through the amblyopic eye (Fig. 5). Apart from these highly significant differences between the synchronization behavior of cells driven through the normal and the amblyopic eye, no other differences were found in the commonly determined response properties of these cells. Thus, cells connected to the amblyopic eye continued to respond vigorously to gratings whose spatial frequency had been too high to be discriminated with the amblyopic eye in the preceding behavioral tests. These results suggest that disturbed temporal coordination of responses such as reduced synchrony may be one of the neuronal correlates of the amblyopic deficit. Indeed, if synchronization of responses at a millisecond time scale is used by the system to tag and identify the responses of cells that code for the same feature or contour, disturbance of this temporal patterning could be the cause for the crowding phenomenon. If responses evoked by nearby contours can no longer be associated unambiguously with either one or the other contour but become confounded, perceptual deficits are expected that closely resemble the crowding phenomenon. As a possible reason for the reduced synchronization among cells driven by the amblyopic eye, one might consider abnormalities in the network of cortico-cortical connections linking cell groups dominated by this eye. It is conceivable that the continuous suppression of the signals provided from this eye has impeded the experience-dependent specification of the respective intracortical synchronizing connections. Because reduced synchrony also impairs the transmission of responses and hence their saliency (see below), the present results can further account for the fact that amblyopic patients have difficulties attending to the signals conveyed by the amblyopic eye when both eyes are open. In that case signals from the amblyopic eye are usually eliminated from further processing and are not perceived.

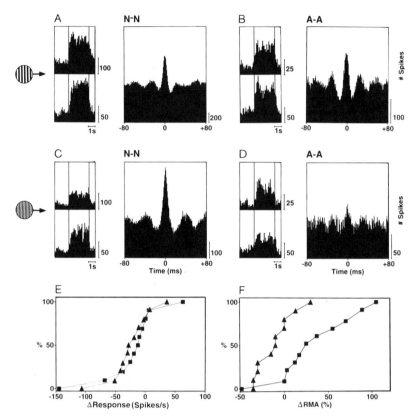

FIG. 5. Amplitudes and synchronization of responses to gratings of different spatial frequencies recorded from cats with strabismic amblyopia. (A–D) Responses to low (A and B) and high (C and D) spatial frequency gratings, recorded simultaneously from two cell groups driven by the normal eye (N sites; A and C) and two cell groups driven by the amblyopic eye (A sites; B and D), respectively. The left and right panels show the response histograms and the corresponding cross-correlograms, respectively. Note that response amplitudes decrease at the higher spatial frequency in both cases, whereas the relative modulation amplitude increases for the N–N pair but decreases for the A–A pair. (E) Cumulative distribution functions of the differences between the amplitude of responses to low and high spatial frequency gratings of optimal orientation. ■, N sites ($n = 53$); ▲, A-sites ($n = 35$). Abscissa, responses to high spatial frequency minus responses to low spatial frequency gratings. Note the similarity of the two distributions ($P > 0.1$). (F) Cumulative distribution functions of the differences between relative modulation amplitudes (ΔRMA) of cross-correlograms obtained for responses to high and low spatial frequency gratings of N–N pairs (■, $n = 24$) and A–A pairs (▲, $n = 11$). ΔRMA values (abscissa) were calculated by subtracting the relative modulation amplitude obtained with the low spatial frequency from that obtained with the high spatial frequency. The difference between the ΔRMA distributions of N–N pairs and A–A pairs is highly significant (from Roelfsema *et al.*, 1994).

X. Duration of Coherent States

It has been argued that synchronous oscillatory activity is unlikely to serve a function in visual processing because the time required to establish and to evaluate synchrony would be incompatible with the short recognition times common in visual perception (Tovee and Rolls, 1992). The following considerations suggest that such time constraints are probably not critical. In a study by Gray *et al.* (1992) recordings of field potential and unit activity were performed at two sites in cat visual cortex having a separation of at least 4 mm. Chosen for analysis were those field potential responses that displayed a particularly close correlation to the simultaneously recorded unit activity. The following variables were determined: (1) the onset latency of the synchronous activity, (2) the time-dependent changes in phase, frequency, and duration of the synchronous episodes within individual trials, and (3) the intertrial variation in each of these parameters.

The results, combined with previous observations (Engel *et al.*, 1990), demonstrated that correlated responses in cat visual cortex exhibit a high degree of dynamic variability. The amplitude, frequency, and phase of the synchronous events vary over time. The onset of synchrony is variable and bears no fixed relation to the stimulus. Multiple epochs of synchrony can occur on individual trials and the duration of these events also fluctuates from one stimulus presentation to the next. Most importantly, the results demonstrated that response synchronization can be established within 50–100 msec, a time scale consistent with behavioral performance on visual discrimination tasks (Gray *et al.*, 1992).

Similar, rapid fluctuations between synchronous and asynchronous states have been observed in other systems, and recent methodological developments have made possible a quantitative assessment of these rapid changes. Using the joint-PSTH and gravitational clustering algorithms (Gerstein *et al.*, 1985; Gerstein and Aertsen, 1985; Aertsen *et al.*, 1991), it has been possible to examine the time course of correlated firing among pairs and larger groups of neurons, respectively. These findings clearly indicate that the formation of coherently active cell assemblies is a dynamic process. Patterns of synchronous firing can emerge from seemingly nonorganized activity within tens of milliseconds, and can change as a function of stimulus and task conditions within similarly short time intervals. These findings suggest that the temporal constraint imposed by perceptual performance can be met by the dynamic processes that underlay the organization of synchronously active cell assemblies.

Theoretical considerations point in the same direction. Assemblies defined by synchronous discharges need not oscillate at a constant frequency over prolonged periods of time. Rather, it is likely that neuronal networks that have been shaped extensively by prior learning processes can settle very rapidly into a coherent state when the patterns of afferent sensory activity match with the architecture of the weighted connections in the network. Such a good match can be expected to occur for familiar patterns that during previous learning processes had the opportunity to mold the architecture of connections and to optimize the fit. If what matters for the nervous system is the simultaneity of discharges in large arrays of neurons, a single synchronous burst in thousands of distributed neurons may actually be sufficient for recognition. Obviously, the nervous system can evaluate and attribute significance to coherent activity even if synchrony is confined to a single burst because its parallel organization allows for simultaneous assessment of highly distributed activity.

Especially if no further ambiguities have to be resolved, or if no further modifications of synaptic connectivity are required, it would actually be advantageous if the system would not enter into prolonged cycles of reverberation after having converged toward an organized state of synchrony. Rather, established assemblies should be erased by active desynchronization as soon as possible in order to allow for the buildup of new representations. Thus, when processing highly familiar patterns or executing well-trained motor acts that raise no combinatorial problem, the system would function nearly as fast as a simple feedforward network. The differential and flexible routing of activity that is required in order to organize the appropriate assemblies could be achieved by the weighted association fibers within only a few reentrant cycles, if there are no ambiguities. The duration of such reentrant cycles would be of about the same order of magnitude as the delays for simple feedforward processing, as the parallel organization of the system allows for simultaneous exchange of signals between distributed processes. It is even conceivable that the organization of a pattern characterized by simultaneous discharges of distributed neurones can be achieved faster than expected from the addition of conduction and integration times in single feedforward architectures. The reason is that the cortical network is already active and continuously exchanging signals between neurons when new visual signals become available. In order to organize a synchronous state it is thus not necessary to collect sufficient excitatory drive to reach in succession the thresholds of serially connected neurons. Rather, it appears to be sufficient to only shift the time of occurrence of action potentials to establish synchrony, and this might be less time consuming.

XI. Significance of Synchrony in Neuronal Processing and Read-Out Mechanisms

If response synchronization is used by the nervous system to tag response episodes, synchronous discharges must be distinguishable from asynchronous events and hence should be of particular significance for cortical processes. Recent data on principles of cortical connectivity and on the properties of cortical synapses suggest that synchronization of responses on a time scale of milliseconds may indeed be an event that is highly significant for cortical processing and may be even more salient than the increase of the discharge rate of individual neurons. Cortical cells receive many thousand synaptic inputs but on the average a particular cell contacts any of its target cells only with a few synapses (Braitenberg and Schütz, 1991). *In vitro* studies from cortical slices indicate that the efficacy of individual synapses is low and that not every presynaptic action potential triggers the release of transmitter (Stevens, 1987). Moreover, synapses of cortical cells tend to be rather frequency sensitive and undergo a reduction of their efficacy with repetitive stimulation. The amplitude of excitatory postsynaptic potentials (EPSPs) decreases markedly already with stimulation frequencies as low as 1 Hz (A. Thomson, personal communication; A. Artola and M. Volgushev, unpublished observations). Thus, if a signal needs to be relayed across a chain of cortical cells, transmission cannot be assured solely by raising discharge rates. A complementary and probably more effective way of increasing the safety factor of transmission is to synchronize the discharges in converging pathways, as proposed previously by Abeles [for an extensive theoretical treatment of this issue, see Abeles (1991)]. It follows from this that activation patterns characterized by a high degree of synchrony are more likely than uncorrelated activity to be propagated. In networks such as neocortex, synchronization is thus equivalent with and complementary to rate increases because the impact of the responses of a particular cell on target neurons can be enhanced either by raising its discharge rate or by synchronizing the response of this cell with other responses. Because synchronization, in contrast to mere rate increases, necessarily establishes a relation between several cells, it always enhances not only the saliency of an individual response but that of a whole response pattern. Apart from that difference, however, the "read-out" of synchronous states can occur in the same way as the read-out of rate-coded population activities. In both cases read-out consists of the selective propagation of the most salient activation patterns and it should not matter whether saliency is achieved by rate increases or synchronization or both. However, if synchronization occurs on the basis of oscillatory signals, the read-out mechanism could be made particularly selective if its resonant properties are tuned to the time structure of the input signals. Ultimately, synchrony will of course be retranslated into rate codes because synchronous inputs will produce stronger responses in the respective target cells, compared to asynchronous inputs. Thus, both rate and synchrony can be used in combination to achieve selective routing of activity.

Even more cooperativity than is necessary for reliable signal transmission is required for the induction of use-dependent synaptic modifications, such as long-term potentiation and long-term depression. In the neocortex these modifications have high thresholds and require substantial postsynaptic depolarization (for review, see Artola and Singer, 1993). Temporal coordination of cortical responses appears thus necessary both for successful transmission across successive processing stages and for the induction of use-dependent synaptic modifications.

At present we ignore whether the observed synchronization of responses has a functional role in cortical processing. The data reviewed in this chapter are compatible with this possibility because they support predictions derived from hypotheses that assign a functional role to synchrony. But we are still lacking direct experimental evidence for causal relations between synchronization at the neuronal level, and behavioral correlates. Utilizing synchrony as a code in addition to rate and place codes would be advantageous because it provides the important option to define in a flexible and dynamic way relations among distributed neurons and to enhance simultaneously the saliency of the ensemble of cells distinguished by these relations.

References

Abeles, M., ed. (1991). "Corticonics." Cambridge Univ. Press, Cambridge, UK.

Aertsen, A., Vaadia, E., Abeles, M., Ahissar, E., Bergmann, I. I., Carmon, B., Lavner, Y., Margalit, E., Nelken, I., and Rotter, S. (1991). Neural interactions in the frontal cortex of a behaving monkey. Signs of dependence on stimulus context and behavioral states. *J. Hirnforsch.* **32,** 735–743.

Artola, A., and Singer, W. (1987). Long-term potentiation and NMDA receptors in rat visual cortex. *Nature (London)* **330,** 649–652.

Artola, A., and Singer, W. (1993). Long-term depression of excitatory synaptic transmission and its relationship to long-term potentiation. *Trends Neurosci.* **16,** 480–487.

Artola, A., Bröcher, S., and Singer, W. (1990). Different voltage-dependent thresholds for the induction of long-term depression and long-term potentiation in slices of the rat visual cortex. *Nature (London)* **347,** 69–72.

Barlow, H. B. (1972). Single units and cognition: A neurone doctrine for perceptual psychology. *Perception* **1,** 371–394.

Baylis, G. C., Rolls, E. T., and Leonard, C. M. (1985). Selectivity between faces in the responses of a population of neurons in the cortex in the superior temporal sulcus of the monkey. *Brain Res.* **342**, 91–102.

Blakemore, C., and Vital-Durand, F. (1992). Different neural origins for 'blur' amblyopia and strabismic amblyopia. *Ophthalmol. Physiol. Opt.* **12.**

Braitenberg, V. (1978). Cell assemblies in the cerebral cortex. *Lect. Notes Biomath.* **21,** 171–188.

Braitenberg, V., and Schütz, A. (1991). "Anatomy of the Cortex." Springer-Verlag Berlin and New York.

Bullier, M. J., Munk, M. H. L., and Nowak, L. G. (1992). Synchronization of neuronal firing in areas V1 and V2 of the monkey. *Soc. Neurosci. Abstr.* 11.7.

Callaway, E. M., and Katz, L. C. (1990). Emergence and refinement of clustered horizontal connections in cat striate cortex. *J. Neurosci.* **10**, 1134–1153.

Callaway, E. M., and Katz, L. C. (1991). Effects of binocular deprivation on the development of clustered horizontal connections in cat striate cortex. *Proc. Natl. Acad. Sci. U.S.A.* **88**, 745–749.

Crewther, D. P., and Crewther, S. G. (1990). Neural sites of strabismic ambylopia in cats: Spatial frequency deficit in primary cortical neurons. *Exp. Brain Res.* **79**, 615–622.

Crick, F. (1984). Function of the thalamic reticular complex: The searchlight hypothesis. *Proc. Natl. Acad. Sci. U.S.A.* **81**, 4586–4590.

Crick, F., and Koch, C. (1990). Towards a neurobiological theory of consciousness. *Semin. Neurosci.* **2**, 263–275.

Desimone, R., Albright, T. D., Gross, C. G., and Bruce, C. (1984). Stimulus-selective properties of inferior temporal neurons in the macaque. *J. Neurosci.* **4**, 2051–2062.

Desimone, R., Schein, S. J., Moran, J., and Ungerleider, L. G. (1985). Contour, color and shape analysis beyond the striate cortex. *Vision Res.* **24**, 441–452.

Eckhorn, R., Bauer, R., Jordan, W., Brosch, M., Kruse, W., Munk, M., and Reitboeck, H. J. (1988). Coherent oscillations; A mechanism for feature linking in the visual cortex? *Biol. Cybernet.* **60**, 121–130.

Eckhorn, R., Schanze, T., Brosch, M., Salem, W., and Bauer, R. (1992). Stimulus-specific synchronizations in cat visual cortex: Multiple microelectrode and correlation studies from several cortical areas. *In* "Induced Rhythms in the Brain" (E. Basar and T. H. Bullock, eds.), pp. 47–80. Birkhäuser, Boston.

Eckhorn, R., Frien, A., Bauer, R., Woelbern, T., and Kehr, H. (1993). High frequency (60–90 Hz) oscillations in primary visual cortex of awake monkey. *NeuroReport* **4**, 243–246.

Edelman, G. M. (1987). "Neural Darwinism: The Theory of Neuronal Group Selection." Basic Books, New York.

Edelman, G. M. (1989). "The Remembered Present: A Biological Theory of Consciousness." Basic Books, New York.

Edelman, G. M., and Mountcastle, V. B., eds. (1978). "The Mindful Brain." MIT Press, Cambridge, MA.

Engel, A. K., König, P., Gray, C. M., and Singer, W. (1990). Stimulus-dependent neuronal oscillations in cat visual cortex: Intercolumnar interaction as determined by cross-correlation analysis. *Eur. J. Neurosci.* **2**, 588–606.

Engel, A. K., Kreiter, A. K., König, P., and Singer, W. (1991a). Synchronization of oscillatory neuronal responses between striate and extrastriate visual cortical areas of the cat. *Proc. Natl. Acad. Sci. U.S.A.* **88**, 6048–6052.

Engel, A. K., König, P., Kreiter, A. K., and Singer, W. (1991b). Interhemispheric synchronization of oscillatory neuronal responses in cat visual cortex. *Science* **252**, 1177–1179.

Engel, A. K., König, P., and Singer, W. (1991c). Direct physiological evidence for scene segmentation by temporal coding. *Proc. Natl. Acad. Sci. U.S.A.* **88,** 9136–9140.

Engel, A. K., König, P., Kreiter, A. K., Schillen, T. B., and Singer, W. (1992). Temporal coding in the visual cortex: New vistas on integration in the nervous system. *Trends Neurosci.* **15,** 218–226.

Gallant, J. L., Braun, J., and van Essen, D. C. (1993). Selectivity for polar, hyperbolic and cartesian gratings in macaque visual cortex. *Science* **259,** 100–103.

Garraghty, P. E., and Kaas, J. H. (1992). Dynamic features of sensory and motor maps. *Curr. Opin. Neurobiol.* **2,** 522–527.

Georgopoulos, A. P. (1990). Neural coding of the direction of reaching and a comparison with saccadic eye movements. *Cold Spring Harbor Symp. Quant. Biol.* **55,** 849–859.

Gerstein, G. L., and Aertsen, A. M. H. J. (1985). Representation of cooperative firing activity among simultaneously recorded neurons. *J. Neurophysiol.* **54**(6), 1513–1528.

Gerstein, G. L., and Perkel, D. H. (1972). Mutual temporal relationship among neuronal spike trains. Statistical techniques for display and analysis. *Biophys. J.* **12,** 453–473.

Gerstein, G. L., Perkel, D. H., and Dayoff, J. E. (1985). Cooperative firing activity in simultaneously recorded populations of neurons: Detection and measurement. *J. Neurosci.* **5**(4), 881–889.

Ghose, G. M., and Freeman, R. D. (1992). Oscillatory discharge in the visual system: Does it have a functional role? *J. Neurophysiol.* **68**(5), 1558–1574.

Gray, C. M., and Singer, W. (1987). Stimulus-specific neuronal oscillations in the cat visual cortex: A cortical functional unit. *Soc. Neurosci. Abstr.* **13,** 404.3.

Gray, C. M., and Singer, W. (1989). Stimulus-specific neuronal oscillations in orientation columns of cat visual cortex. *Proc. Natl. Acad. Sci. U.S.A.* **86,** 1698–1702.

Gray, C. M., and Viana di Prisco, G. (1993). *Soc. Neurosci. Abstr.* **19,** 359.8.

Gray, C. M., König, P., Engel, A. K., and Singer, W. (1989). Oscillatory responses in cat visual cortex exhibit inter-columnar synchronization which reflects global stimulus properties. *Nature (London)* **338,** 334–337.

Gray, C. M., Engel, A. K., König, P., and Singer, W. (1990). Stimulus-dependent neuronal oscillations in cat visual cortex: Receptive field properties and feature dependence. *Eur. J. Neurosci.* **2,** 607–619.

Gray, C. M., Engel, A. K., König, P., and Singer, W. (1992). Synchronization of oscillatory neuronal responses in cat striate cortex: Temporal properties. *Visual Neurosci.* **8,** 337–347.

Gross, C. G., Rocha-Miranda, E. C., and Bender, D. B. (1972). Visual properties of neurons in inferotemporal cortex of the macaque. *J. Neurophysiol.* **35,** 96–111.

Grossberg, S. (1980). How does the brain build a cognitive code? *Psychol. Rev.* **87,** 1–51.

Hebb, D. O. (1949). "The Organization of Behavior." Wiley, New York.

Innocenti, G. M. (1981). Growth and reshaping of axons in the establishment of visual callosal connections. *Science* **212,** 824–827.

Innocenti, G. M., and Frost, D. O. (1979). Effects of visual experience on the maturation of the efferent system to the corpus callosum. *Nature (London)* **280,** 231–234.

König, P., and Schillen, T. B. (1991). Stimulus-dependent assembly formation of oscillatory responses. I. Synchronization. *Neural Comput.* **3,** 155–166.

König, P., Engel, A. K., Löwel, S., and Singer, W. (1990). Squint affects occurrence and synchronization of oscillatory responses in cat visual cortex. *Soc. Neurosci. Abstr.* **16,** 523.2

König, P., Engel, A. K., Löwel, S., and Singer, W. (1993). Squint affects synchronization of oscillatory responses in cat visual cortex. *Eur. J. Neurosci.* **5,** 501–508.

Kreiter, A. K., and Singer, W. (1992). Oscillatory neuronal responses in the visual cortex of the awake macaque monkey. *Eur. J. Neurosci.* **4,** 369–375.

Kreiter, A. K., Engel, A. K., and Singer, W. (1992). Stimulus-dependent synchronization of oscillatory neuronal activity in the superior temporal sulcus of the macaque monkey. *Eur. Neurosci. Abstr.* **15**, 1076.

Lehky, S. R., and Sejnowski, T. J. (1990). Neural model of stereoacuity and depth interpolation based on distributed representation of stereo disparity. *J. Neurosci.* **10**, 2281–2299.

Livingstone, M. S. (1991). Visually evoked oscillations in monkey striate cortex. *Soc. Neurosci. Abstr.* **17**, 73.3.

Llinas, R., and Ribary, U. (1993). Coherent 40-Hz oscillation characterizes dream state in humans. *Proc. Natl. Acad. Sci. U.S.A.* **93**, 2078–2081.

Löwel, S., and Singer, W. (1992). Selection of intrinsic horizontal connections in the visual cortex by correlated neuronal activity. *Science* **255**, 209–212.

Luhmann, H. J., Martinez-Millan, L., and Singer, W. (1986). Development of horizontal intrinsic connections in cat striate cortex. *Exp. Brain Res* **63**, 443–448.

Luhmann, H. J., Singer, W., and Martinez-Millan, L. (1990). Horizontal interactions in cat striate cortex. I. Anatomical substrate and postnatal development. *Eur. J. Neurosci.* **2**, 344–357.

Milner, P. M. (1974). A model for visual shape recognition. *Psychol. Rev.* **81**, 521–535.

Miyashita, Y. (1988). Neuronal correlate of visual associative long-term memory in the primate temporal cortex. *Nature (London)* **335**, 817–820.

Munk, M. H. J., Nowak, L. G., Chouvet, G., Nelson, J. I., and Bullier, J. (1992). The structural basis of cortical synchronization. *Eur. J. Neurosci., Suppl.* **5**, 21.

Mussa-Ivaldi, F. A., Giszter, S. F., and Bizzi, E. (1990). Motor-space coding in the central nervous system. *Cold Spring Harbor Symp. Quant. Biol.* **55**, 827–835.

Nelson, J. I., Salin, P. A., Munk, M. H. J., Arzi, M., and Bulleir, J. (1992a). Spatial and temporal coherence in cortico-cortical connections: A cross-correlation study in areas 17 and 18 in the cat. *Visual Neurosci.* **9**, 21–38.

Nelson, J. I., Nowak, L. G., Chouvet, G., Munk, M. H. J., and Bullier, J. (1992b). Synchronization between cortical neurons depends on activity in remote areas. *Soc. Neurosci. Abstr.* **18**, 11.

Neuenschwander, S., and Varela, F. J. (1990). Sensory-triggered oscillatory activity in the avian optic tectum. *Soc. Neurosci. Abstr.* **16**, 47.6.

Palm, G. (1982). "Neural Assemblies." Springer-Verlag, Berlin and New York.

Palm, G. (1990). Cell assemblies as a guideline for brain research. *Concepts Neurosci.* **1**, 133–137.

Perrett, D. I., Mistlin, A. J., and Chitty, A. J. (1987). Visual neurones responsive to faces. *Trends Neurosci.* **10**, 358–364.

Pinault, D., and Deschênes, M. (1992a). Voltage-dependent 40-Hz oscillations in rat reticular thalamic neurons *in vivo*. *Neuroscience* **51**, 245–258.

Pinault, D., and Deschênes, M. (1992b). Control of 40-Hz firing of reticular thalamic cells by neurotransmitters. *Neuroscience* **51**, 259–268.

Price, D. J., and Blakemore, C. (1985a). The postnatal development of the association projection from visual cortical area 17 to area 18 in the cat. *J. Neurosci.* **5**, 2443–2452.

Price, D. J., and Blakemore, C. (1985b). Regressive events in the postnatal development of association projections in the visual cortex. *Nature (London)* **316**, 721–724.

Raether, A., Gray, C. M., and Singer, W. (1989). Intercolumnar interactions of oscillatory neuronal responses in the visual cortex of alert cats. *Eur. Neurosci. Abstr.* **12**, 72.5.

Ribary, U., Joannides, A. A., Singh, K. D., Hasson, R., Bolton, J. P. R., Lado, F., Mogilner, A., and Llinas, R. (1991). Magnetic field tomography of coherent thalamocortical 40 Hz oscillations in humans. *Proc. Natl. Acad. Sci. U.S.A.* 88, 11037–11041.

Roe, A. W., and Ts'o, D. Y. (1992). Functional connectivity between V1 and V2 in the primate. *Soc. Neurosci. Abstr.* **18**, 11.4.

Roelfsema, P. R., König, P., Engel, A. K., Sireteanu, R., and Singer, W. (1994). Reduced neuronal synchrony: A physiological correlate of strabismic amblyopia in cat visual cortex. *Eur. J. Neurosci.* (in press).

Rolls, E. T. (1991). Neural organization of higher visual functions. *Curr. Opin. Neurobiol.* **1**, 274–278.

Sakai, K., and Miyashita, Y. (1991). Neural organization for the long-term memory of paired associates. *Nature (London)* **354**, 152–155.

Schillen, T. B., and König, P. (1990). Coherency detection by coupled oscillatory responses—Synchronization connections in neural oscillator layers. In "Parallel Processing in Neural Systems and Computers" (R. Eckmiller, ed.), pp. 139–142. Elsevier, Amsterdam.

Schuster, H. G., and Wagner, P. (1990a). A model for neuronal oscillations in the visual cortex. 1. Mean-field theory and derivation of the phase equations. *Biol. Cybernet.* **64**, 77–82.

Schuster, H. G., and Wagner, P. (1990b). A model for neuronal oscillations in the visual cortex. 2. Phase description of the feature dependent synchronization. *Biol. Cybernet.* **64**, 83–85.

Schwarz, C., and Bolz, J. (1991). Functional specificity of the long-range horizontal connections in cat visual cortex: A cross-correlation study. *J. Neurosci.* **11**, 2995–3007.

Shimizu, H., Yamaguchi, Y., Tsuda, I., and Yano, M. (1986). Pattern recognition based on holonic information dynamics: Towards synergetic computers. In "Complex Systems-Operational Approaches" (H. Haken, ed.), pp. 225–240. Springer-Verlag, Berlin and New York.

Singer, W. (1985). Activity-dependent self-organization of the mammalian visual cortex. In "Models of the Visual Cortex" (D. Rose and V. G. Dobson, eds.), pp. 123–136. Wiley, Chichester.

Singer, W. (1990). Search for coherence: A basic principle of cortical self-organization. *Concepts Neurosci.* **1**, 1–26.

Singer, W. (1993). Synchronization of cortical activity and its putative role in information processing and learning. *Annu. Rev. Physiol.* **55**, 349–374.

Singer, W. (1994). Putative functions of temporal correlations in neocortical processing. In "Large Scale Neuronal Theories of the Brain" (C. Koch and J. Davis, eds.), pp. 201–237. MIT Press, Cambridge, MA.

Softky, W. R., and Koch, C. (1993). The highly irregular firing of cortical cells is inconsistent with temporal integration of random EPSPs. *J. Neurosci.* **13**, 334–350.

Sparks, D. L., Lee, C., and Rohrer, W. H. (1990). Population coding of the direction, amplitude and velocity of saccadic eye movements by neurons in the superior colliculus. *Cold Spring Harbor Symp. Quant. Biol.* **55**, 805–811.

Sporns, O., Gally, J. A., Reeke, G. N., Jr., and Edelman, G. M. (1989). Reentrant signaling among simulated neuronal group leads to coherency in their oscillatory activity. *Proc. Natl. Acad. Sci. U.S.A.* **86**, 7265–7269.

Sporns, O., Tononi, G., and Edelman, G. M. (1991). Modeling perceptual grouping and figure–ground segregation by means of active reentrant conditions. *Proc. Natl. Acad. Sci. U.S.A.* **88**, 129–133.

Steriade, M., Curro-Dossi, R., Paré, D., and Oakson, G. (1991). Fast oscillations (20–40 Hz) in thalamocortical systems and their potentiation by mesopontine cholinergic nuclei in the cat. *Proc. Natl. Acad. Sci. U.S.A.* **88**, 4396–4400.

Steriade, M., Curro-Dossi, R., and Contreras, D. (1993). Electrophysiological properties of intralaminar thalamocortical cells discharging rhythmic ($\approx$40 Hz) spike-bursts at $\approx$1000 Hz during waking and rapid eye movement sleep. *Neuroscience* **56**, 1–9.

Stevens, C. F. (1987). Specific consequences of general brain properties. *In* "Synaptic Function" (J. M. Edelman and W. E. Gall, eds.), Chapter 24, pp. 699–709. Wiley, New York.

Tanaka, K., Saito, H., Fukada, Y., and Moriya, M. (1991). Coding visual images of objects in the inferotemporal cortex of the macaque monkey. *J. Neurophysiol.* **66,** 170–189.

Tovee, M. J., and Rolls, E. T. (1992). The functional nature of neuronal oscillations. *Trends Neurosci.* **15,** 387.

Ts'o, D. Y., Gilbert, C. D., and Wiesel, T. N. (1986). Relationship between horizontal interactions and functional architecture in cat striate cortex as revealed by cross-correlation analysis. *J. Neurosci.* **6,** 1160–1170.

von der Malsburg, C. (1985). Nervous structures with dynamical links. *Ber. Bunsenges. Phys. Chem.* **89,** 703–710.

von der Malsburg, C., and Schneider, W. (1986). A neural cocktail-party processor. *Biol. Cybernet.* **54,** 29–40.

von Noorden, G. K. (1990). "Binocular Vision and Ocular Motility: Theory and Management of Strabismus." Mosby, St. Louis, MO.

TEMPORAL MECHANISMS IN PERCEPTION

Ernst Pöppel

Forschungszentrum Jülich GmbH
D-52425 Jülich, Germany

I. Primary Consciousness: Constituent Parts and Characteristics

This paper can be viewed as a commentary to some ideas presented in Chapter 9 of "The Remembered Present" (1989) by Gerald Edelman. The chapter treats primary consciousness as Edelman defines it. Primary consciousness is characterized by three components. "The first component emerges as a result of the evolution of close linkages between systems mediating concept formation in various areas (frontal, temporal, parietal, and cingulate cortex) and interoceptively determined value systems mediated by circuits related to hedonic responses" (p. 153). The second component is a separate form of memory emerging as a result of the functioning of these linkages. There would be "an adaptive advantage in evolving a conceptually based memory system that correlated the continual ongoing interactions between categorized exteroceptive signals and interoceptive signals that reflect homeostatic needs" (p. 154). The third component "provides the *sufficient* condition for consciousness to appear. Consistent with the ideas of neuronal group selection, the model proposes that special circuits evolved that carry out a continual re-entrant signaling between the second component (mediating 'value-category memory') and the ongoing real-time exteroceptive global mappings that are concerned with perceptual categorization of *current* exteroceptive stimuli *before* they can form part of the value-category memory (p. 154)." "The re-entrant interaction between a special form of memory with strong conceptual components . . . and a stream of perceptual categorizations would generate primary consciousness. Phenomenally this function would appear as a 'picture' of ongoing categorized events or a 'mental image' " (p. 154). And a little later Edelman states "given that the extended theory is based on the TNGS [theory of neuronal group selection], the categorizations perforce involve motor acts, and actions and responses are therefore a key part of the model" (p. 155).

Thus, the repertoire of primary consciousness is based on neuronal programs in four different domains, implementing perceptions, memories, evaluations, and actions (Pöppel, 1989a). Neuropsychological evidence suggests that elementary functions within these domains are represented in a modular fashion; the main support for such a conclusion comes from neuroanatomical studies in the visual system (Zeki, 1978). Because of spatial segregation of function, the brain has to deal with intermodular binding of neuronal activities to construct unified and coherent percepts. Powerful models have been developed to solve the problem of spatial binding on the cellular and areal level of analysis (Sporns et al., 1989; Tononi et al., 1992a,b).

It is certainly useful to distinguish between different levels of binding (Pöppel et al., 1991). At a primary level we may discuss spatial binding of identical features within one sensory modality. Taking, for instance, the visual system, this level of binding is characterized by linking activities that represent identical features in different regions. Such binding is presumably presemantic and automatic and may be the prerequisite to establish contours or surfaces (i.e., topological primitives) throughout the visual field. There is experimental evidence suggesting that this kind of binding may be provided by the synchronization of oscillating neuronal activities (Gray et al., 1989). On another level one deals with binding within one sensory modality for different qualities (e.g., Tononi et al., 1992a). At this level one already has to think of semantic aspects. If different qualities are linked together, such as colors and surfaces giving rise to perceived objects, then the system presumably has to define which qualities are bound together. Thus, a scheme or an a priori internal representation of the perceived object should be centrally available, against which sensory information is compared. On a third level of binding one deals with the problem of how activities from different sense modalities are linked together. Objects perceived are often characterized visually, auditorally, and sometimes by information from other modalities; obviously, intersensory binding must transcend intrasensory operations. It has been suggested that for the binding operations at the indicated three levels, a common temporal mechanism based on excitability cycles may be used that provides a temporal frame for further operations being responsible for binding (Pöppel et al., 1990a).

In his analysis of primary consciousness Edelman (1989) often refers to time or temporal aspects of information processing, for instance when he mentions continual ongoing interactions, a continual reentrant signaling, an ongoing real-time exteroceptive global mapping, current exteroceptive stimuli, a stream of perceptual categorization. How can these processes be related to temporal mechanisms of perception? This brings us again to another level of binding that no longer is responsible for the connection of spatially distributed activities but for the connection of successive events. I would like to suggest that primary consciousness is embedded in time on two hierarchically related levels, the general idea being that central information processing is quantized. One level is the temporal domain of approximately 30 msec; this level is related to the first three levels of binding as indicated above and it serves the definition of "primordial events." The other level is the temporal domain of approximately 3 seconds, where temporal binding sets in, i.e., at this level the primordial events are linked with each other. For both these operational domains there is a large corpus of evidence from different experimental paradigms (e.g., Pöppel, 1978, 1988). Primary consciousness proper is conceived of being implemented in a temporal window of approximately 3 seconds duration.

II. System States in the 30-msec Domain: A Temporal Window for Linking Distributed Activities

At first some experimental evidence for the 30-msec domain is given. If one measures choice reaction time, for instance presenting visual and auditory stimuli in a random sequence to a subject, one often observes multimodal distribution of the response times if measurements are obtained under stationery experimental conditions (Harter and White, 1968; Ilmberger, 1986; Jokeit, 1990; Pöppel, 1968, 1970, 1988). Even for simple reaction times, multimodal response distributions have been observed (Wynn, 1977). In all these cases the intermodal distance is close to 30 msec. This observation implies that whenever a decision has to be made to initiate a movement, the response is not programmed in a continuous fashion; either one or a successive time window is selected for the response. The decision process seems to be dependent on an underlying neuronal process that is characterized by sequential quanta of approximately 30 msec duration.

It is important to note that multimodalities in response histograms can only be observed if the response is temporally related to stimulus onset. If one would assume a continuously oscillating neuronal process underlying for central processing of sensory information (a scansion process), it would not be possible to explain multimodalities in response histograms. In such a case stimuli would appear at any phase of the oscillation, and an internal temporal segmenting process would no longer be visible on the observational level (Pöppel, 1970). Thus, the motor response must be triggered by the stimulus, or a continuously running oscillation must be entrained instantaneously by stimulus onset.

Temporal segmentation in the domain of 30 msec is also typical in the control of oculomotor behavior. If saccadic or pursuit eye movements are recorded in humans or lower primates (Frost and Pöppel, 1976; Fuchs, 1967; Pöppel and Logothetis, 1986; Ruhnau and Haase, 1993), multimodal response histograms are often observed if the measurements are obtained under strictly controlled conditions. The intermodal distance in these cases is similar to those observed with manual responses in reaction time tasks. If a visual target slowly starts to move, one observes that the pursuit movement does not start according to a continuous mode of temporal processing but with preference of latencies that differ by 30 to 40 msec; such preferred latencies would be, for instance, 130, 160, or 190 msec.

The reason why such multimodalities are not regularly observed is manyfold. Sometimes fatigue of the subjects and time of day, which are known to influence reaction time in an unspecific way, are not controlled properly. Another problem in such experiments producing instationarities is intraexperimental learning, in particular if choice reaction is measured. In such cases the variance of the initial measurements is so high that underlying systematic effects indicating quantal processing of information usually are masked. One experiment on intrahemispheric choice reaction time may illustrate this point (Pöppel et al., 1990b). Visual stimuli were presented to the right visual field, auditory stimuli to the right ear, and responses had to be given by the right hand. The sequence of the stimuli and the interstimulus interval were randomized. For each experimental session response histograms were obtained either for the visual or the auditory stimuli. The histograms for the first experimental session showed noisy distributions with no indication of systematic multimodalities; already by the second day clear bimodal response distributions were, however, visible. These response peaks were observed for several successive days and they stayed exactly at the same latency windows; finally learning of this task resulted in a unimodal response histogram with very small variability, the position of this response peak coinciding with those peaks of shortest latency observed throughout the successive preceding sessions. Apparently, one temporal window for a shortest response was set up early during the experiment and served as a final attractor; during the learning phase a discretely separated temporal window served as a competitive attractor, which resulted in the bimodal distributions during the learning phase.

Thus, this experiment showed three qualitatively different response modes. At first an irregular and noisy response mode was tapped (many experiments in cognitive psychology stay at this observational level if subjects are asked to participate just once in an experiment); second, during a learning phase different response windows were selected, and finally after completing learning one response window remained. Interestingly, in these experiments, which mainly reflect intrahemispheric processing, the intermodal distance of the temporal windows was between 60 and 70 msec, and not 30 msec as observed in the previously mentioned experiments.

A prolongation of intermodal distance in response histograms can also be observed if brain-injured patients are studied (Pöppel et al., 1978). In one such case an intermodal distance of approximately 100 msec was observed. This observation illustrates the fact that brain injury usually results in a slowing down of neuronal processes, as is, for instance, also reflected in a selective reduction of critical flicker fusion (Pöppel et al., 1975). A similar phenomenon of slowing down has been observed in studies in which the effect of alcohol on reaction time was measured (Pöppel and Steinbach, 1986). In the alcohol study it could be demonstrated that during the drunk state right hemisphere functioning deteriorates with respect to visual processing and left hemisphere functioning deteriorates with respect to auditory processing; this result suggests a certain independence of temporal processing within the two cerebral hemispheres.

Insight into temporal processing at the level of system states with 30 msec duration also comes from studies on temporal order threshold. In a now classic paper by Hirsh and Sherrick (1961) it could be demonstrated that temporal order threshold in three sense modalities (visual, auditory, and tactile sense) is approximately the same. In such tasks the subject has to indicate in what temporal succession two stimuli appear. Using this paradigm it could be demonstrated that auditory order threshold is approximately 30 msec, corresponding to the intermodal distance in response histograms of reaction time or oculomotor latency distributions (von Steinbüchel and Pöppel, 1991). In these studies it was also observed that brain-injured patients with agrammatism suffer a severe prolongation of auditory order threshold, suggesting a slowing down of neuronal analysis. Often order thresholds longer than 100 msec in these patients were observed.

Because acoustic information necessary to distinguish between voiced and unvoiced sounds or characterizing consonants themselves can be as short as some tens of milliseconds, it is reasonable to assume that some aspects of aphasia can be explained on the basis of slowed down brain processes. Because successive consonants would fall into one time window, their before–after relationship can no longer be determined if order threshold is pathologically prolonged. Therefore we attempted to improve temporal order threshold and to test whether a potentially improved order threshold may generalize toward linguistic tasks. With a simple training using a feedback procedure, auditory order threshold in a treatment group of patients was brought back to almost normal values between 30 and 40 msec. These patients with improved temporal processing showed also a functional gain in the speech domain. When asked to distinguish between voiced and unvoiced stop-consonant–vocal syllables, the treatment group showed much better performance compared to patients without temporal training. These observations may have some practical importance (von Steinbüchel and Pöppel, 1993): In patients who have suffered brain injury resulting in aphasic problems, most often the therapy is linguistically oriented; one tries to improve the lexical, pragmatic, syntactic, semantic, phonetic, or prosodic competences. What is often overlooked is that lesions also result in a significant change in temporal processing. It is suggested to put more emphasis on their domain in neuropsychological rehabilitation.

The catalog providing support for system states of 30 msec can be extended by a number of further studies. Memory studies suggest that the scanning process throughout short-term memory is successive, with each step taking between 30 and 40 msec (Sternberg, 1966). Latour (1967) observed that visual thresholds oscillate with a period close to 30 msec. If two random patterns that together form a word are shown for 6 msec, each with temporal intervals of 25 msec, 50 msec, etc., the words will be recognized perfectly with a 25-msec interval but much less often with a 50-msec interval (Erikson and Collins, 1968). Two experiences that can be distinguished from each other are reported when the overall duration of two color stimuli is 60 msec, i.e., if 30 msec for each of the temporally contiguous events is available (Efron, 1967).

Complementary evidence for the existence of system states with a duration of approximately 30 msec can be derived from neurophysiological studies on single cells and cell assemblies. Such observations come from the somatosensory, auditory, and visual system. For instance, temporal integration in the somatosensory system seems to operate in the domain of 30 msec (Gardner and Costanzo, 1980), a conclusion that is also supported by observations on oscillations with approximately the same period (Murthy and Fetz, 1992). In particular, the 40-Hz component in evoked potentials or the electroencephalogram can be interpreted with respect to system states provided by the brain to process information in a temporally contiguous fashion (Baser *et al.*, 1976; Galambos *et al.*, 1981; Ribary *et al.*, 1991). Especially after the work of Galambos and his colleagues a lot of evidence on the 40-Hz activity has been collected using the midlatency response of the auditory-evoked potential (Mäkelä and Hari, 1987; Pantev *et al.*, 1991).

The 40-Hz component in the midlatency response of the auditory-evoked potential representing theoretical system states of approximately 30 msec duration plays also an interesting role in anesthesiological studies (Madler and Pöppel, 1987; Schwender *et al.*, 1993). General anesthesia is characterized by the fact that information no longer is processed; as it turns out this is only the case if the oscillatory components in the midlatency response are no longer present. Auditory information is still picked up, as can be seen from brain stem potentials, which are still visible during the anesthetic state; integrated neuronal activity, however, as indicated by the oscillatory components, is lost during the anesthetic state. It appears that the theoretical system states with a duration of 30 msec are a necessary condition to establish the raw material of consciousness, the "primordial events." The typical anesthetic condition has an interesting subjective corollary. Often patients waking up from anesthesia report that no time at all since the beginning of anesthesia has elapsed, i.e., the state of anesthesia is like "dead time," which is a categorically different situation compared to regular sleep.

The 40-Hz oscillatory activity on the level of single-cell activity has obtained particular importance by new observations in the visual system, and these oscillations have been discussed with respect to the binding of distributed activities (Gray *et al.*, 1989). Oscillations that are stimulus locked—and not induced after a rather long latency—have been observed already at earlier processing stages in the visual system, such as the lateral geniculate nuleus (Podvigin, 1972). Using a well-established technique by moving around a complex scene in front of a receptive field, it was possible to reconstruct the spatial properties, in particular the outline of an object at the level of the lateral geniculate nucleus, by stimulus-triggered neuronal oscillations in the 40-Hz domain (Podvigin *et al.*, 1992).

It appears that in the different sensory systems, after a constant time of stimulus transduction, neuronal oscillations are initiated. One period of such oscillatory responses can be interpreted as providing a system state of approximately 30 msec duration, which may determine "primordial events." This conclusion is supported by the psychophysical evidence that indicates such a temporal window by a number of different experimental paradigms.

If one relates neuronal oscillations to system states of 30 msec duration, it has to be clarified what kind of oscillation one is talking about. There are at least two kinds of oscillations in neuronal systems that are principally different, namely pendulum versus relaxation oscillations (e.g., Wever, 1965). A relaxating system in the technical sense is an oscillator that can be entrained instantaneously; this is a principal distinction between the relaxation and the pendulum oscillator. Most of the observations reported here refer to stimulus-triggered or instantaneously entrained system states or oscillations and, thus, to relaxating systems. These system properties also imply that the oscillations are damped, i.e., dependent on a damping factor, the oscillations disappear after several periods (in the extreme case after only one period). Furthermore, other than in the case of pendulum oscillations, the period of relaxation oscillations is more variable and not a fixed constant.

With respect to temporal representation one has to conclude that within one period, time in a subjective sense does not exist because the before–after relationship of successive stimuli cannot be defined, as has been suggested by the experiments on temporal order threshold. Thus, system states are characterized by the fact that information is treated as cotemporal, which means the states are *atemporal*. Such atemporal kernels can be conceived of as the building blocks of events. A separate question is how successive system states are neuronally represented; a new model suggests a discrete spatial representation of such states (Schill and Zetzsche, 1994), which would allow a separate mechanism to have instantaneous access to discrete temporal events. Before turning to such an implied separate mechanism, which integrates successive events into perceptual units, a still open question in visual processing and a potentially functional use of system states shall be addressed.

In object perception different parts that characterize an object have to be integrated. Normally these different parts are characterized by different reflectances. It is often overlooked that this produces a problem for spatial integration because different optical flux results in different transduction time at the retinal level. Thus, the central availability of the different parts of an object is usually nonsimultaneous (Pöppel et al., 1990a). One solution for this "temporal diplopia" could be the initiation of system states by using neuronal oscillations as discussed here. A system state can be set up by the leading stimulus, i.e., the one with the highest light intensity; later stimuli, which still would fall into the just-created system state, would be treated as cotemporaneous with the leading stimulus. Thus, by using system states, the logistical problem the brain has to deal with (because of biophysical mechanisms at the transduction level) could be overcome. The temporally "leading" stimulus triggers a relaxation oscillation and the "lagging" information is read into the same temporal window. Because system states are atemporal the visual system can free itself from flux differences that are necessary to define objects physically in perception.

Interestingly, the first mention of 30 msec as an elementary time unit can be found in the last century. In 1865 Ernst Mach demonstrated that perceptual time intervals shorter than 30 msec do not exist, because one does not have a feeling of duration for intervals shorter than this interval. This early report on an elementary temporal phenomenon in perception gives the opportunity to indicate that most concepts in this field of research were formulated more than 100 years ago, actually in the seventh decade of the last century. In addition to the discovery of Mach there appeared in 1864 a now famous paper by Karl Ernst von Baer; this paper is based on a talk von Baer delivered in 1860 in St. Petersburg. Here he introduced the theoretical notion of a perceptual moment, i.e., the smallest sensible time interval, and von Baer suggested that the perceptual moment has to be thought of being different in different animal species. Because of this one may conclude that the subjective flow of time in these species is probably also different. A third essential paper was published by Donders (1868) wherein he described the paradigm of reaction time and its different variations to study mental processes; the chronometric analysis of decision or thought processes in general as performed in cognitive psychology, in particular in evoked-potential studies, goes back to Donders. A fourth key paper setting the stage for studies on temporal mechanisms of perception for more than a century is a dissertation by Karl Vierordt (1868); he demonstrated in experiments on reproduction of temporal intervals that short intervals tend to be overestimated and long intervals are usually underestimated. The experimental paradigm of temporal reproduction brings us to the level of temporal integration or temporal binding.

III. Presemantic Temporal Integration in the 3-second Domain: An Operational Window for Primary Consciousness

As has been outlined above, system states with a duration of approximately 30 msec provide temporal windows, within which binding spatial operations can be implemented; these operations are thought of as providing primordial events. The discreteness of such events is a necessary but not a sufficient condition for time tags being attached to such constructed events. In order to come to sequences of events, an additional neuronal mechanism that provides time tags has to be assumed. The experiments on order threshold (e.g., Hirsh and Sherrick, 1961) allow only to infer a mechanism that codes the before–after relationship of two events. Such binary order information may, however, be used as input by a further mechanism to set up longer sequences. Such a neuronal mechanism to construct sequences can presently only be speculated about, although the left frontal cortex is believed to be involved in these processes because patients with lesions in these areas often have problems in time tagging.

Time tags of sucessive events could theoretically be used for temporal binding, i.e., to construct the coherence of temporal patterns, because time tags are markers of events. Experimental observations, however, suggest that temporal binding, at least in the domain up to a few seconds, is presemantic and, thus, independent from concrete events. Converging evidence on the basis of a great number of different experimental paradigms leads one to conclude that the limit of temporal binding is approximately 3 seconds. Because of the independence of what is processed, the term "binding" may be misleading because it implies the idea that binding is secondary to event perception; thus, the term "presemantic temporal integration" (PTI) will be preferred.

What is the experimental support for PTI in the temporal domain of 3 seconds? Studies using the paradigm of reproduction of intervals (e.g., Vierordt, 1868) provide results that can be interpreted with respect to PTI (Pöppel, 1978). If a subject has the task to reproduce the duration of intervals, one observes that such intervals up to approximately 3 seconds are reproduced accurately (often with a tendency of a slight overestimation), and longer intervals are reproduced shorter than the standard (Pöppel, 1971; Elbert et al., 1991). The transition from over- to underestimation (the "indifference interval") can be looked at as a border for a qualitative change of temporal processing. Up to the indifference interval, information can be represented accurately; beyond this interval a temporal leakage leads to a subjective compression of an interval in retrospect. Up to approximately 3 seconds, information can apparently be treated as a unit; beyond this interval a qualitatetively different mechanism has to deal with sucessive information. If the temporal capacity of integration is limited there may be a natural tendency that successive information disintegrates into parts if longer lasting stimulus sequences have to be processed. Direct evidence for this hypothesis comes from observations on ambiguous figures (Pöppel, 1988; Radilova et al., 1990) or binocular rivalry (unpublished observations, Gómez et al., 1994).

One such example is the Necker cube, which can be perceived in two different perspectives. If a viewer can see the two perspectives, it is impossible while looking at the cube to see only one perspective continuously. Automatically after some time there is an automatic reversal to the other perspective. The sponanteous reversal rate of the Necker cube and other ambiguous figures shows values close to 3 seconds for each discrete percept. The condition for this reversal rate is, however, that the viewer mentally has represented a cube. Similar experiments on auditory ambiguous "figures" have given similar results for the reversal rate (Radilova et al., 1990). As stimulus sequences, computer-generated sounds such as "CU" and "BA" or "SO" and "MA" have been used; the perceived verbal or quasi-verbal syllable sequences were either CUBA or BACU or SOMA and MASO. Automatically after approximately 3 seconds the listener switches to the alternative interpretation. It is as if the brain, after an exhaust period of 3 seconds, asks the question to the sensory system what might be new in the environment. In case of ambiguous figures or sound sequences, the alternative interpretation will then be self-generated.

An automatic reversal in visual perception has also been described for binocular rivalry (Gómez et al., 1994). Without conscious influence or effort, either one or the other eye takes control over perception with a period of approximately 3 seconds if the stimuli contradict each other. Binocular rivalry with a much longer period for either monocular percept has been described in a brain-damaged patient who suffered a lesion in the occipital lobe (Pöppel et al., 1978). This observation supports the notion that lesions in the nervous system result in a slowing down of processing.

The capacity to hold stimuli for only up to approximately 3 seconds is demonstrated also in experiments on short-term memory (Peterson and Peterson, 1959). If rehearsal is not allowed after presentation of new information, the accuracy of what has been represented is lost dramatically after a 3-second interval.

The 3-second window of neuronal processing as demonstrated in experiments on temporal integration, visual and auditory reversal timing, or short-term memory can also be demonstrated in motor timing. If a regular stimulus sequence has to be synchronized with motor taps, one observes usually an anticipation of stimulus occurrence by some tens of milliseconds. But this is observed only if the interstimulus interval is shorter than the 3-second window. Beyond 3 seconds stimuli can no longer be accurately anticipated, i.e., the initiation of a motor program can be extended only up to 3 seconds (Mates et al., 1994).

Further support for a temporal window of 3 seconds dominating motor programming comes from studies on the duration of intentional acts (Schleidt et al., 1987). As has been demonstrated in these studies, homolog movement patterns in different cultures, also in those that still belong to the stone age (for instance, Yanomami Indians or Kalahari bushmen), have a duration of approximately 3 seconds. Thus, it can be concluded using the experimental and observational evidence that not only perception and cognition but also movement control, in particular with respect to intentional movements, share similar temporal mechanisms.

Electrophysiological experiments have also given evidence for underlying temporal processes of a 3-second window of neuronal integration. Slow cortical potentials as measured in experiments on temporal reproduction show qualitatively different results in brain activity for tasks up to approximately 3 seconds and beyond (Elbert *et al.*, 1991). In experiments on mismatch negativity using the magnetic mismatch field (Sams *et al.*, 1993), it was shown that the biggest mismatch field is obtained at interstimulus intervals of 3 seconds. These experiments are a first hint for neurophysiological mechanisms underlying a 3-second window of processing. It should be stated that from the observational level such a temporal limit has always been stressed by Fraisse (e.g., 1984). It is necessary that the neuronal mechanisms setting up temporal windows will be integrated into theoretical models (e.g., Pöppel and Schill, 1994), which are, however, at present still at a qualitative level.

IV. Philosophic and Aesthetic Implications

The temporal mechanisms underlying perceptual, motor, and cognitive processes have some interesting philosophical and also aesthetic implications. In philosophical discourse one question discussed since antiquity pertains to what the "present" could be. If one argues on an abstract level, the present can be considered as a timeless border between past and future. Such a view is typical for classical psychophysics, which has been dominated since the middle of last century by an orientation toward Newtonian physics. One basic idea in psychophysics is that mental processes are a direct reflection of physical processes; by knowing the transformation rules (the "psychophysical laws") that have to be applied to physical properties of stimuli, one can reconstruct the mind. With respect to time this leads to the situation that phenomenally there is no present directly given—it has to be reconstructed secondarily. In spite of efforts by James (1890) and others to introduce the "specious present," it has taken almost another century to free oneself from the burden of classical psychophysics.

This new reasoning has actually an old philosophical root. If one goes back to the philosopher Aurelius Augustinus and his work "Confessions" (book 11, 397/398), one can argue that the present is a temporal interval with finite duration. I am suggesting that the temporal integration interval that automatically binds processed information together to a perceptual or conceptual unit of approximately 3 seconds can be interpreted as the basis of what we call in the Augustinian tradition "present." Because of the historical importance of this alternative thought, which is in a way orthogonal to ideas of classical physics, the original quotation of Augustinus is given:

> Nec futura "sunt" nec praeterita, nec proprie dicitur: tempora "sunt" tria, praeteritum, praesens et futurun, sed fortasse proprie diceretur. tempora "sunt" tria, praesens de praeteritis (*memoria*), praesens de praesentibus (*contuitus*), praesens de futuris (*expectatio*). [Neither the future nor the past "is," and one actually cannot say that there "are" three times, past, present, and future, but one should correctly say: there "are" three times, the present of the past (memory), the present of the present (conscious perception), the present of the future (expectation).]

The idea that there is only present—or primary consciousness—and that we reconstruct past and future from a temporal window of presence can also be found in poetry. T.S. Eliot says it in these words:

> Time past and time future
> what might have been and what has been
> points to one end which is always present.

These connotations are meant to clarify one point: If one uses the word "present," one easily runs into equivocations. On one level of discourse that appears to be related to classical physics, the present is an extensionless point in time separating the facticity of past from the potentiality of future. On another level of discourse in which phenomenal reality is taken as an axiomatic basis, the present has a duration, and because of this the time of present can be measured. In neuroscience we want to understand the neuronal processes that determine phenomenal reality. Thus, it is obviously preferable to use the "present" in the Augustinian sense and by doing so stay away from a traditional equivocation (or semantic muddle).

Another domain that is related to temporal binding of approximately 3 seconds is the arts, namely, poetry and music. Temporal segmentation of the apparently continuous flow of information is also observed in language. Spontaneous speech is characterized by a rhythmical organization, i.e., temporal segments with a duration of 2 to 3 seconds follow each other (Vollrath *et al.*, 1992), and this dynamic structuring of speech seems to be independent of age (Kowal *et al.*, 1975). The phenomenon of temporal segmentation of spontaneous speech is also reflected in poetry. Analyses of many poems in several languages have shown that the duration of a single verse nicely blends into a temporal unit of approximately 3 seconds (Turner and Pöppel, 1983). As an example, some lines of a famous sonnet from Shakespeare are given; each line lasts approximately 3 seconds:

> Shall I compare thee to a summer's day?
> Thou art more lovely and more temperate,
> Rough winds do shake the darling buds of May,
> And summer's lease hath all too short a date.

If a verse is longer, as in the hexameter, automatically a caesura is introduced within a line. Thus, independent of historic tradition, cultural background, or the linguistic rules of a language, the duration of a verse seems to be a universal phenomenon. This suggests the hypothesis that poets of all ages and all languages automatically embed their poetic phrases within temporal units provided by brain mechanisms. Because of the close link to short-term memory (e.g., Peterson and Peterson, 1959), the chosen time window for verses in poetry presumably also allows optimal storage.

The observation that spoken verses in different languages tend to last approximately 3 seconds can actually be used as a further support for the existence of automatic temporal integration. Only if such a neuronal mechanism is very powerful can it survive constraints derived from the special syntax of a language or traditional rules that have been developed possibly independently in the different cultures.

Another aesthetic domain in which temporal segmentation becomes apparent is music (Pöppel, 1989b). Musical themes often have a temporal limit of about 3 seconds. The famous theme from Beethoven's *Fifth Symphony* or the Dutchman's theme from Wagner's *The Flying Dutchman* can serve as representative examples. At least in the tradition of occidental music, there seems to be a universal phenomenon at work here that cannot be ignored by the composer or the performing musician. If one hears music in which the temporal structure, as it is referred to here, is abandoned, then the aesthetic effect is also altered. Apparently, mechanisms of the human brain define temporal constraints that are also applied for aesthetic evaluation. If the biologically predetermined temporal framework is violated or ignored, the aesthetic frame of reference within which the music generally is judged is also changed.

Poetic verses or musical motives, thus, tend to be temporally located within integration units of approximately 3 seconds duration. Subjective reality is also characterized, however, by the sense of continuity. How does the brain produce subjective continuity in time if the representation at the level of primary consciousness is discontinuous? It is suggested that temporal continuity is provided by semantic binding of what is represented in successive 3-second temporal windows; the contents of successive segments are linked with each other. Neuronally this linking operation may be provided by the rather long time constants in the domain of stimulus evaluation (Pöppel and Schwender, 1993). The observation that continuity can break down, as in the case of some schizophrenic states or after brain injury (E. Pöppel, N. V. Steinbüchel, and M. Kashabi, unpublished observations), implies that under normal circumstances a specific neuronal program is responsible for the effectiveness of semantic binding.

I want to finish with a poem by the German poet Heinrich Heine, which in a way is also a comment on this paper. Technically, however, the poem shall demonstrate two aspects that have been discussed here: every line should last approximately 3 seconds, and there should be a semantic connection between successive lines for the poem to make sense.

Zu fragmentarisch ist Welt und Leben,
ich will mich zum deutschen Professor begeben,
der weiss das Leben zusammenzusetzen,
und er macht ein verständlich System daraus,
mit seinen Nachtmützen und Schlafrockfetzen
stopft er die Lücken des Weltenbaus.

References

Aurelius Augustinus: "Confessiones," Book 11, 397/398.
Basar, E., Gönder, A., and Ungan, P. (1976). Important relation between EEG and brain evoked potentials. II. A systems analysis of electrical signals from the human brain. *Biol. Cybernet.* **25,** 41–48.
Donders, F. C. (1868). On the speed of mental processes. *Acta Psychol.* **30,** 412–431 (1969).
Edelman, G. M. (1989). "The Remembered Present: A Biological Theory of Consciousness." Basic Books, New York.
Efron, R. (1967). The duration of the present. *Ann. N. Y. Acad. Sci.* **138,** 713–729.
Elbert, T., Ulrich, R., Rockstroh, B., and Lutzenberger, W. (1991). The processing of temporal intervals reflected by CNV-like brain potentials. *Psychophysiology* **28,** 648–655.
Erikson, C. W., and Collins, J. F. (1968). Sensory traces versus the psychological moment in the temporal organization of form. *J. Exp. Psychol.* **77,** 376–382.
Fraisse, P. (1984). Perception and estimation of time. *Annu. Rev. Psychol.* **35,** 1–36.
Fraser, J. T., Haber, F. C.,, and Müller, G. H., eds. (1972). "The Study of Time," pp. 219–241. Springer-Verlag, Heidelberg.
Frost, D., and Pöppel, E. (1976). Different programming modes of human saccadic eye

movements as a function of stimulus eccentricity: Indications of a functional subdivision of the visual field. *Biol. Cybernet.* **23**, 39–48.

Fuchs, A. F. (1967). Saccadic and smooth pursuit eye movements in the monkey. *J. Physiol. (London)* **191**, 609–631.

Galambos, R., Makeig, S., and Talmachoff, P. J. (1981). A 40-Hz auditory potential recorded from the human scalp. *Proc. Natl. Acad. Sci. U.S.A.* **78**, 2643–2647.

Gardner, E. P., and Costanzo, R. M. (1980). Temporal integration of multiple-point stimuli in primary somatosensory cortical receptive fields in alert monkeys. *J. Neurophysiol.* **43**, 444–468.

Gómez, C., Argandona, E. D., Solier, R. G., Angulo, J. C., and Vazquez, M. (1994). Timing and competition in networks representing ambiguous figures. *Brain Cognition* (Unpublished manuscript).

Gray, C., König, P., Engel, A. K., and Singer, W. (1989). Oscillatory responses in cat visual cortex exhibit inter-columnar synchronization which reflects global stimulus properties. *Nature (London)* **338**, 334–337.

Harter, R., and White, C. T. (1968). Periodicity within reaction time distributions and electromyograms. *Q. J. Exp. Psychol.* **20**, 157–166.

Hirsh, I. J., and Sherrick, C. E., Jr. (1961). Perceived order in different sense modalities. *Q. J. Exp. Psychol.* **62**, 423–432.

Ilmberger, J. (1986). Auditory excitability cycles in choice reaction time and order threshold. *Naturwissenschaften* **73**, 743–744.

James, W. (1890). "The Principles of Psychology." Holt, New York.

Jokeit, H. (1990). Analysis of periodicities in human reaction times. *Naturwissenschaften* **77**, 289–291.

Kowal, S., O'Connell, D. C., and Sabin, E. J. (1975). Development of temporal patterning and vocal hesitations in spontaneous narratives. *J. Psycholinguistic Res.* **4**, 195–207.

Latour, P. L. (1967). Evidence of internal clocks in the human operator. *Acta Psychol.* **27**, 341–348.

Mach, E. (1865). Untersuchungen über den Zeitsinn des Ohres. *Sitzungsber. Mathe.-Natur-wiss. Kl. Kaiserl. Akad. Wiss.*, Abt. 2 **51**, (1–5), 133–150.

Madler, C., and Pöppel, E. (1987). Auditory evoked potentials indicate the loss of neuronal oscillations during general anaesthesia. *Naturwissenschaften* **74**, 42–43.

Mâkelä, J. P., and Hari, R. (1987). Evidence for cortical origin of the 40-Hz auditory evoked response in man. *Electroencephalogr. Clin. Neurophysiol.* **66**, 539–546.

Mates, J., Müller, U., Radil, T., and Pöppel, E. (1994). Temporal integration in sensorimotor synchronization. *J. Cognit. Neurosc.* (in press).

Murthy, V. N., and Fetz, E. E. (1992). Coherent 23- to 35-Hz oscillations in the sensorimotor cortex of awake behaving monkeys. *Proc. Natl. Acad. Sci. U.S.A.* **89**, 5670–5674.

Pantev, C., Makeig, S., Hoke, M., Galambos, R., Hampson, S., and Gallen, C. (1991). Human auditory evoked gamma-band magnetic fields. *Proc. Natl. Acad. Sci. U.S.A.* **88**, 8996–9000.

Peterson, L. B., and Peterson, M. J. (1959). Short-term retention of individual items. *J. Exp. Psychol.* **58**, 193–198.

Podvigin, N. F. (1972). On the mechanism of operative memory in the visual system. *Sechenov Physiol. J. USSR* **58**, 592–594.

Podvigin, N. F., Jokeit, H., Pöppel, E., Chizh, A. N., and Kiselyeva, N. B. (1992). Stimulus-dependent oscillatory activity in the lateral geniculate body of the cat. *Naturwissenschaften* **79**, 428–431.

Pöppel, E. (1968). Oszillatorische Komponenten in Reaktionszeiten. *Naturwissenschaften* **55**, 449–450.

Pöppel, E. (1970). Excitability cycles in central intermittency. *Psychol. Forsch.* **34**, 1–9.

Pöppel, E. (1971). Oscillations as possible basis for time perception. *Stud. Gen.* **24**, 85–107. (reprinted in Fraser *et al.*, 1972).

Pöppel, E. (1978). Time perception. *In* "Handbook of Sensory Physiology" (R. Held, H. W. Leibowitz, and H.-L. Teuber, eds.), pp. 713–729. Springer-Verlag, Heidelberg.

Pöppel, E. (1988). "Mindworks: Time and Conscious Experience." Harcourt Brace Jovanovich, Boston.

Pöppel, E. (1989a). Taxonomy of the subjective: An evolutionary perspective. *In* "Neuropsychology of Visual Perception" (J. W. Brown, ed.), pp. 219–232. Erlbaum, Hillsdale, NJ.

Pöppel, E. (1989b). The measurement of music and the cerebral clock: A new theory. *Leonardo* **22**, 83–89.

Pöppel, E., and Logothetis, N. (1986). Neuronal oscillations in the brain. Discontinuous initiations of pursuit eye movements indicate a 30-Hz temporal framework for visual information processing. *Naturwissenschaften* **73**, 267–268.

Pöppel, E., and Schill, K. (1994). Time perception. *In* "The Handbook of Brain Theory and Neural Networks" (M. A. Arbib, ed.). Bradford Books, MIT Press, Cambridge, MA (in press).

Pöppel, E., and Schwender, D. (1993). Temporal mechanisms of consciousness. *Int. Anesthesiol. Clin.* **31**, 27–38.

Pöppel, E., and Steinbach, T. (1986). Selective vulnerability of the two cerebral hemispheres under alcohol. *Naturwissenschaften* **73**, 327–328.

Pöppel, E., von Cramon, D., and Backmund, H. (1975). Eccentricity-specific dissociation of visual functions in patients with lesions of the central visual pathways. *Nature (London)* **256**, 489–490.

Pöppel, E., Brinkmann, R., von Cramon, D., and Singer, W. (1978). Association and dissociation of visual functions in a case of bilateral occipital lobe infarction. *Arch. Psychiatry Neurol. Sci.* **225**, 1–21.

Pöppel, E., Schill, K., and von Steinbüchel, N. (1990a). Sensory integration within temporally neutral system states: A hypothesis. *Naturwissenschaften* **77**, 89–91.

Pöppel, E., Schill, K., and von Steinbüchel, N. (1990b). Multistable states in intrahemispheric learning of a sensorimotor task. *NeuroReport* **1**, 69–72.

Pöppel, E., Chen, L., Glünder, H., Mitzdorf, U., Ruhnau, E., Schill, K., and von Steinbüchel, N. (1991). Temporal and spatial constraints for mental modelling. *In* "Frontiers in Knowledge-Based Computing" (V. P. Bhatkar and K. M. Rege, eds.), pp. 57–68. Narosa Publ. House, New Delhi.

Radilova, J., Pöppel, E., and Ilmberger, J. (1990). Auditory reversal timing. *Act. Nerv. Super.* **32**, 137–138.

Ribary, U., Ioannides, A. A., Singh, K. D., Hasson, R., Bolton, J. R. P., Lado, F., Mogilner, A., and Llinas, R. (1991). Magnetic field tomography of coherent thalamocortical 40-Hz oscillations in humans. *Proc. Natl. Acad. Sci. U.S.A.* **88**, 11037–11041.

Ruhnau, E., and Haase, V. G. (1993). Parallel distributed processing and integration by oscillations. *Behav. Brain Sci.* **16**, 587–588.

Sams, M., Hari, R., Rif, J., and Knuutila, J. (1993). The human auditory sensory memory trace persists about 10 sec.: Neuromagnetic evidence. *J. Cognit. Neurosc.* **5**, 363–370.

Schill, K., and Zetzsche, C. (1994). A model of visual spatio-temporal memory. The icon revisited. *Psychol. Res.* (in press).

Schleidt, M., Eibl-Eibesfeldt, I., and Pöppel, E. (1987). A universal constant in temporal segmentation of human short-term behavior. *Naturwissenschaften* **74**, 289–290.

Schwender, D., Klasing, S., Madler, C., Pöppel, E., and Peter, K. (1993). Midlatency auditory evoked potentials and cognitive function during general anesthesia. *Int. Anesthesiol. Clin.* **31**(4), 89–106.

Sporns, O., Gally, J. A., Reeke, G. N., Jr., and Edelman, G. M. (1989). Reentrant signaling among simulated neuronal groups leads to coherency in their oscillatory activity. *Proc. Natl. Acad. Sci. U.S.A.* **86**, 7265–7269.

Sternberg, S. (1966). High-speed scanning in human memory. *Science* **153**, 652–654.

Tononi, G., Sporns, O., and Edelman, G. M. (1992a). Reentry and the problem of integrating multiple cortical areas: Simulation of dynamic integration in the visual system. *Cereb. Cortex* **2**, 310–335.

Tononi, G., Sporns, O., and Edelman, G. M. (1992b). The problem of neural integration: Induced rhythms and short-term correlations. *In* "Induced Rhythms in the Brain" (E. Basar and T. H. Bullock, eds.), pp. 367–395. Birkhäuser, Boston.

Turner, F., and Pöppel, E. (1983). The neural lyre. Poetic meter, the brain and time. *Poetry*, August, pp. 277–309.

Vierordt, K. (1868). "Der Zeitsinn nach Versuchen." Laupp, Tübingen.

Vollrath, M., Kazenwadel, J., and Krüger, H.-P. (1992). A universal constant in temporal segmentation of human speech. *Naturwissenschaften* **79**, 479–490.

von Baer, K. E. (1864). Welche Auffassung der lebenden Natur ist die richtige? Und wie ist diese Aufassung auf die Entomologie anzuwenden? St. Petersburg 1860. In (H. Schmitzdorff, ed.), pp. 237–284. Verlag der Kaiserl. Hofbuchhandl., St. Petersburg.

von Steinbüchel, N., and Pöppel, E. (1991). Temporal order threshold and language perception. *In* "Frontiers in Knowledge-Based Computing" (V. P. Bhatkar and K. M. Rege, eds.), pp. 81–90. Narosa Publ. House, New Delhi.

von Steinbüchel, N., and Pöppel, E. (1993). Domains of rehabilitation: A theoretical perspective. *Behav. Brain Res.* **56**, 1–10.

Wever, R. (1965). Pendulum vs. relaxation oscillation. *In* "Circadian Clocks" (J. Aschoff, ed.), pp. 74–83. North-Holland Publ., Amsterdam.

Wynn, V. T. (1977). Simple reaction time—Evidence for two auditory pathways to the brain. *J. Audit. Res.* **17**, 175–181.

Zeki, S. M. (1978). Functional specialisation in the visual cortex of the rhesus monkey. *Nature (London)* **274**, 423–428.

SECTION III
DISCUSSION

The problem of integration discussed in this section emerged in parallel with the discovery of functional segregation in the brain, that is, with the discovery of localization of function. At first, functional segregation was demonstrated in very broad terms; for example, the back of the brain was associated with sensation and the front with motion or thought. Subsequently it became clear that different modalities were represented in different regions of the cerebral cortex and of subcortical structures. Both "horizontal" and "vertical" subdivisions were proposed: different submodalities were localized to specific cortical areas, and different levels of processing were attributed to primary, secondary, and tertiary areas. More recently, neurophysiology has demonstrated finer and finer parcellations within each cortical area; for example, neighboring neuronal groups tend to be specialized for different stimulus attributes or different values of the same attribute. In terms of development and activity-dependent processes, it appears that localization of function results from the tendency of axons carrying correlated signals to group together and segregate from other axons (Singer's *dictum:* what fires together, wires together). This process of grouping and segregation seems to be a key organizational principle that allows temporal correlations in the input to be converted into spatial proximity of synaptic terminals, resulting in the formation of axonal patches.

Though the presence of specialized neuronal groups is advantageous from a functional point of view, it is evident that the activity of these specialized groups and areas has to be integrated to yield a coherent perceptual scene. This is quite obvious in terms of phenomenology: despite the diversity of elements and relations, each perceptual scene has an undeniable unity and coherence. Functionally, a unified perceptual scene is essential to drive adaptive behavior, which is necessarily integrated. In addition, a glance at the anatomical organization of the brain, especially of the cerebral cortex, reveals that reciprocal and parallel connectivity is the rule rather than the exception, indicating that ongoing mutual interactions among neuronal groups and areas are not just possible but unavoidable.

The phenomenological unity of perceptual scenes, the behavioral requirement for coherent actions, and the structural substrate for widespread interactions among cortical regions explain why, coexisting with views emphasizing the specificity and modularity of brain organization, there have always been antilocalizationist, or holistic, views that have stressed global functions and Gestalt phenomena. For instance, Gestalt psychologists maintained that the whole (or Gestalt) comes before the parts; the parts have no meaningful independent existence but exist only through their mutual relationships and their relationship to the whole. The general idea behind these positions is that the activity of individual elements is essentially meaningless without the context within which they are arranged, or the ensemble of relationships in which they are embedded. Much of the research program of Gestalt psychologists consisted in the demonstration of regularities or "laws" according to which integrated wholes play an organizing role in perception. These Gestalt laws determine how elements are unified to form objects, and how objects are related to each other to form scenes. The demise of the Gestalt school as a main force in psychology was partly due to the inability of its proponents to point to a consistent neuroanatomical or neurophysiological foundation for the rules of integration; the Gestalt notion of isomorphic fields was soon to be dismissed.

The antithetical but intuitively appealing idea of an integration center in the brain can also be ruled out. There are many conceptual problems with this idea, including the so-called combinatorial explosion, the difficulty in accounting for both generalization and categorization, and the implausibility of the required developmental schemes. Empirically, a universal integration center has never been found. Clearly, any proposal as to how the problem of integration is solved in the brain must not only be logically consistent, but also consistent with anatomical, physiological, and psychological facts.

It is therefore highly significant that a solution to the integration or binding problem framed in selectionist terms seems to fit all of these requirements. The demonstration that the integration of functionally segregated areas can be achieved in time and space through the process of reentry, as elaborated in the chapter by Tononi, is directly based on our knowledge of the anatomical and physiological characteristics of the visual system. It is also significant that Gestalt phenomena and various categories of perceptual illusions find natural explanations in this context. The computer simulations used to illustrate these ideas go hand in hand with the experimental evidence summarized by Singer. His results reveal the local cooperativity within a neuronal group and the emergence of specific intra- and interareal correlations mediated by reciprocal cortico-cortical connections. Although computer models have been used, as we have seen, to make a strong argument for the effectiveness on behavior of short-term correlations brought about by reentry, it will be crucial to obtain a direct experimental demonstration of their behavioral relevance. In this respect, the data obtained from strabismic cats are an extremely promising beginning.

The three chapters in this section raise a number of other points that are relevant to an understanding of integration in the brain. First, there is the issue of clarifying what is meant by *integration*, a term that has been rather loosely defined and used in the neuroscientific literature. At the end of the chapter by Tononi, a suggestion is made as to how to define and measure integration. The general idea is that a measure of integration corresponds to the deviation from statistical independence among the elements of a system. The system, in this case, is the brain, and the elements could be, for example, specialized groups of neurons. By making certain assumptions, such deviation from independence, which, in essence, is a measure of the simultaneous degree of correlation among multiple variables, can be assessed quantitatively. A distinction between functional segregation and integration can then be made in terms of the size of the subsets of neuronal groups that are being considered. Functional segregation corresponds to substantial independence when considering small subsets of neuronal groups within the brain, because such groups will, on average, perform different, specialized tasks. On the other hand, taken as a whole, or in large subsets, the brain should show a significant deviation from independence or integration, because many neuronal groups and areas engage in cooperative activities that lead to a coherent, adaptive output. Finally, within this theoretical framework, one can define a measure, *neural complexity*, that is high if a neural system displays simultaneously functional segregation and global integration. Conversely, systems that are composed of either completely independent or completely dependent elements have low complexity. This perspective allows a theoretical resolution or synthesis of the "dialectic" apposition of local and global, or of localizationism and holism. Consistent with this notion, both computer simulations and some preliminary results from functional neuroimaging seem to indicate that the peculiar organization of the cerebral cortex in terms of specialized elements linked by reentrant connectivity is associated with high complexity.

This theoretical framework also helps us to explain the fact that, in the brain, integration takes place at many *different levels of organization*, as discussed in the chapters by Tononi and Pöppel. A fundamental level is the functional integration of single cells into neuronal groups. Another level is the "linking" of the responses of neuronal groups belonging to the same (sensory) feature domain within a single cortical area. Examples of integration at this early level are phenomena of perceptual grouping within a single submodality. Still another level is the "binding" of the responses of neuronal groups from different feature domains involving different cortical areas. An example is the integration of neuronal responses to a particular contour with those resulting from its direction of movement or to its color. This distinction of multiple levels of integration closely corresponds to levels of anatomical organization (intragroup, intraareal, and interareal). At a higher level, the integration of perceptual and conceptual components is required to categorize objects. Furthermore, several objects can be integrated into a coherent scene, and several modalities, thoughts, memories, and feelings are integrated into a conscious state referring to a single self. Finally, as we have seen, integration has to be achieved over time, so as to connect one instant with the next in the constant stream of consciousness, as recognized by William James. Although the structures and mechanisms responsible for these higher levels of integration remain to be clarified, it is a reasonable assumption that no radically new principles are involved.

A visual scene requires integration in that it derives its full meaning only when all its elements are put in context. At the same time, it is essential to maintain some degree of "differentiation" between the various elements. The realization that neurons can show correlated activity at several time scales suggests a way to solve this problem. Neurons that exhibit an increase in mean firing rate, i.e., a correlation on a time scale of hundreds of milliseconds, can signal the presence of various features in a visual scene that occur within that time frame. On the other hand, as demonstrated by Singer, correlations over shorter time scales, i.e., milliseconds, allow neurons with increased mean firing rate to group and segregate differentially, e.g., to bind selectively the various attributes of different objects simultaneously present in the visual scene. Thus, both the simultaneous presence and the relationships between the elements can be preserved.

Another important point is that integration of functionally segregated areas and neuronal groups can occur both in the presence of various visual stimuli and during spontaneous activity. The spontaneous patterns of correlations among neuronal groups are presumably determined by the specific connectivity among them. Such patterns of cortico-cortical connectivity are determined, in turn, by natural selection and by processes of activity-dependent selection that occur during development and experience, as demonstrated for horizontal connections in primary visual areas. Ultimately, therefore, spontaneous patterns of correlations should reflect some of the regularities present in the signals sampled from the environment. It is tempting to suggest that specific patterns of activity triggered by extrinsic stimuli can rapidly (within tens of milliseconds) select among a repertoire of spontaneous patterns of correlations and result in a quick, integrated response.

There is another sense in which the problem of integration is particularly interesting from a selectionist perspective. From an instructionist perspective, it would be difficult to understand how the brain can coordinate the activity of so many disparate neuronal groups and areas in a coherent way. An elaborate system of tags and addresses would be needed, as computer scientists faced with similar problems in parallel computing know only too well. In addition, such a precise system of tags and cross-references would be very unlikely to arise through known developmental processes. In a selectionist framework, by contrast, the process is reversed. Whenever there are correlations between the activity of neuronal groups, and these correlations match those sampled by interacting with the environment, connections subserving those correlations become selectively enhanced over others. Coherent patterns of activity that fit well with correlations in the input would be strongly favored under value constraint, no matter at how many levels. Given the highly reentrant architecture of the cerebral cortex, patterns of activity resulting from cooperative interactions in multiple areas can influence local synaptic changes at any given site, making them context dependent. Thus, whereas an integrated system is exceedingly difficult to manage from an engineering or instructionist point of view, it is a powerful substrate for selection, because *selection can act at all places and levels simultaneously.*

SECTION IV
MEMORY AND MODELS

The three chapters in this section illuminate the problem of human memory from different perspectives, each contributing to the formulation of a new view of memory solidly based on our present-day knowledge of brain physiology and circuitry.

George Reeke takes issue with "classical" cognitivist formulations of how the mind/brain works. He rejects functionalism on the grounds that it does not solve the "homunculus problem," a problem that arises every time a human programmer or instructor (sometimes cleverly disguised) enters the stage of cognitive theory. Selectionism's concern with biological foundations of cognition, the emphasis on development as well as on adaptation and population aspects of brain function, provides a viable alternative to functionalist or computationalist proposals. Reeke illustrates his points by reviewing a series of automata designed to perform perceptual categorization and motor tasks. He focuses on memory as a system property as opposed to localized storage of information.

In his chapter, Larry Squire observes a possible conceptual connection between effects at the level of developmental neuroanatomy and certain characteristics of long-term memory in humans. More precisely, competition between developing axons can lead to elimination of some and selective strengthening of others, whereas gradual changes in human memory may involve the elimination of some memories together with the selective enhancement of others. At first this appears to be purely an analogy, but there is the intriguing possibility (insufficiently explored so far) that the synaptic and neuronal mechanisms underlying global changes in human memory over time are selectional in nature. Squire reviews the phenomenon of retrograde amnesia and presents evidence that suggests that the memory system of the medial temporal lobe is engaged at an early stage of memory formation but that more permanent memories are established elsewhere, presumably in neocortex. Though coherent cortical activity is sufficient for immediate perception of some forms of short-term memory, later retrieval is made possible by activity in the medial temporal lobe. At even later stages of memory formation and consolidation the role of the medial temporal lobe in maintenance and retrieval diminishes.

Recall of memories can be conscious, as well as implicit or nonconscious; this is the subject of Dan Schacter's contribution. In some cases, human patients with brain damage or normal subjects are unable consciously to recollect previous events or perceptions, whereas there are objective signs that they have nonconscious or implicit access to knowledge of these events or perceptions. This is not due to psychiatric conditions but comprises examples of neuropsychological dissociations between implicit and explicit knowledge. These dissociations range over a wide arena of subjects, tasks, and knowledge domains. Schacter argues that this dissociation is not limited to a few aberrant and pathological cases but represents an aspect of "normal" brain function as well. The explanation of such dissociations may emphasize the resemblance of the phenomenon across various domains; in this case, one can postulate a common mechanism for all such phenomena. Alternatively, there could be separate mechanisms for individual dissociations involving different modalities and brain regions. Whether unified accounts or domain-specific theories are more adequate to describe the data is, according to Schacter, as yet unknown.

SELECTION VERSUS INSTRUCTION: USE OF COMPUTER MODELS TO COMPARE BRAIN THEORIES

George N. Reeke, Jr.

The Rockefeller University
New York, New York 10021

I. Introduction

In this article, the main features of the functionalist theory of mind that underlies most current research in cognitive science and artificial intelligence are reviewed. The strongly reductionist outlook of this theory leads to a class of brain models in which abstract data representations and processing algorithms are emphasized in preference to biological realism. In contrast, selectionist approaches give primacy to the observed properties of real nervous systems. They attempt to explicate brain function in terms of self-contained evolutionary and developmental processes that do not require the intervention of an external observer or teacher to give meaning to patterns of neuronal activity. Such processes provide a possible route to understanding how symbolic representational systems can arise in organisms interacting with an unlabeled world.

The selectionist paradigm is illustrated with two synthetic model organisms, Darwin III and Darwin IV, which interact respectively with a simulated two-dimensional world and with our own everyday world. Analysis of the behavior of these models under different assumptions permits selectionist theories to be refined and compared with alternative, functionalist theories. We conclude that functionalism, though it may provide helpful descriptions of many aspects of signal processing in the mature brain, does not provide a satisfactory account of the processes by which intelligent systems come to exist and to display adaptive behavior in the real world.

The term "functionalism" arises in discussions of the philosophy of mind, wherein many divergent definitions may be found. The common element that will concern us here is the notion that the important thing about mental states is their interactions with one another [see Bechtel (1988) for a more complete definition and a discussion of the varieties of functionalism].[1] Functionalism holds that the mind arises as a functional property of the arrangement of component parts in the nervous system, and does not depend in any fundamental way on the particular material composition or history of those parts. It is a specialized form of materialism, the assumption that all the properties of the mind arise from a particular arrangement of ordinary matter that is accessible to scientific study. Taken at face value, the functionalist assumption is unexceptionable to most scientists, and indeed, it is the accepted basis for most current work in cognitive science and artificial intelligence. Functionalism provides the necessary philosophical underpinning for these fields in the form of the beliefs that the relevant things to study in order to understand intelligent behavior are (1) abstract representations of information ("representations" in this context are generally taken to be synonymous with symbolic "encodings") and (2) the manipulation of such encoded information by procedures that operate on symbolic representations without direct reference to the things represented. In short, this theory holds that the basis of intelligent behavior is computation.

As the term "computation" is ordinarily understood, the encodings and procedures referred to above are assumed to be devised by human programmers. Evidently, the types of intelligent systems we are considering, whether biological or (putatively) artifactual, are distinguished by forms of self-organization in which such programming by external agents is unnecessary.[2] The essential question for any science of such systems

[1] Functionalist philosophy of mind is related to, but should not be confused with, functionalist psychology, which emphasizes the functional nature of responses to stimuli and is uncommitted with respect to neural mechanisms (a suggestion of these ideas can be found, for example, in Dewey, 1896).

[2] It is an open debate whether such self-organizing systems should properly be called "computational" (Edelman, 1992; Churchland and Sejnowski, 1992). The definition of the term can be bent to exclude the elements of planned representation and procedures, but when this is done, not much is left of computer science but an information-processing metaphor that is of questionable explanatory value when applied to the brain (Reeke, 1994).

is to explain how this self-organization can take place. As we shall show later in this paper, however, many models of brain function that are intended to be taken seriously do not provide such an explanation, but instead postulate organization through training procedures ("supervised learning") that effectively depend on the prior existence of another intelligent system of the kind being studied. Learning then becomes a process of replicating the internal structure of a preexisting teacher, not of developing intelligent capabilities anew in each newborn animal according to the possibilities latent in its genetic heritage. Such models effectively hide the mind in an infinite regress of teachers (an example of the "homunculus problem" described below) and can explain nothing about its origins. Following Edelman (1978), I refer to such systems of explanation as "instructional," because they depend on the explicit or implicit transfer of information from a preexisting instructor to the naive nervous system. This terminology emphasizes what we shall identify as the principal defect in functionalism, and avoids the term "computationism," which has become effectively meaningless in present usage.[3]

A. THE HOMUNCULUS PROBLEM

The brain is unique as an object of scientific study in being the very organ by which that study is carried out. This fact has led some to postulate the impossibility that a brain can ever understand its own mechanisms of operation (e.g., McGinn, 1991), or even to deny the existence of mental states (this is the essence of behaviorism). However, in view of the uncertain epistemological foundations of these beliefs, it seems best to take a more pragmatic stance and proceed with the chase in the hope that scientifically acceptable descriptions of brain function will emerge. Nonetheless, prudence dictates a most careful attention to methodological issues in these studies.

One of the best known, yet most frequent and most pernicious of the traps that bedevil the interpretation of brain models is the "homunculus problem" (Reeke and Edelman, 1988). In its most basic form, the homunculus problem arises when any critical cognitive aspect of the neural processing involved in a particular task is postulated to occur in unspeci-

---

[3] For example, Hopfield (1994) says: "we view a computer as an input–output device, with the input and output signals in the same general medium or format. . . . The computer produces a transformation on the inputs to generate the outputs. Within this view, the brain is a computer." This definition, unfortunately, contributes a metaphorical description, and nothing more, to our understanding of the brain, because almost none of the theoretical results of computer science apply to such general devices. It is for this reason that Hopfield's definition and others like it may be said to be essentially meaningless.

fied "higher centers" or "other areas" that are not included in the model at hand. To the extent that their unspecified functions incorporate part of the neural function to be explained, these "other areas" take on the aspect of "little men," or homunculi, that must in turn be explained to complete the theory. The danger of an infinite regress in this situation is obvious.

The homunculus problem is found in nearly all early theories of the brain. Such theories were usually dualist, and it was difficult to avoid placing a homunculus in the immaterial side of the mind. Perhaps Descartes' connection of the optic nerve to the homunculus (res cogitans) via the pineal gland is the best known example (Descartes, 1664). Today, functionalism continues this tradition, actively encouraging the development of models with hidden homunculi. The reason for this has already been pointed out—the currency of functionalist computations is encoded information, and, as yet, no one has found a way for computational systems to represent what it is their codes actually signify in the world. This is essentially the problem referred to by Searle (1984) as the "intentionality" problem, and by Harnad (1990) as the "symbol-grounding" problem. Under functionalism, this state of affairs is acceptable, because the code *is* the information; the observer who defines the meaning of the symbols is seen as being *outside* the system, and not as an essential part of what must be explained about the mind (Bickhard, 1993). A few authors have sought to solve this problem within the symbol-processing paradigm (Kolers and Smythe, 1984), but for most, the functionalist world view has made it natural and acceptable to put these critical mechanisms aside in a homunculus that need never be explained.

B. Artificial Intelligence

Functionalism has developed in two major streams. In artificial intelligence (AI), symbolic representations are manipulated explicitly. In connectionism, such representations arise implicitly as a result of the interaction of a suitably configured computational system with the world. AI customarily involves models for cognitive processes that are specified and tested in the form of computer programs. Because of the limited power of the first computers, early AI models typically dealt with limited areas of competence, known as "toy worlds." For example, Winograd's celebrated program SHRDLU (Winograd, 1972) was able to carry out natural-language commands relating to the "block world," a space containing only colored geometric shapes. Progress with such models was encouraging, but the techniques were less successful when applied to real-world problems, such as vision and unconstrained natural language [see Mammone (1994) for a summary of recent research in these areas].

Some workers continue to attack these problems by appealing to more powerful computers and more extensive "knowledge bases" of facts and procedures (Guha and Lenat, 1991). Others have noted the need to model the mechanisms by which symbolic descriptions become available to cognitive systems. Most influential has been the approach of Marr (1982), who proposed an essentially bottom-up theory of vision leading from a raw image, via a series of increasingly abstract descriptions (called "sketches"), to a symbolic description. In Marr's approach, vision itself is a "blind" mechanical process, separated from reason, which occurs at a "higher" level according to traditional AI algorithms. This separation is contrary to what is now known of the connectivity of visual cortex, which participates in massive reentrant loops with the "higher" cortical areas where reason is supposed to be found (Van Essen *et al.*, 1992; Zeki and Shipp, 1988). In retrospect, it can be seen that, in his preoccupation to reduce vision to an approachable stand-alone process, Marr introduced a homunculus to receive the output of his visual system and thereby separated the inseparable parts of a unitary cognitive process.

Minsky (1985), in his "Society of Mind" (reviewed in Reeke, 1991), went beyond Marr to propose that all cognitive function, including conscious awareness, could be understood as arising from the interaction of numerous independent processing elements having individually no more capability than simple computers. By treating the entire mind as a single system, Minsky avoided the homunculus problem, but his Society is nonetheless instructional, because it lacks mechanisms for the self-organization of its components and the self-acquisition of meaning for its symbolic codes. The Society of Mind is of particular interest because, in its parallel arrangement of simple processing elements, it closely resembles connectionist systems and thereby illustrates the fundamental unity of the two main branches of functionalist modeling.

C. CONNECTIONISM

"Connectionism" refers to a class of models in which information is stored in the states of connections between computing elements. Connectionism arose from attempts to model perceptual categorization and other decision-making processes in neural systems. The "perceptron" of Rosenblatt (1958) is an early example; the more recent flowering of the paradigm has been described in Rumelhart *et al.* (1986a) and McClelland *et al.* (1986). The basic organization of connectionist systems is familiar and will not be reviewed here. However, it should be noted that there is no unanimity of view as to the significance of the components of connectionist systems. For most authors, the cells are intended to be taken literally as abstractions of real neurons; for others, they express a subsymbolic level of description of information that can support symbolic computation (Smolensky, 1988); for still others, networks of neurons are metaphors for networks of concepts (Anderson, 1983a) (Fig. 1) and no direct affinity with biological neurons is intended. Thus, connectionism is not a single theory, and each connectionist model must be evaluated on its own merits.

Although connectionism has often been lauded as an approach to eliminating the need for the human programmer, which is the greatest weakness in AI systems, it in fact accepts the basic functionalist assumption that what is important is the abstract description of data-processing tasks, rather than any particular physical mechanism for supporting the underlying information-processing system. Accordingly, conformity of connectionist models with neurobiological facts has not generally been considered very important (Churchland and Sejnowski, 1992). Connectionism is also instructionalist because it assumes its network mappings can be formed by an algorithm. The usual mechanism of training is

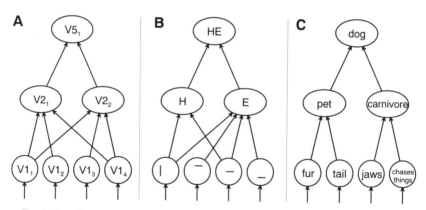

FIG. 1. Levels of representation employed for units in neural or connectionist networks. Each panel represents a small portion of a much larger network model. The similar arrangement of units in the three panels suggests the ease with which concepts borrowed from neurobiology may be employed, sometimes inappropriately, in models based on entirely different conceptual structures. (A) Fully distributed representation based on a small subset of the areas in visual cortex (V1, V2, V5). No specific meaning can be attached to the activity of any particular cell. (B) Subsymbolic. Each cell represents a feature or characteristic that forms part of the physical instantiation of a symbol, here the word HE. (c) Symbolic or conceptual. Each cell represents a symbol, idea, or concept.

supervised learning, which, as we have seen, introduces a homunculus as teacher. However, some recent connectionist studies are beginning to avoid this problem (e.g., Mazzoni *et al.*, 1991; Becker and Hinton, 1992; Bullock *et al.*, 1993).

Many models for intelligent behavior are based on one or the other of the main streams of functionalism. Both claim to give a sufficient description of the properties necessary for a system to exhibit such behavior. Connectionist models, in particular, are frequently described as "neurallike" or "brainlike" by virtue of their dependence on computation in networks of simple processing elements designed in some ways to resemble neurons. However, it should be clearly understood that the properties of the model neurons used in these networks (e.g., a scalar state variable calculated as a function of the weighted sum of the inputs to the neuron) have typically been selected because of their useful computational properties, and not because there is compelling evidence that these properties are the most relevant ones in real nervous systems, or even that they work best in model nervous systems. Many other properties of neurons, such as spiking outputs interspersed with refractory periods, are often ignored, but may play important, if not critical, roles in the function of real brains (Gerstner *et al.*, 1993).

D. SELECTIONISM

As we shall try to show, functionalism is unsatisfactory as a basis for the study of the mind just because it encourages research that focuses on data representations and computations, and discourages research that would examine the actual connectivity of cells in the brain, the actual dynamics of the signals in the brain, and the developmental processes by which the brain becomes organized to produce adaptive behavior. Functionalism neglects these properties as "mere details of the implementation." It is not interested in origins, only in performance. However, in biology, history counts. Biological parts have an evolutionary past that must often be known to understand their present function. The Darwinian outlook that provides the basis for modern biology demands that we seek an alternative to functionalism that will remove the brain from abstract computational space and place it firmly in an evolutionary and organismic framework.

When this is done, the overwhelming anatomical variability seen everywhere in neural systems suggests that selective processes may be at work, creating organization from variation just as they do in evolution at large. The operation of such mechanisms in nonbiological decision-making systems was explored by Selfridge (1959) at about the same time as the first connectionist models, and some of the principles were later presented in a biological context by Young (1979) and by Changeux *et al.* (1973). However, a full selectionist theory of brain function, the theory of neuronal group selection (TNGS), was first put forward in detailed form by Edelman (1978, 1987, 1989). Edelman and his colleagues have also presented large-scale computer models (Edelman and Reeke, 1982; Reeke *et al.* 1990a,b) demonstrating the consistency and performance of the theory.

Selectionism provides a population-based theory of the brain that accounts for perceptual categorization, motor control, and conscious awareness. It addresses the origins of adaptive behavior in terms of the common evolutionary history and unique experiential history of each individual animal. It suggests that the primary mechanism of self-organization in the brain is selection operating on populations of neural circuits formed with a high degree of *a priori* variation during development. Because neurons do not generally divide after they have differentiated, the mechanism of selection is proposed to be changes in the strengths of synapses connecting neural circuits rather than differential reproduction as in natural selection. This mechanism changes the relative contribution of each such circuit, or neuronal group, to behavior, depending on the *ex post facto* evaluation of that behavior by innate mechanisms known as value systems.

A further important component of the TNGS is the role assigned to the extensive parallel connections, known as reentrant connections, that link different brain areas. Reentrant connections provide a mechanism for correlation, and, through selection, common mapping of associated sensory features in different neural pathways. These associations obviate the need for neural signals to have preassigned meanings, and provide the basis for associative memory and learning.

Selection requires no prior labeling of objects or events in the world and no external teacher to provide error feedback signals. Selectionism insists that the mechanisms by which information is created and processed in the nervous system must satisfy constraints derived not only from theories of information and computation, but also constraints derived from biology. Because of this larger corpus of available constraints, selectionist brain theories are better delineated and more readily subject to experimental test than are the more abstract functionalist theories.

The goal of the remainder of this paper will be to clarify the differences between functionalist and selectionist theories of the brain with the aid of models. I shall try to show that the differences are pivotal to further advances in our understanding, and not merely alternative descriptions of the same processes, as some have claimed (Crick, 1989; see reply in Reeke, 1990). The reader should consult the work by Sporns in this volume for a history and more detailed description of selectionist theory.

II. Models as a Tool in Neurobiology

The importance of modeling as a tool for understanding complex phenomena hardly requires comment. Computer models can predict the consequences of a theory, even in situations wherein experimentation may be difficult. Computer models are particularly valuable when analytic solutions are unavailable (perhaps due to nonlinearity) or when a system contains many independent interacting components. All of these conditions are, of course, characteristic of the nervous system, and that is why most neural models today are computer models.

Computer modeling cannot be done without a theory. In fact, construction of a computer model forces the theoretician to specify every relevant detail of a theory, including those that might well escape attention in a narrative description. The very act of successfully running a model provides a strong consistency check on a nascent theory. Therefore, the ability to serve as the foundation for a successful computer model might well be considered one criterion for evaluating theories of the brain.

However, this is not enough. Successful performance has often provided the basis for claims that a particular model is relevant to understanding how the nervous system accomplishes a given task (Churchland and Sejnowski, 1992), even though it is well known and has often been pointed out that mere replication of some behavior does not, in the absence of other evidence, tell us anything about how animals accomplish that behavior (Gyr et al., 1966; Webb, 1991).

In the absence of such evidence, models can still be used to distinguish contrasting theories, because they can generate testable predictions for them. However, this is not often done in practice. Different models are seldom tested under identical conditions, or even on the same behavioral task. Instead, models are judged in isolation, on the basis of performance of some task. Because of this lack of published comparative data on models, I shall in this work merely point out a number of biological constraints that may be applied to the judgment of models and cite a number of models that are incompatible with each of these constraints.

To avoid the homunculus problem, care must be taken in the choice of both theories and tests. It is not enough just to ensure that no explicit action by a programmer is involved in assigning codes and procedures within a model system; one must also ensure that no observer is involved in inferring the connection between signals inside that system and the subjective perceptions the system might experience or the behaviors it might display as a result of those signals. Such an observer becomes part of the loop, a homunculus whose actions must be explained to understand the whole system. The only test paradigm that can eliminate the possibility of this kind of hidden homunculus is one in which the observer has access only to the sensory inputs provided to the system and to the behavioral outputs it produces. Synthetic neural modeling (Reeke *et al.*, 1990a; see also Mulloney and Perkel, 1988, for a related proposal) is one approach to this problem, in which a simulated organism with a nervous system and a phenotype is allowed to behave in a simulated world or in the real world. The behavior of the simulated organism can be recorded in detail by the simulation software and the results evaluated by comparison with data for real animals in comparable experimental situations. This approach will be discussed in more detail after some criteria for evaluating models have been identified.

A. THE APPROPRIATE ELEMENTARY UNIT FOR NEURAL MODELING

Models of behaving systems can be constructed at various levels of description, ranging from the purely psychological to the neural system or local circuit, and even to the individual neurons, synapses, and ion channels (Shepherd, 1990). In all cases, the goal is to understand more complex levels in terms of simpler ones, but the choice of level depends on a judgment as to the lowest level that can reasonably be connected with behavioral events. Quite exact models based on channel conductances and cable properties of neurites have been constructed for simple behaviors, such as swimming in the lamprey (Grillner *et al.*, 1990), but the computational demands of such models make it unlikely that they will soon be extended to embrace higher-level cognitive functions. Thus, a suitable abstract neuron and synapse are needed to provide a basis for neural-level behavioral modeling.

The search for such an abstract neuron began with McCulloch and Pitts (1943), who first showed that neurons could be viewed as logical elements, of the same kind as those being used to fashion the first digital computers (Fig. 2). McCulloch and Pitts were not the first to relate "thinking" to computation, but their concrete approach did much to

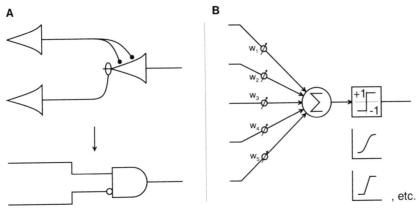

Fig. 2. Abstract neurons used in neural network models. (A) AND-NOT circuit constructed from McCulloch–Pitts neurons and its equivalent in modern electronic notation. The filled circles represent excitatory connections, of which two are required to fire the target unit. The open circle represents an inhibitory connection that vetoes firing of the target unit. (B) Conventional model neuron. This unit responds according to a continuous response function (several examples are shown) when the sum of its weighted inputs exceeds a given threshold. The weights (w_1, ...) can be adjusted according to a specified "learning rule."

popularize functionalism as a valid paradigm for neuropsychology. They were daring in their conclusions: "Thus, in psychology, introspective, behavioristic or physiological, the fundamental relations are those of two-valued logic. . . . Thus, both the formal and final aspects of that activity which we are wont to call *mental* are rigorously deducible from present neurophysiology" (McCulloch and Pitts, 1943).

This bold vision has not been so quickly fulfilled, whether because more work simply needs to be done, as functionalists would have us believe, or because the basic premise is false at its foundations. In either case, however, the McCulloch and Pitts neuron, or a very similar continuous-valued cousin, is at the heart of nearly every neural model that pitches itself above the channel and cable level (Fig. 2). Some of the relative advantages and deficiencies of these various model neurons will be pointed out in the next section.

B. Criteria for Comparing Models

Connectionist and AI models have made valuable contributions to the effort to understand the function of the brain. Some have tackled problems of self-organization, others have introduced information-processing constraints, and still others have helped to clarify issues of representation and learning. Nonetheless, many of these models do not meet basic criteria of biological verisimilitude. Rather than examine any one model in detail, we enumerate a few of these criteria here and in Table I and cite some models that are inconsistent with them:

1. Does the model provide an explanation for acts of perception or behavior? If the input or output of a model is in the form of encoded information or patterns of neural firing that must be interpreted by an observer, rigorous care must be exercised to ensure that the observer does not inadvertently act as a homunculus to complete the model.

2. Does the model function in the presence of background noise and variant stimuli? Can it perform different tasks according to context?

3. Does the model address representative cognitive tasks? Perceptual categorization and motor control are suitable tasks, whereas chess playing and solving college physics problems are not, because the latter tasks and others like them operate in restricted formal realms that disguise real problems of meaning and ambiguity that animals must face in the real world.

4. Does the model provide memory with properties, including error patterns, primacy and recency effects, etc., similar to those of humans or other animals? Exact, replicative memory is characteristic of systems in which information is stored in symbolic form. The actual performance of humans and other animals in memory tasks is suggestive of a much more complicated arrangement with multiple submodalities of memory (Squire, 1986; Tulving and Schacter, 1990; Baddeley, 1992).

5. Is the model compatible with known facts about the nervous system? A number of anatomical, physiological, and developmental facts of neurobiology are collected in Table I. Above all, the model must be consistent with development through genetic inheritance plus individual experience.

Having stated these criteria, we now proceed to a description of some synthetic neural models based on the theory of neuronal group selection. At the end, we consider how well these models meet the suggested criteria and some implications for the comparison of functionalist and selectionist theories.

III. Selectionism and Synthetic Neural Models

The general outline of the synthetic neural modeling discipline has already been presented. Beginning with a theory of organization and

TABLE I
BIOLOGICAL CRITERIA FOR EVALUATING BRAIN MODELS

Constraint or criterion	Characteristics of models excluded by the constraint or criterion	Examples of models that violate the criterion
Anatomical constraints		
Simple discrete units operating in parallel	Von Neumann architecture; continuous models	"Traditional" AI; Wilson and Cowan (1973)
Unidirectional connections	Symmetric connections	Hopfield (1982)
Arborizations varied	Regular arrays of duplicated elements	Kohonen (1984); Silverman et al. (1986)
Number of connections $\ll n^2$	Full connectivity	Rumelhart et al. (1986a); McClelland et al. (1986); Kohonen (1984)
Physiological constraints		
Noisy analog responses	Precise arithmetic	Kohonen (1984)
Millisecond unit speed	Extensive iterations	Boltzmann machine (Hinton et al., 1984; Ackley et al., 1985); conventional robotics
Input and responses continually changing	Relaxation to a steady state	Boltzmann machine; Hopfield (1982)
Homeostatic medium	Simulated annealing	Kirkpatrick et al. (1983); Kienker et al. (1986)
Cells cannot be clamped to desired output; error signals not communicated from output to specific connections	Back propagation	Rumelhart et al. (1986b); Lehky and Sejnowski (1988); Zipser and Andersen (1988); Lockery et al. (1989); Shapiro and Hetherington (1993); etc.
Developmental constraints		
No exact connectivity	Prewired models	Braitenberg (1984); Brooks (1989, 1991)
Adapts to growing body	Fixed algorithms	Conventional robotics
No neuron is indispensable	Concepts represented by single neurons	Anderson (1983b); Rumelhart and McClelland (1986); Hinton and Shallice (1991)
DNA specifies structures, not processes	"Genetic" algorithms	Holland (1975); Holland et al. (1986); Brady (1985)
World is unlabeled	Supervised learning	Most connectionist models

learning in the nervous system (in the examples to be presented here, the TNGS), one constructs a synthetic organism with a suitable nervous system and phenotype (a collection of sensors and effectors), and simulates, in a biologically realistic manner, the behavior and development of that organism as it interacts with the world. Because there is no observer in the behavioral loop, the homunculus problem is avoided.

Very general simulation software is needed for the construction of synthetic neural models. The program must be able to simulate complex networks of neurons of multiple kinds, along with a variety of sensors and effectors, as well as an environment including stimuli, backgrounds, and noise. The program used to generate the models Darwin III and Darwin IV presented here is called CNS, or Cortical Network Simulator (Reeke and Edelman, 1987; Reeke *et al.* 1990a): [The earlier models Darwin I (Edelman, 1981) and Darwin II (Edelman and Reeke, 1982) dealt with aspects of pattern recognition and reentrant perceptual categorization in selective systems, but they were not synthetic organisms.]

A. DARWIN III

Darwin III (Reeke *et al.*, 1990a,b) was designed to test ideas of the TNGS in a simple behaving automaton. The tasks addressed include visual tracking of moving objects, reaching to objects with a multijointed arm, and responding to those objects according to a value determined by their categorization based on reentrant interaction between visual and tactile senses. An outline schematic of the principal systems of Darwin III is shown in Fig. 3. Darwin III is equipped with simulated senses of vision in a single eye, touch at the tip of the movable arm, and kinesthesia relating to its own muscle movements. Simulated motor outputs include those necessary to move the eye across a visual array corresponding to the environment, and to move the arm in the same two-dimensional world. The model nervous system includes the simulated brain regions needed to couple these senses and movements: an oculomotor system for generating tracking eye movements, a reach system including a model cerebellum for study of gestural selection, and a categorization system in which visual and kinesthetic responses are correlated by reentrant mappings. The output of the categorization system is expressed behaviorally by means of coupling to a "reflex" swatting movement of the arm by which "noxious" stimuli are removed from the immediate surround. The details of the construction of Darwin III and its world, including all relevant anatomical and dynamical parameters, are given in Reeke *et al.* (1990a,b). Here, we only summarize some of the experimental results

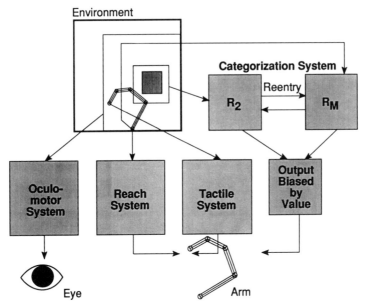

FIG. 3. Principal neuronal and functional subsystems of Darwin III. Environment (heavy square outline at upper left) contains stimulus objects (for example, the shaded square). Visual fields of Darwin III's eye are indicated by the small (foveal vision) and larger (peripheral vision) squares centered on the stimulus object. The four-jointed arm is attached at bottom center. Neuronal subsystems (see Reeke *et al.*, 1990a,b for more details) subserve (left-to-right) saccades and visual tracking (oculomotor system), reaching, tactile exploration of objects, and categorization. Categorization is accomplished by a reentrant pair of areas that receive input, respectively, from vision (R_2) and kinesthesia (R_M). (Reproduced with permission from Reeke *et al.*, 1990a.)

obtained with this model, so that the differences between the functionalist and selectionist approaches may be clearly seen.

In Fig. 4 are shown the results of a typical run in which Darwin III was presented with moving geometric shapes in its visual field. Connections between the visual and oculomotor areas were selectively modified according to a value measure that was derived simply from the overall level of response in the primary visual area. Thus, connections were strengthened that were active just before a movement occurred that happened to increase the illumination on the retina, and connections were weakened in the opposite case. Movement occurred initially by chance according to the level of spontaneous activity in the oculomotor system. Because the moving objects served as sources of light, those movements that brought the eye toward them were selected, and after about 5000 cycles of training, the eye made a saccade to any new object

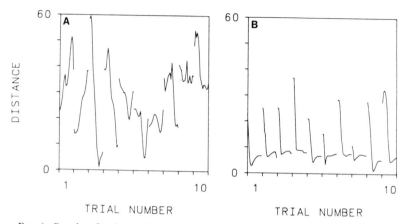

FIG. 4. Results of training the oculomotor system of Darwin III. The ordinates display the distance of the center of the visual field from the center of the stimulus (in pixels) as a function of time, before (A) and after (B) training for 313 trials of 16 cycles each. At the start of each new trial (tick marks on abscissae), the stimulus jumps to a new position and tracking is disrupted. Before training, eye movements do not follow stimulus motion and most of the time there is no decrease of eye–object distance following a jump. After training, a characteristic "comb" pattern emerges. Following each random jump the eye quickly moves toward the new stimulus position, the object is kept foveated (radius of the foveal region is 10 pixels), and, if the object moves, it is tracked. (Reproduced with permission from Reeke *et al.*, 1990a.)

that was introduced, and then tracked the movement of that object as shown in the figure. Both saccades and tracking were obtained with no teacher and no error feedback, beginning only with a suitable anatomy and innate value scheme.[4] As we shall see in the next example, these are the typical requirements for successful performance in selective systems.

Reaching to touch objects with its four-jointed arm is for Darwin III a similar task to visual tracking, even though the geometry of the two tasks is quite different. Relevant sensory input comes from vision, which responds to both target and arm, and from kinesthesia, which responds to joint movements. Responses to these inputs project through a series of connected neural areas, eventually reaching a motor cortex that drives the opposing "muscle" pairs that move the joints of the arm. As a result of spontaneous activity in this motor cortex, the arm initially executes apparently aimless gestures. Neurons of an innate value system respond more actively as the hand is seen to approach the target object, and this activity modulates synaptic change throughout the cascaded areas that

[4] In a real animal, the value system used here would need to be inhibited by excessively strong illumination to prevent damage from tracking the sun.

control the arm. As a result, neuronal groups are selected which generate gestures that are effective in bringing the arm closer to the target, and the arm gradually acquires a greater ability to touch objects presented in the visual field.

Results of a typical training run are shown in Fig. 5. In the left panel, traces of the paths taken by the tip of the arm are shown before training; shown in the right panel are corresponding paths after 300 object presentations. Gestures that lead to close approach of the tip to the object are clearly favored. More detailed analysis (Sporns and Edelman, 1993) shows that training results in the selection of synergies, or correlated movements of joint assemblies, effectively reducing the number of degrees of freedom that must be controlled to obtain purposeful arm movement. This mode of control, which arises quite spontaneously in Darwin III as a result of the chosen neural architecture and value scheme, provides an approach to the problem of coordinating movement in motor systems with redundant degrees of freedom, which was pointed out and extensively discussed by Bernstein (1967).

The ability of Darwin III to categorize geometrical shapes according to their visual (stripy vs. uniformly colored) and tactile (smooth vs. bumpy) features emerges from the reentrant connectivity between visual and tactile sensory channels sketched in Fig. 3. Visual response required successful foveation of the target object by the visual tracking system,

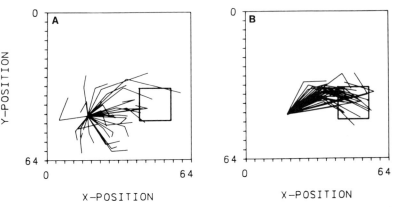

FIG. 5. Traces of paths taken by the distal tip of Darwin III's arm before (A) and after (B) 300 training trials. Before each trial, the arm was placed in a standard position (common origin of traces at left). The target area was the square at right. The results indicate that selection at the behavioral level is occurring: after training (B), movements that reached the object have been selected from a preexisting repertoire of possible movements with only some tuning of the individual trajectories. There is still variability in the exact paths taken. (Reproduced with permission from Reeke and Edelman, 1988b.)

and tactile response required successful contact of the arm with the object by the reaching system. For demonstration purposes, cells responding to a combination of stripy and bumpy features were connected in such a way as to excite cells in the arm's motor cortex that generated a reflexive swatting motion that would usually remove the object from the vicinity of the automaton. Figure 6 shows results obtained with eight presenta-

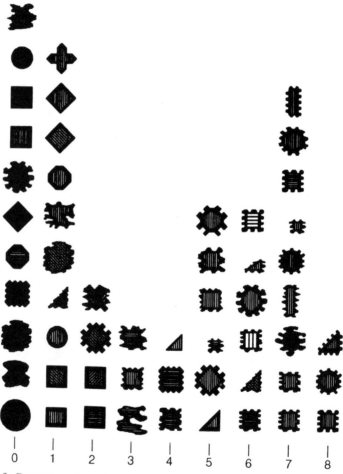

FIG. 6. Frequency of swatting responses to eight presentations of each of 55 stimulus objects, showing groupings generated by Darwin III's categorization system. A negative response was scored if swatting did not occur within 50 time steps after presentation of the stimulus. Objects are arranged in columns according to the frequency with which they met with a swatting (rejection) response (numbers on abscissa). (Reproduced with permission from Reeke et al., 1990a.)

tions of each of 55 different objects displaying various degrees of stripiness and bumpiness. Categorization was not absolute, that is, the response was not always identical for the same object. However, the distribution of responses indicates that the inconstancies were not random—objects were effectively classified along a scale according to the degree of their membership in the class stripy/bumpy. The number of swatting responses to each object was larger for objects that a human observer might classify as "more stripy" or "more bumpy," a form of probabilistic categorization consistent with many studies of human and animal categorization (e.g., Rosch, 1978; Mervis and Rosch, 1981; Smith and Medin, 1981; Herrnstein et al., 1976; Herrnstein, 1984, 1985).

In a final experiment, the fixed connectivity between the categorization area and the swatting reflex cells in the motor cortex was replaced with a set of plastic connections. Changes in synaptic strength in these connections were modulated (see Reeke and Edelman, 1987, for equations) according to activity in cells of a value system that responded to a simulated "taste" that was assigned to the test objects. Taste could be sensed only when the arm made contact with the object, not during saccade or reaching. This arrangement permitted a form of classical conditioning to be demonstrated in Darwin III by experimental manipulation of the tastes assigned to different test objects (Fig. 7). Objects were of two kinds, designated by the open and filled circles in the figure. Visual appearance corresponded to conditioned stimulus, taste to unconditioned stimulus. Initially, the probability of a swatting response was approximately equal for the two classes. When "good taste" was assigned to one class (filled circles) and "bad taste" to the other (open circles), Darwin III became conditioned, after only a few presentations, to generate the swatting response with much larger probability to the "bad tasting" objects. After 16 presentations, the assignment of taste to the two object classes was arbitrarily reversed. Extinction of the original conditioning then occurred, and after a further 16 presentations, the probabilities of swatting responses were effectively reversed. Thus, the synthetic nervous system of Darwin III was able to exhibit classical conditioning, making it possible to relate behavior to neural activity in a simple, but realistic, computer model based on neuronal group selection.

B. DARWIN IV

As we have seen, Darwin III was successful in demonstrating that a synthetic organism could be constructed with a nervous system that develops with experience according to selectionist principles, and that such an

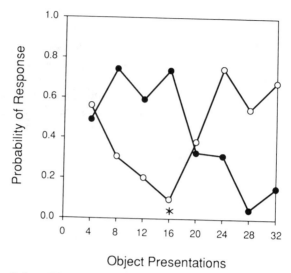

Object Presentations

Fig. 7. Classical conditioning and extinction in Darwin III. Two stimuli, represented, respectively, by open circles and closed circles, were presented in separate sequences of 32 trials each. The probability of a rejection response (swatting) was scored for each set of 4 trials (ordinates). Initially, "good taste" was arbitrarily assigned to the object represented by the open circles, and "bad taste" to the object represented by the closed circles. After 16 trials, the "tastes" were reversed (asterisk).

organism could exhibit interesting motor and categorization behaviors. Nonetheless, it was necessary to recognize that there are significant limitations on the degree of realism that can be achieved with simulations of this kind. For example, objects in the environment of Darwin III were two-dimensional and had no inertia or friction. The visual input had limited spatial resolution and distracting background elements were carefully controlled. In order to demonstrate conclusively that these simplifications had not introduced inadvertent biases that might have been critical to the success of Darwin III, we decided to place a similar synthetic nervous system in an artifact that would interact with the real world.

This artifact is called NOMAD (Neurally Organized Mobile Adaptive Device), and the entire system, including NOMAD and its model nervous system, is Darwin IV (Edelman *et al.*, 1992). NOMAD was designed to be able to move about in an experimental area of limited size under guidance of visual input from a small charge-coupled device (CCD) video camera, and to grasp and carry small objects. The characteristics of the device were chosen to permit, in time, comparison with some of the animal experiments in the psychological literature. Here, we will show only two simple behaviors that can be compared with similar behaviors of Darwin III: tracking a moving light source and segregating small metal objects by color.

The experimental arrangement is shown in Fig. 8. NOMAD is seen at the center of an 8 foot × 12 foot experimental floor. Its components may be seen more clearly in labeled schematic view in Fig. 9. The floor may be covered with either opaque or translucent material, and is supported 2 feet above the normal room floor so that an illuminated tracking target can be deployed underneath. The dark enclosure walls seen here may be replaced, if desired, by reflecting screens on which images of objects may be projected. Objects, such as the colored cubes and the rectangular homing target seen in Fig. 8, can be placed on the floor or walls as desired. Thus, a great deal of flexibility is possible in the experiments that can be carried out. A video camera placed in the ceiling at

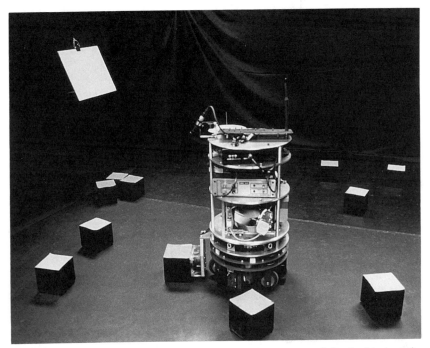

FIG. 8. Photograph of NOMAD in its environment as arranged for the block sorting experiments. The floor may be translucent or opaque (as seen here); the walls may be white projection screens or black curtains (as seen here). Blocks were cubes constructed of sheet steel and covered with either conducting or insulating plastic film. The tops of the blocks were colored blue or red. The rectangular object at upper left is a green cardboard homing target. Components of NOMAD are shown in Fig. 9. (Reproduced with permission from Edelman *et al.*, 1992.)

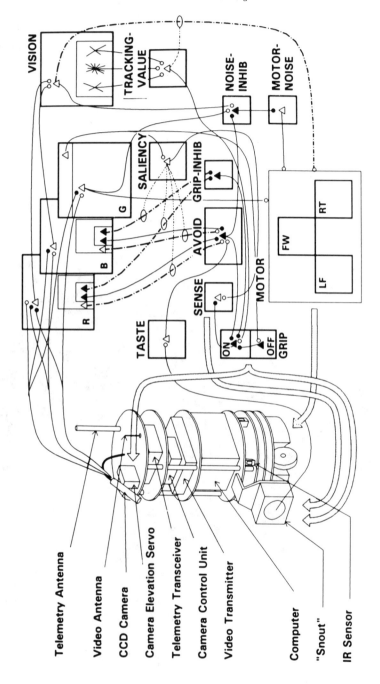

the center of the enclosure records the behavior of NOMAD in these experiments for later analysis.

The mechanical arrangement of NOMAD and the connections of its components to its nervous system are shown in Fig. 9. NOMAD is constructed on a three-wheeled, 15-inch-diameter base (RWI Inc., Dub-

---

FIG. 9. Schematic diagram of Darwin IV showing the major components of NOMAD (left) and the simulated nervous system used for the block sorting task (right). Boxes represent neuronal repertoires. Open and filled triangles denote excitatory and inhibitory cells, respectively. Lines connecting cells or repertoires indicate neuronal pathways (only a few representative cells and connections are shown); heavy arrows indicate efferent motor pathways. Open and filled circles indicate excitatory and inhibitory synapses, respectively. Synaptic pathways subject to value-dependent selective amplification are indicated by dot–dash lines. Dashed lines originating at the value systems involved end in loops around the affected pathways. Beginning at the upper left, the red (R), blue (B), and green (G) channels from the CCD video camera provide input to color-opposition cells in areas R, B, and G, respectively. Areas R and B jointly provide input to the VISION repertoire (top right), which directly excites MOTOR areas FW (for forward motion), LF (for left motion), and RT (for right motion), bottom center (see also Fig. 10). These areas in turn activate NOMAD's wheels to produce locomotion. MOTOR neurons also receive noise input from the MOTOR-NOISE area, which generates spontaneous (exploratory) motions of NOMAD. MOTOR-NOISE is inhibited by activity in NOISE-INHIB, which is excited by VISION, thereby reducing spontaneous locomotion when a potential tracking target is in sight. Connections from VISION to MOTOR are amplified under the selective influence of the TRACKING-VALUE repertoire. TRACKING-VALUE responds most strongly to light falling directly in front of NOMAD, which excites the rectangular area near the bottom of the VISION repertoire, corresponding to the proximal region of the field of view. Cells in the foveal and perifoveal regions of R and B (smaller rectangles at bottoms of R and B repertoires) are also connected via selectively modified synapses (see below) to excite area AVOID and to inhibit area GRIP-INHIB when an object is sighted at a moderate distance. After training, these areas are responsible, respectively, for initiating the avoidance and preventing the gripping reflexes discussed in the text. GRIP-INHIB is normally active, leading to inhibition of GRIP. When GRIP-INHIB is inhibited, GRIP is released from inhibition and can activate the snout magnet and camera elevation effectors, but only when excitatory input is received at the same time from TRACKING-VALUE, causing NOMAD to pick up objects that have been foveated. AVOID acts by inhibiting both NOISE-INHIB and GRIP, causing NOMAD to move randomly without activating its gripping magnet. The green (G) visual repertoire is responsible for recognition of the green home area. When the camera has been elevated and the green target is seen from a distance (when cells at bottom of G are active), MOTOR and NOISE-INHIB are excited, causing NOMAD to move toward the green target. When the target is reached, other cells (top of G) become active, exciting GRIP-OFF cells and providing the SALIENCY signal. SALIENCY immediately excites SENSE neurons, activating the conductivity sensor in the snout. "Bad taste" activates TASTE cells, which excite reflex avoidance via a direct pathway to AVOID. Activation of AVOID by this mechanism while SALIENCY is still active leads to strengthening of connections from R or B (whichever was active when the object was recently viewed) to AVOID; as a consequence, after training, avoidance can be activated directly by visual signals without need for the object to be tasted. (Reproduced with permission from Edelman et al., 1992.)

lin, NH). The upper portion, which carries a series of circular metal plates that provide mounting surfaces for the electronic components, rotates about the center axis, permitting turns on essentially zero radius. A CCD camera mounted on an elevation servo on the topmost plate provides three-color visual input to the nervous system. A magnetic "snout" (bottom, front) enables NOMAD to pick up and carry small ferrometallic objects. The snout carries a sensor that responds to the conductivity of objects picked up by the electromagnet. This provides NOMAD's analog for the sense of taste, which is used in the conditioning experiments to be described.

The remaining equipment on the NOMAD platform comprises a camera control unit, video and digital telemetry, a control computer, and batteries. The control computer translates sensory inputs into simulated neuronal firings for input to the simulated nervous system, and similarly translates motor neuron firings from the nervous system into the necessary signals to control the motors and other effectors on the base. This computer plays no role in determining the behavior of the device, except that it is able to override locomotion commands from the neural simulation when the IR sensors indicate that a collision is imminent.

The nervous system of Darwin IV is simulated using CNS on an NCUBE parallel supercomputer connected to NOMAD via either cable or telemetry. The overall organization of this simulation is described in the legend to Fig. 9. Note particularly the two value systems: "Tracking value" is derived from visual input immediately in front of NOMAD and modulates selection events in the connections between visual and motion areas, enabling Darwin IV to acquire the ability to track moving objects. "Saliency" is derived from the same signals that activate the conductivity sensor in the snout, and modulates changes in connection strength between visual and reflex motion centers, providing the necessary anatomical prerequisites for classical conditioning to occur. Behavior as a whole is thus a combination of ongoing, sensory-guided movements, such as tracking illuminated targets, and reflex actions, such as carrying an object to a base position. Selection changes the relative probabilities of these behaviors in accord with criteria of adaptive value expressed physically in the activity of units in the two value systems.

1. Tracking Task

Results of two typical training sessions for the tracking task are shown in Fig. 10. A light source is placed under the translucent floor and programmed to move in a random pattern. In NOMAD's nervous system, connections between the VISION and MOTOR areas (Fig. 9) are plastic, subject to selective modification when cells in the TRACKING-VALUE area are active. The motor area has cells controlling forward (FW), left

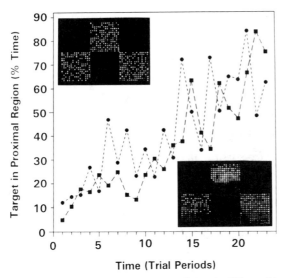

FIG. 10. Training curve for two individual runs of Darwin IV's tracking system. Time is given in trial periods, with each trial period lasting for 250 time steps. The success rate is given as the percentage of total time that the target was in the proximal part of NOMAD's visual field. Insets show strength of connections between VISION and MOTOR areas before (upper left) and after (lower right) training. Stronger connections are indicated by larger and lighter squares (see text). (Reproduced with permission from Edelman *et al.*, 1992.)

(LF), and right (RT) motion of NOMAD. Connections to these areas are shown before and after training in the insets in Fig. 10. Movements are initially disorganized, the result of spontaneous activity in the MOTOR-NOISE area (Fig. 9). When one of these movements happens to bring the target light into the near visual field, thus activating TRACKING-VALUE, connections between active units in the VISION and MOTOR areas are strengthened, increasing the probability that the same motion will occur again when the target is visible in the same position. Initially the target is visible approximately 10% of the time, corresponding to the 14% of the floor area that is in the visual field of the camera at any one time. After 25 periods of 250 time steps each, NOMAD tracks the target, which remains in the proximal visual region from 60 to 85% of the time (Fig. 10). (This percentage is substantially reduced by the fact that when tracking is lost, it cannot be regained until the target accidentally reenters NOMAD's rather small visual field.)

The connections shown in the insets in Fig. 10 are mapped according to the location of the receptive field of the source cell for each connection. As can be seen, the connections are initially random (upper left inset), but after training (lower right inset), connections are strengthened (brighter color) from areas directly in front of NOMAD to the forward motor cells, and to a lesser extent from areas on the left to the left motor cells and from areas on the right to the right motor cells. In addition, connections from visual areas directly in front of NOMAD to all three types of motor cells are weakened (darker color), because no motion is needed when the target is already in position.

2. Block Sorting Task

For the block sorting task, an opaque floor was used. The blocks served as lighted targets, and NOMAD approached any block that appeared in its visual field by use of the same visuo-motor connections that were trained in the visual tracking experiments just described. Blocks were either conducting ("bad taste" analog) or nonconducting ("good taste" analog). Unbeknown to Darwin IV, all conducting blocks were red and all nonconducting blocks were blue. Blocks of the two types were placed randomly on the floor. To provide readily assayed behavioral outputs, the nervous system of NOMAD was constructed with four built-in "reflex" behaviors. (1) A "gripping reflex" activated the snout magnet when a block entered proximal visual space. (2) The camera was elevated to a horizontal position during gripping so that NOMAD could more easily search for the green "home" position seen in Fig. 8. (3) When NOMAD reached the home position, it would stop moving, lower the camera, and activate the conductivity sensor. (This may be thought of as analogous to an animal that brings food to its lair before tasting it.) (4) When a conductive object was sensed, an "aversive reflex" caused NOMAD to drop the object and move away in an arbitrary direction.

The combined action of these "reflex" behaviors led to the following overall behavioral pattern without any training other than that required for visual tracking and approach: when a block was sighted, NOMAD would approach the block, grasp it with the magnetic snout, then search for the home position. On reaching home, NOMAD would taste the object and flee rapidly from any objects that were conductive.

Connectivities between visual areas and motor areas controlling these various reflex behaviors were provided as indicated in Fig. 9. Initially all such connections were weak, but selective modification was possible when the SALIENCY value system was active. These arrangements provided the anatomical and physiological preconditions for classical conditioning to occur. As a result of conditioning, blue color became recognized as a conditioned stimulus predictive of bad taste, and after a few trials, NOMAD picked up and carried home only red blocks, avoiding any blue blocks that it encountered. Typical results from an experiment of this kind are shown in Table II. As expected, conditioning occurs only if the appropriate value systems are present and active. Otherwise, no distinction is made between red and blue blocks other than that which is inherent in the reflex response to conductive (blue) ones. This conditioned response is in no way built into the construction of NOMAD's nervous system, but is instead a consequence of selective processes acting during experience.

IV. Discussion and Conclusions

The experiments with Darwin III and Darwin IV presented here demonstrate that selection in neural populations is a possible mechanism for the acquisition of simple physical skills, such as visual tracking and reaching, cognitive skills such as perceptual categorization, and classical conditioned behavior. These demonstrations were all carried out without violating any of the biological constraints listed in Table I. Selectionism therefore constitutes a theory of the brain that is both biologically accept-able and psychologically relevant. Further verification of the theory will require more detailed simulations of behaviors that can be directly com-pared with their animal counterparts. The NOMAD device, perhaps augmented with additional, more realistic sensors and effectors, provides an excellent platform for such tests.

Further development of these ideas may well be expected to suggest possible means of improving the ability of computers to interact with humans in a way that is more like the way humans interact with each other. Attempts to emulate natural language in computers will naturally be of the greatest interest in this regard. Such attempts will provide an important test of competing theories of brain function, inasmuch as selectionism suggests that such capability will not be possible until artifi-cial systems can be constructed that are able to create symbolic representa-

TABLE II
RESPONSE FREQUENCIES IN THE BLOCK SORTING TASK

Task	Color	Contact	Grip	Home	Avoid
Block collection (value disabled)	Red	24	15	11	0
	Blue	34	16	13	0
Block sorting (value enabled)	Red	30	30	21	0
	Blue	0	0	0	32

tions, the meaning of which is apprehended within the system, not just by an external observer. Functionalism, on the other hand, makes no such claim.

It is characteristic of selective neural systems that complex patterns of adaptive behavior are constructed from simple spontaneous elements, such as gestures, that in themselves require no learning. In this way, the need for a programmer or teacher is eliminated. Edelman (1989) has outlined in detail how these mechanisms can be recursively iterated to provide a basis for concept formation, syntax, and language, and in their ultimate flowering, for conscious awareness. Selectionism thus appears to provide an approach to understanding how biological symbol-processing systems can arise in nervous systems that are formed from components of essentially the same kind as those required for simpler perceptual and motor control skills. In this regard, selectionism differs most fundamentally from functionalism, which has not yet provided a satisfactory explanation for the self-organization of symbol-processing systems.

In conclusion, it is now possible to construct biologically realistic computer models of the nervous system that can provide meaningful tests of competing theories of behavior. Such models can help test ideas that are not currently accessible to laboratory experimentation, provided a paradigm such as synthetic neural modeling is used to avoid the inadvertent introduction of homunculi acting through the observer who interprets the models. In devising such models, it is not necessary to assume that information exists *a priori* in the world, that learning processes exist to transmit such information into the brain, or that the brain processes information symbolically. Models incorporating these assumptions, which are derived from functionalism, have been extremely difficult to implement consistent with what is known of the neurobiology of the brain. Perhaps it is time for functionalism itself to be subjected to critical reassessment.

Acknowledgments

The work reported here was performed as part of the Institute Fellows in Theoretical Neurobiology program at The Neurosciences Institute, which is supported by the Neurosciences Research Foundation. The Darwin III model was constructed in collaboration with G. M. Edelman, L. H. Finkel, and O. Sporns, and Darwin IV, in collaboration with G. M. Edelman, W. E. Gall, O. Sporns, G. Tononi, and D. W. Williams.

References

Ackley, D. H., Hinton, G. E., and Sejnowski, T. J. (1985). A learning algorithm for Boltzmann machines. *Cognit. Sci.* **9,** 147–169.

Anderson, J. R. (1983a). "The Architecture of Cognition." Harvard Univ. Press, Cambridge, MA.

Anderson, J. R. (1983b). A spreading activation theory of memory. *J. Verbal Learning Verbal Behav.* **22,** 261–295.

Baddeley, A. (1992). Working memory. *Science* **255,** 556–559.

Bechtel, W. (1988). "Philosophy of Mind: An Overview for Cognitive Science." Erlbaum, Hillsdale, NJ.

Becker, S., and Hinton, G. E. (1992). Self-organizing neural network that discovers surfaces in random-dot stereograms. *Nature (London)* **355,** 161–163.

Bernstein, N. A. (1967). "The Coordination and Regulation of Movements." Pergamon, Oxford.

Bickhard, M. H. (1993). Representational context in humans and machines. *J. Exp. Theor. Artif. Intell.* **5,** 285–333.

Brady, R. M. (1985). Optimization strategies gleaned from biological evolution. *Nature (London)* **317,** 804–806.

Braitenberg, V. (1984). "Vehicles: Experiments in Synthetic Psychology." MIT Press, Cambridge, MA.

Brooks, R. A. (1989). A robot that walks: Emergent behaviors from a carefully evolved network. *Neural Comput.* **1,** 253–262.

Brooks, R. A. (1991). New approaches to robotics. *Science* **253,** 1227–1232.

Bullock, D., Grossberg, S., and Guenther, F. H. (1993). A self-organizing neural model of motor equivalent reaching and tool use by a multijoint arm. *J. Cognit. Neurosci.* **5,** 408–435.

Changeux, J.-P., Courrége, P., and Danchin, A. (1973). A theory of the epigenesis of neuronal networks by selective stabilization of synapses. *Proc. Natl. Acad. Sci. U.S.A.* **70,** 2974–2978.

Churchland, P. S., and Sejnowski, T. J. (1992). "The Computational Brain." MIT Press, Cambridge, MA.

Crick, F. H. C. (1989). Neural Edelmanism. *Trends Neurosci.* **12,** 240–248.

Descartes, R. (1664). "Treatise on Man." Paris.

Dewey, J. (1896). The reflex arc concept in psychology. *Psychol. Rev.* **111,** 357–370.

Edelman, G. M. (1978). Group selection and phasic reentrant signaling; A theory of higher brain function. *In* "The Mindful Brain" (G. M. Edelman and V. B. Mountcastle, eds.), pp. 51–100. MIT Press, Cambridge, MA.

Edelman, G. M. (1981). Group selection as the basis for higher brain function. *In* "The Organization of the Cerebral Cortex" (F. O. Schmitt, F. G. Worden, G. Adelman, and S. G. Dennis, eds.), pp. 535–563. MIT Press, Cambridge, MA.

Edelman, G. M. (1987). "Neural Darwinism: The Theory of Neuronal Group Selection." Basic Books, New York.

Edelman, G. M. (1989). "The Remembered Present: A Biological Theory of Consciousness." Basic Books, New York.

Edelman, G. M. (1992). "Bright Air, Brilliant Fire: On the Matter of the Mind." Basic Books, New York.

Edelman, G. M., and Reeke, G. N., Jr. (1982). Selective networks capable of representative transformations, limited generalizations, and associative memory. *Proc. Natl. Acad. Sci. U.S.A.* **79,** 2091–2095.

Edelman, G. M., Reeke, G. N., Jr., Gall, W. E., Tononi, G., Williams, D., and Sporns, O. (1992). Synthetic neural modeling applied to a real-world artifact. *Proc. Natl. Acad. Sci. U.S.A.* **89,** 7267–7271.

Gerstner, W., Ritz, R., and von Hemmen, J. L. (1993). Why spikes? Hebbian learning and retrieval of time-resolved excitation patterns. *Biol. Cybernet.* **69,** 503–515.

Grillner, S., Wallén, P., Brodin, L., Lansner, A., Ekeberg, Ö., Tråven, H., Matsushima, T., and Christenson, J. (1990). Neuronal network generating lamprey locomotion—Experiments and simulations—Supraspinal, intersegmental mechanisms. *Soc. Neurosci. Abstr.* **16,** 726 (abstr.).

Guha, R. V., and Lenat, D. B. (1991). Cyc: A mid-term report. *Appl. Artif. Intell.* **5,** 45–86.

Gyr, J. W., Brown, J. S., Willey, R., and Zivian, A. (1966). Computer simulation and psychological theories of perception. *Psychol. Bull.* **65,** 174–192.

Harnad, S. (1990). The symbol grounding problem. *In* "Emergent Computation" (S. Forrest, ed.), pp. 335–346. North-Holland Publ., Amsterdam.

Herrnstein, R. J. (1984). Objects, categories, and discriminative stimuli. *In* "Animal Cognition" (H. L. Roitblat, T. G. Bever, and H. S. Terrace, eds.), pp. 233–261. Erlbaum, Hillsdale, NJ.

Herrnstein, R. J. (1985). Riddles of natural categorization. *Philos. Trans. R. Soc. London, Ser. B* **308,** 129–144.

Herrnstein, R. J., Loveland, D. H., and Cable, C. (1976). Natural concepts in pigeons. *J. Exp. Pscyhol.: Anim. Behav. Processes* **2,** 285–302.

Hinton, G. E., and Shallice, T. (1991). Lesioning an attractor network: Investigations of acquired dyslexia. *Psychol. Rev.* **98,** 74–95.

Hinton, G. E., Sejnowski, T. J., and Ackley, D. H. (1984). Boltzmann machines: Constraint satisfaction networks that learn. *Carnegie-Mellon Univ. Tech. Rep.* **CMU-CS-84-119.**

Holland, J. H. (1975). "Adaptation in Natural and Artificial Systems: An Introductory Analysis with Applications to Biology, Control, and Artificial Intelligence." University of Michigan, Ann Arbor.

Holland, J. H., Holyoak, K. J., Nisbett, R. E., and Thagard, P. R. (1986). "Induction: Processes of Inference, Learning, and Discovery." MIT Press, Cambridge, MA.

Hopfield, J. J. (1982). Neural networks and physical systems with emergent collective computational abilities. *Proc. Natl. Acad. Sci. U.S.A.* **79,** 2554–2558.

Hopfield, J. J. (1994). Neurons, dynamics and computation. *Phys. Today,* February, pp. 40–46.

Kienker, P. K., Sejnowski, T. J., Hinton, G. E., and Schumacher, L. E. (1986). Separating figure from ground with a parallel network. *Perception* **15,** 197–216.

Kirkpatrick, S., Gelatt, C. D., Jr., and Vecchi, M. P. (1983). Optimization by simulated annealing. *Science* **220,** 671–680.

Kohonen, T. (1984). "Self-Organization and Associative Memory." Springer-Verlag, Berlin.

Kolers, P. A., and Smythe, W. E. (1984). Symbol manipulation: Alternatives to the computational view of mind. *J. Verbal Learning Verbal Behav.* **23,** 289–314.

Lehky, S. R., and Sejnowski, T. J. (1988). Network model of shape-from-shading: Neural function arises from both receptive and projective fields. *Nature (London)* **333,** 452–454.

Lockery, S. R., Wittenberg, G., Kristan, W. B., and Cottrell, G. W. (1989). Function of identified interneurons in the leech elucidated using neural networks trained by back-propagation. *Nature (London)* **340,** 468–471.

Mammone, R. J., ed. (1994). "Artificial Neural Networks for Speech and Vision." Chapman & Hall, London.

Marr, D. (1982). "Vision." Freeman, San Francisco.

Mazzoni, P., Andersen, R. A., and Jordan, M. I. (1991). A more biologically plausible learning rule than backpropagation applied to a network model of cortical area 7a. *Cereb. Cortex* **1**, 293–307.

McClelland, J. L., Rumelhart, D. E., and The PDP Research Group (1986). "Parallel Distributed Processing: Explorations in the Microstructure of Cognition," Vol. 2. MIT Press, Cambridge, MA.

McCulloch, W. S., and Pitts, W. (1943). A logical calculus of the ideas immanent in nervous activity. *Bull. Math. Biophys.* **5**, 115–133.

McGinn, C. (1991). "The Problem of Consciousness: Essays Towards a Resolution." Basil Blackwell, Oxford.

Mervis, C. B., and Rosch, E. (1981). Categorization of natural objects. *Annu. Rev. Psychol.* **32**, 89–115.

Minsky, M. (1985). "The Society of Mind." Simon & Schuster, New York.

Mulloney, B., and Perkel, D. H. (1988). The roles of synthetic models in the study of central pattern generators. *In* "Neural Control of Rythmic Movements in Vertebrates" (A. H. Cohen, S. G. Rossignol, and S. Grillner, eds.), pp. 415–453. Wiley, New York.

Reeke, G. N., Jr. (1990). Neural Edelmanism. *Trends Neurosci.* **13**, 11–12.

Reeke, G. N., Jr. (1991). Book review: Marvin Minsky, *The Society of Mind. Artif. Intell.* **48**, 341–348.

Reeke, G. N., Jr. (1994). Book review: Patricia S. Churchland and Terrance J. Sejnowski, *The Computational Brain. Artif. Intell.* (in press).

Reeke, G. N., Jr., and Edelman, G. M. (1987). Selective neural networks and their implications for recognition automata. *Int. J. Supercomput. Appl.* **1**, 44–69.

Reeke, G. N., Jr., and Edelman, G. M. (1988). Real brains and artificial intelligence. *Daedalus (Boston)* **117**, 143–173.

Reeke, G. N., Jr., and Edelman, G. M. (1988b). Recognition automata based on neural Darwinism. *Forefronts* **3**, 3–6 (Cornell University, Ithaca, NY).

Reeke, G. N., Jr., Finkel, L. H., Sporns, O., and Edelman, G. M. (1990a). Synthetic neural modeling: A multilevel approach to the analysis of brain complexity. *In* "Signal and Sense: Local and Global Order in Perceptual Maps" (G. M. Edelman, W. E. Gall, and W. M. Cowan, eds.), pp. 607–706. Wiley, New York.

Reeke, G. N., Jr., Sporns, O., and Edelman, G. M. (1990b). Synthetic neural modeling: The 'Darwin' series of automata. *Proc. IEEE* **78**, 1498–1530.

Rosch, E. (1978). Principles of categorization. *In* "Cognition and Categorization" (E. Rosch and B. B. Lloyd, eds.), pp. 27–48. Erlbaum, Hillsdale, NJ.

Rosenblatt, F. (1958). The perceptron: A probabilistic model for information storage and organization in the brain. *Psychol. Rev.* **65**, 386–408.

Rumelhart, D. E., and McClelland, J. L. (1986). On learning the past tenses of English verbs. *In* "Parallel Distributed Processing" (J. L. McClelland and D. E. Rumelhart, eds.), Vol. 2, pp. 216–271. MIT Press, Cambridge, MA.

Rumelhart, D. E., McClelland, J. L., and The PDP Research Group (1986a). "Parallel Distributed Processing: Explorations in the Microstructure of Cognition," Vol. 1. MIT Press, Cambridge, MA.

Rumelhart, D. E., Hinton, G. E., and Williams, R. J. (1986b). Learning representations by back-propagating errors. *Nature (London)* **323**, 533–536.

Searle, J. (1984). "Minds, Brains, and Science." Harvard Univ. Press, Cambridge, MA.

Selfridge, O. G. (1959). Pandemonium: A paradigm for learning. *In* "Mechanization of Thought Processes," Vol. 1, pp. 511–526. H. M. Stationery Office, London.

Shapiro, M. L., and Hetherington, P. A. (1993). A simple network model simulates hippocampal place fields: Parametric analysis and physiological predictions. *Behav. Neurosi.* **107**, 34–50.

Shepherd, G. M. (1990). The significance of real neuron architectures for neural network simulations. *In* "Computational Neuroscience" (E. L. Schwartz, ed.), pp. 82–96. MIT Press, Cambridge, MA.

Silverman, D. J., Shaw, G. L., and Pearson, J. C. (1986). Associative recall properties of the Trion model of cortical organization. *Biol. Cybernet.* **53**, 259–271.

Smith, E. E., and Medin, D. L. (1981). "Categories and Concepts." Harvard Univ. Press, Cambridge, MA.

Smolensky, P. (1988). On the proper treatment of connectionism. *Behav. Brain Sci.* **11**, 1–74.

Sporns, O., and Edelman, G. M. (1993). Solving Bernstein's problem: A proposal for the development of coordinated movement by selection. *Child Dev.* **64**, 960–981.

Squire, L. R. (1986). Mechanisms of memory. *Science* **232**, 1612–1619.

Tulving, E., and Schacter, D. L. (1990). Priming and human memory systems. *Science* **247**, 301–306.

Van Essen, D. C., Anderson, C. H., and Felleman, D. J. (1992). Information processing in the primate visual system: An integrated systems perspective. *Science* **255**, 419–423.

Webb, B. H. (1991). Do computer simulations really cognize? *J. Exp. Theor. Artif. Intell.* **3**, 247–254.

Wilson, H. R., and Cowan, J. D. (1973). A mathematical theory of the functional dynamics of cortical and thalamic nervous tissue. *Kybernetik* **13**, 55–80.

Winograd, T. (1972). "Understanding Natural Language." Academic Press, New York.

Young, J. Z. (1979). Learning as a process of selection and amplification. *J. R. Soc. Med.* **72**, 801–814.

Zeki, S., and Shipp, S. (1988). The functional logic of cortical connections. *Nature (London)* **335**, 311–317.

Zipser, D., and Andersen, R. A. (1988). A back-propagation programmed network that simulates response properties of a subset of posterior parietal neurons. *Nature (London)* **331**, 679–684.

MEMORY AND FORGETTING: LONG-TERM AND GRADUAL CHANGES IN MEMORY STORAGE*

Larry R. Squire

Veterans Administration Medical Center, San Diego, California 92161 and
Departments of Psychiatry and Neurosciences, University of California School of
Medicine, San Diego, California

I. Introduction

This essay focuses on two related aspects of memory: consolidation and forgetting. These topics have a long and interesting history in psychology and neuroscience. It has often been supposed that memory can be usefully viewed as a continuation of the developmental program. During development, competitive synaptic events underlie the strengthening of some connections, the elimination of others, and provide for the sculpting out of the adult pattern of connectivity (Purves, 1988). The specific pattern of connectivity that is achieved is dependent on endogenous, patterned neural activity. These same events, it is supposed, could remain effective in adulthood and operate according to the same rules, such that connections could be strengthened or weakened as a result of behavioral experience.

* Portions of this paper are adapted and reprinted by permission of American Psychological Association, *Psychological Review*, **99**, 195–231, (1992).

243

The synaptic events of interest are the parallel competitive gains and losses in synaptic strength that occur during development. Two well-known examples illustrate these phenomena. In the submandibular ganglion of the newborn rat, an average of five axons initially terminate on each ganglionic neuron (Purves and Lichtman, 1980). During the first 4 weeks of life, pruning occurs such that eventually only one axon terminates on each ganglion. In addition, and in parallel to the elimination of inputs, the surviving axons expand their terminal arbors and increase the number of synapses that each axon makes on its target neuron. In the developing lateral geniculate of the carnivore, retinal ganglion axons from each eye initially terminate in appropriate as well as inappropriate zones, i.e., they terminate both in lamina that in the adult receive retinal input from one eye and in lamina that receive retinal input from the other eye. During development, two events occur (Goodman and Shatz, 1993; Shatz and Sretavan, 1986). First, there is regression and withdrawal of retinal axon terminals from inappropriate layers. Second, there is an exuberance of growth of retinal axons into the appropriate layers. Both of these examples make the point that development should not be characterized simply as an oversupply of connections that is then corrected by pruning out of the surplus. Rather, there is competition for target sites, and both gains and losses occur during development.

This same theme is useful for thinking about certain aspects of memory. The beginning point for this discussion lies in a paradox about memory that has long interested psychologists; namely, that as time passes after learning, memory grows weaker in one sense (it becomes less accessible to retrieval), and in another sense it becomes stronger (it becomes less susceptible to disruption by drugs, convulsive stimulation, and brain lesions). One way to account for this apparent paradox is to suppose that forgetting is associated with the gradual and literal loss of some of the connections that originally served to represent stored information. One could then account for the strengthening of memory across time (what has often been termed memory consolidation) by supposing that those elements that remain within a representation become more strongly connected (Squire, 1987). Unfortunately, there are few data available to illuminate the phenomena of memory storage and forgetting in terms of synaptic events. Indeed, direct information is not yet available at all about the synaptic changes that record memory storage in the mammalian brain.

The only strong evidence about the synaptic basis of behavioral forgetting comes from studies of the marine mollusc *Aplysia california,* in which morphological changes have been recorded in sensory neurons at different times after long-term behavioral sensitization (Bailey and Chen,

1989). The sensory neurons that were sampled were part of the circuitry of the gill- and siphon-withdrawal reflex. This reflex can be potentiated (sensitized) for several weeks following a series of 16 electric shocks to the neck region distributed across 4 days. The finding was that long-term sensitization was accompanied by a persistent increase in the number of presynaptic varicosities per sensory neuron and in the number of active zones contained within the varicosities. The varicosities are the sites of chemical synapses, and the active zones are thought to be regions where neurotransmitter is released. An increase in these measures presumably means that the sensory neurons are extending additional processes and forming additional synapses as a result of behavioral training.

As behavioral forgetting proceeded across a period of 3 weeks, there was a gradual reversal of these changes. Behavioral forgetting was not complete after 3 weeks, and the change in active zone number was only partially reversed. This study provides strong support for the general idea that behavioral forgetting can reflect in part a literal loss of information from storage and a corresponding loss of some of the synaptic changes that initially represented the stored information.

II. Memory Consolidation and Forgetting from a Brain-Systems Perspective

Much of what we currently understand about gradual changes in memory storage in the vertebrate brain comes from studies of the structure and function of the medial temporal lobe. The medial temporal lobe was first implicated in memory function through study of the noted amnesic patient H.M. (Scoville and Milner, 1957). This work established the fundamental principle that memory could be dissociated from other intellectual functions. Studies of other amnesic patients, and cumulative study of an animal model of human amnesia in the monkey (Mishkin, 1982; Squire and Zola-Morgan, 1983; Mahut and Moss, 1984), have led to the identification of the brain structures and connections that constitute the medial temporal lobe memory system (Squire and Zola-Morgan, 1991). Damage to this system in monkeys causes circumscribed memory impairment, and the memory impairment observed in monkeys has many points of similarity with human amnesia (Zola-Morgan and Squire, 1990b). The system consists of the hippocampus proper (together with the dentate gyrus and subicular complex), as well as certain adjacent and anatomically related cortical structures (entorhinal, perirhinal, and parahippocampal cortex).

This brain system, working in conjunction with neocortical areas involved in analyzing and processing incoming information, is essential for a specific kind of memory (here termed declarative memory). The important point is that memory is not a single entity. Medial temporal lobe structures and anatomically related structures in the medial diencephalon are essential for establishing long-term memory for facts and events, which are then available as conscious recollections. This system is not required for short-term (immediate) memory or for a variety of nondeclarative forms of learning, whereby acquired information is expressed through performance. Thus, amnesic patients are capable of acquiring a wide variety of nondeclarative forms of memory, despite their severe impairment of declarative memory (Table I). Nondeclarative memory includes skillful behavior and stimulus-response habits, simple conditioning (including emotional learning), the phenomenon of priming, and other instances whereby experience changes the facility for operating in the world but without affording conscious access to past episodes. Whereas declarative memory concerns recollection, nondeclarative memory concerns behavioral change. In nondeclarative memory, information is acquired as changes within specific perceptual or response systems, independently of memory for the prior encounters that led to behavioral change.

TABLE I

KINDS OF INFORMATION THAT CAN BE SUPPORTED BY NONDECLARATIVE (IMPLICIT) MEMORY AND ACQUIRED BY AMNESIC PATIENTS[a]

Specific information	Novel information	New associations
One-trial learning		
Word identification (Cermak et al., (1985)	Novel melodies (Johnson et al., 1985)	—
Word completion (Graf et al., 1984)	Nonfamous names (Squire and McKee, 1992)	—
Modality-sensitive priming (Graf et al., 1985)	Unfamiliar objects (Schacter et al., 1991); nonwords (Haist et al., 1991)	—
Multiple-trial learning		
Text-specific reading skill (Musen et al., 1990)	Reading nonwords (Musen and Squire, 1991)	Word pairs (Musen and Squire, 1993)
Serial-reaction skill (Nissen and Bullemer, 1987)	Artificial grammar learning (Knowlton et al., 1992)	Classical conditioning (Daum et al., 1989; Weiskrantz and Warrington, 1979)

[a] References are to representative studies and are not exhaustive.

III. Time-Limited Role of the Medial Temporal Lobe Memory System

The main issue to be explored in this essay is the idea that the medial temporal lobe memory system has only a temporary role in the formation and maintenance of declarative memory. Memory is gradually reorganized as time passes after learning. It is initially dependent on this system, but its role diminishes as more permanent memory is established elsewhere, presumably in neocortex. The relevant facts come from studies of retrograde amnesia, i.e., the impairment of memories that were acquired prior to damage within the medial temporal lobe. The theoretical significance of retrograde amnesia was first appreciated in the context of human memory disorders. In 1881, Theodule Ribot compiled a large number of case reports with the objective of developing principles of normal memory (Ribot, 1881, 1882). He noted that recent memory is typically lost more readily than remote memory and formulated a Law of Regression that in memory "the new perishes before the old." Quantitative studies of retrograde amnesia in humans began relatively recently (Sanders and Warrington, 1971). Since that time, a great deal has been learned, despite the fact that the available methods for assessing remote memory objectively in humans are imperfect in a number of ways.

The following sections explore the phenomenon of retrograde amnesia in some detail, beginning with studies of amnesic patients and ending with more recent work, where retrograde amnesia has been studied prospectively in experimental animals following selective brain lesions.

A. QUANTITATIVE STUDIES OF RETROGRADE AMNESIA IN ETIOLOGICALLY DISTINCT PATIENT GROUPS

At the outset, it should be recognized that it has rarely been possible to study retrograde amnesia in patients with selective, histologically confirmed damage. Indeed, it has only recently become possible (with magnetic resonance imaging) to know which patients being studied have damage to the medial temporal lobe region. Although the findings from patients with identified hippocampal formation lesions will be the primary focus here, it will also be useful to consider findings from other patients as well (e.g., patients with diencephalic lesions and cases wherein the anatomical basis of the amnesia is uncertain).

The most useful descriptions of retrograde amnesia have been obtained from quantitative studies of groups of similar patients. The best known and most widely studied example of human amnesia is Korsakoff's syndrome (Albert *et al.*, 1979; Cohen and Squire, 1981; Kopelman, 1989; Meudell *et al.*, 1980; Squire *et al.*, 1989a). The memory impairment in these patients is associated with diencephalic lesions, and the hippocampus is generally intact (for discussion, see Squire *et al.*, 1990a). Unfortunately, this group is not advantageous for studies of retrograde amnesia because the amnesic condition often develops gradually over many years. Accordingly, it is difficult to distinguish retrograde and anterograde amnesia unambiguously. Nevertheless, there is general agreement that remote memory impairment in this group is extensive and temporally graded, affecting the recent past more than the remote past (Fig. 1, top panels). The remote memory impairment most likely reflects true retrograde amnesia, not gradually developing anterograde amnesia. In one notable single-case study (Butters and Cermak, 1986), a patient with Korsakoff's syndrome was observed to have forgotten information that he had written in his autobiography a few years prior to the onset of his amnesia. Extensive retrograde amnesia has also been observed in a severely amnesic patient with Korsakoff's syndrome (patient K7; Squire *et al.*, 1989a), whose family members had witnessed the onset of his amnesia approximately 1 year earlier and could attest to his normal cognitive status prior to that time.

More favorable circumstances for the study of retrograde amnesia occur with patients who became amnesic suddenly on a known calendar day. In this case, there can be no ambiguity about which test items measure retrograde amnesia. Tests of remote memory have now been given to two groups of such patients. One group ($N = 4$) had presumed or confirmed damage to the hippocampal formation [patients AB, GD, WH, and LM from Squire *et al.* (1989a)]. They exhibited extensive and temporally graded retrograde amnesia, covering on average about 15 years of the period prior to the onset of amnesia (Fig. 1, middle panel). In separate tests, it was shown that remote memory was intact even when the test items were so difficult that they could be answered by fewer than 20% of normal subjects (Squire *et al.*, 1989a).

Another group of six patients was studied during and after transient global amnesia (TGA), a neurological syndrome characterized by the sudden onset of severe and selective amnesia that typically lasts 6 to 10 hours. These patients also exhibited extensive, temporally graded retrograde amnesia (Fig. 1, bottom panels; Kritchevsky *et al.*, 1988; Kritchevsky and Squire, 1989). One methodological advantage of this group is that the patients serve as their own control subjects. Thus, the patients were tested while they were amnesic, and at that time they failed questions about public events that they could later answer correctly after recovery from TGA. In addition, as judged by less formal questioning carried out after recovery, permanent memory loss often occurred for informa-

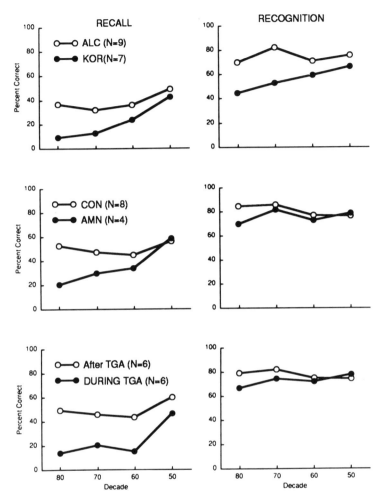

FIG. 1. Remote memory performance of patients with Korsakoff's syndrome (KOR, $N = 7$), alcoholic control subjects (ALC, $N = 9$), amnesic patients with confirmed or suspected damage to the hippocampal formation (AMN, $N = 4$), healthy control subjects (CON, $N = 8$), and patients tested during and after an episode of transient global amnesia (TGA, $N = 6$). Left: recall of past public events that had occurred from 1950 to 1985. Right: performance on a multiple-choice test (four alternatives) involving the same public events (from Squire *et al.*, 1989a; Kritchevsky and Squire, 1989).

tion that had been acquired from a few hours to 1–2 days prior to the episode. Also, memory for the events that had occurred during the period of anterograde amnesia was permanently lost.

The results from these three patient groups (patients with Korsakoff's syndrome, four patients with confirmed or suspected hippocampal formation damage, and TGA patients) show clearly that retrograde amnesia can be extensive and temporally graded. Indeed, all three groups of amnesic patients had similarly extensive and temporally graded retrograde amnesia as measured by the same recall tests of remote memory. Temporally graded remote memory impairment was also detectable, but less severe, when memory was assessed by multiple-choice and yes/no recognition.

B. Retrograde Amnesia in Patients with Hippocampal Formation Lesions

Retrograde amnesia can be less extensive than in the patients just described. Consider, for example, patient RB, who had moderately severe anterograde amnesia in association with ischemic damage that was limited to the CA1 region of the hippocampus bilaterally (Zola-Morgan et al., 1986). For this patient, retrograde amnesia could not be detected in any of six different tests, including the same remote memory test that was given to the three groups of patients discussed above (compare Fig. 1 and top two panels, Fig. 2). It is possible that RB had some retrograde amnesia for a period of a few years or less prior to the onset of his amnesia in 1978 (Fig. 2; detailed recall of public events and the television test). However, the available tests cannot detect such a deficit reliably in a single subject.

Retrograde amnesia appears to vary in its severity and extent as a function of the severity of anterograde amnesia, at least across a considerable range of severity. (For evidence that retrograde and anterograde amnesia can nevertheless be dissociated, see the following section.) Retrograde amnesia is brief when anterograde amnesia is only moderately severe (e.g., patient RB). It is more extensive when anterograde amnesia is more severe than in patient RB, as was the case for the patient groups considered above (the patients with Korsakoff's syndrome, the four amnesic patients with confirmed or suspected pathology of the hippocampal formation, and the six patients with TGA). For example, the group of four patients with hippocampal formation lesions had more severe anterograde amnesia compared to RB (the IQ − MQ difference score for the four patients = 29.0 versus 20 for RB) and also had more severe retrograde amnesia (Fig. 1, middle panels, and Fig. 2, top panels). Correspondingly, these four patients probably have more extensive neuropathology than was found in RB. Indeed, two of the patients in this group have been examined with an improved protocol for imaging the human hippocampus with magnetic resonance (patients LM and WH)

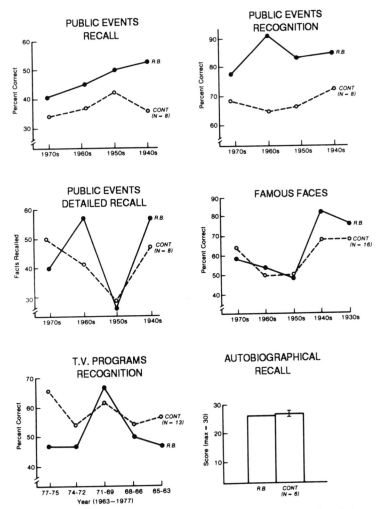

Fig. 2. Performance on six tests of remote memory by amnesic patient RB, compared to control subjects (CONT). The first five tests were given in 1979, 7–10 months following the onset of his amnesia. Recall of personal episodes was tested 2 years after the onset of his amnesia (from Zola-Morgan et al., 1986).

(Press et al., 1989; Squire et al., 1990a). Whereas RB had damage limited to the CA1 field of hippocampus, in both LM and WH the hippocampal formation was markedly reduced in size bilaterally, affecting all the cell fields of the hippocampus, including the CA1 field, together with the dentate gyrus and the subicular complex. These findings suggest that pathology in the hippocampal region, if it involves more than just the CA1 field, can produce relatively severe anterograde and retrograde amnesia. Thus, one can tentatively identify two levels of memory impairment from the human cases: a moderately severe anterograde amnesia and limited retrograde amnesia associated with damage limited to the CA1 field of hippocampus; and more severe anterograde and retrograde amnesia associated with more extensive damage to the hippocampal region.

This proposed link between the severity of anterograde and retrograde amnesia would appear to be contradicted by findings from the well-studied patient HM, who at the age of 27 (in 1953) sustained bilateral removal of the medial temporal lobe for the relief of severe epilepsy. The surgical lesion was intended to include the hippocampal formation, the amygdala, and overlying cortex. Following the surgery, HM developed a more severe anterograde amnesia than is observed in any of the patients discussed above. The extent of his retrograde amnesia is more difficult to judge, in part because quantitative assessments were not undertaken until more than 20 years after he became amnesic. Nevertheless, he is reported to have retrograde amnesia for a period covering only 3 to 11 years prior to his surgery (Corkin, 1984; Marslen-Wilson and Teuber, 1975; Milner *et al.*, 1968; Sagar *et al.*, 1985; Scoville and Milner, 1957). One possibility is that memories from very early life are especially resistant to amnesia. If HM had developed amnesia in middle age, like the majority of amnesic study patients, perhaps he would have exhibited more extensive retrograde amnesia. In any case, more recent findings do support the idea that anterograde amnesia and temporally graded retrograde amnesia are related deficits.

C. Retrograde Amnesia without a Temporal Gradient

It is important to note that some memory-impaired patients have extensive retrograde amnesia with no evidence of a temporal gradient. In such cases, remote memory appears to be severely and similarly impaired across all time periods [for example, following left unilateral temporal lobectomy, and in association with some cases of diencephalic amnesia, Huntington's disease, Alzheimer's disease, encephalitis, or head trauma (Albert *et al.*, 1981; Barr *et al.*, 1990; Beatty *et al.*, 1988; Butters and Stuss, 1989; Cermak and O'Connor, 1983; Damasio *et al.*, 1985; Graf-Radford *et al.*, 1990; Sagar *et al.*, 1988; Stuss *et al.*, 1988; Warrington and McCarthy, 1988; Wilson *et al.*, 1981; Tulving *et al.*, 1988); also see one early report involving a mixed group of amnesic patients (Sanders and Warrington, 1971)]. This type of retrograde amnesia deserves special consideration. One possibility is that ungraded retrograde amnesia is simply the extreme on a continuum of severity. By this view, these patients have both very severe anterograde amnesia (i.e., more severe than any of the patients represented in Fig. 1) and correspondingly severe retrograde amnesia. The difficulty with this view is that not all the patients with extensive and severe retrograde amnesia appear to have severe anterograde amnesia. Perhaps the clearest example of such a dissociation is found in the patients with left temporal lobectomy studied by Barr *et al.* (1990). These patients were only mildly impaired on tests of delayed story recall (not nearly so impaired as the patients whose remote memory scores are shown in Fig. 1), but these same patients had extensive and ungraded retrograde amnesia on several remote memory tests that assessed knowledge of famous persons, public events, and television programs.

Another possibility is that severe and ungraded retrograde amnesia requires damage in addition to (or different from) the medial temporal lobe and midline diencephalic structures usually associated with circumscribed amnesia. This alternative seems plausible because most, if not all, of the clinical conditions in which ungraded retrograde amnesia has been reported are conditions in which additional damage is known to have occurred (e.g., to lateral temporal cortex). This additional damage might impair performance on remote memory tests without contributing proportionally to anterograde amnesia. For example, storage sites for remote memory or access to these sites could be compromised by lateral temporal cortex lesions without destroying the capacity to establish new representations, because new representations could be based on cues and processing strategies that remain intact and that are different from the ones used to establish the memories already in storage. Additional neuropsychological and anatomical information will be needed to identify the determinants of ungraded retrograde amnesia and to confirm that ungraded forms of retrograde amnesia are dissociable from anterograde memory impairment.

D. Retrograde Amnesia for Autobiographical Memory

Most quantitative assessments of retrograde amnesia have been based on tests of public information (e.g., tests of public events and famous faces), because the correct answers can be identified unambiguously. However, tests have also been constructed to assess autobiographical, event-specific memory, e.g., subjects are asked to recollect personal episodes in response to a fixed list of cue words (Crovitz and Schiffman,

1974; Galton, 1879) or to recollect specific episodes in response to structured questions. Frank confabulation is ruled out by determining that subjects are consistent about the telling of the event and its date on two different occasions several weeks apart. On such tests, amnesic patients typically exhibit temporally limited retrograde amnesia (Fig. 3). For example, two patients with confirmed hippocampal formation damage (patients LM and WH), who were normal on tests of factual information for very remote events (Fig. 1), were also able to produce well-formed memories from their early childhood or adolescence (MacKinnon and Squire, 1989). The quality of their memories could not be differentiated from those reported by normal subjects. Moreover, just as was observed in the case of factual information tests, they were impaired when they attempted to recollect more recent events. Altogether, five amnesic patients took both tests, and they had similarly severe autobiographical memory impairment and fact memory impairment.

It has often been reported that memory impairment for factual information and memory impairment for autobiographical material are associated in individual patients (Beatty *et al.*, 1987; Butters and Cermak, 1986; Gabrieli *et al.*, 1988; Kopelman, 1989; Ostergaard, 1987). Importantly, the same patients who exhibit extensive ungraded retrograde amnesia for factual information are also often reported to be unable to produce any autobiographical memories at all (Cermak and O'Connor, 1983; Damasio *et al.*, 1985; Tulving *et al.*, 1988; Warrington and McCarthy, 1988). In general, the findings for autobiographical tests and fact memory tests appear to be in correspondence. Those patients who cannot recollect personal memories also exhibit extensive, ungraded remote memory impairment, whereas those who can recall early personal memo-

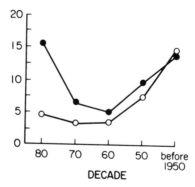

FIG. 3. Time periods from which five amnesic patients (○) and five control subjects (●) recalled well-formed autobiographical memories in response to 75 single-word cues (e.g., tree, flag, window) (from MacKinnon and Squire, 1989).

ries exhibit temporally graded retrograde amnesia for factual information with sparing of very remote memory.

One difficulty in comparing fact memory with autobiographical memory for personal events is that factual knowledge can be acquired through repeated exposure to information. By contrast, remembered events are specific to time and place and cannot be repeated. Whenever amnesia occurs, so long as it is not so severe as to be absolute, one would expect material that has been often repeated to be easier to remember than material that has occurred only once (see Ostergaard and Squire, 1990). This simple difference between facts and events is one reason why event memory can appear to be more affected in amnesia than fact memory. On the one hand, it is clear that both fact memory and event memory are impaired in amnesia, especially if the information was acquired recently. On the other hand, severely amnesic patients have been described who reportedly have some remote fact memory available but no capacity at all for autobiographical, event-specific recall (e.g., Damasio *et al.*, 1985; Tulving *et al.*, 1988). This finding has sometimes been taken to suggest that amnesia especially affects episodic memory. However, the issue is not that such patients can accumulate some semantic (factual) knowledge without acquiring episodic (event) knowledge (Tulving and Schacter, 1990). The issue is whether the ability to acquire factual knowledge is disproportionately spared. Is the ability to recollect autobiographical information disproportionately impaired, beyond the level of impairment that would be expected from the principle that remembering unique events is more difficult than remembering repeated events? At the present time, the evidence favors the simpler view that both kinds of memory are affected in amnesia. This correspondence would be expected if fact memory and event memory are both examples of declarative memory and similarly dependent on the structures damaged in amnesia (also see Squire *et al.*, 1993).

E. Retrograde Amnesia as a Stable Impairment

Everyone has the experience of failing to recollect a piece of information that could then be recalled successfully on some later occasion. Following from this observation, it seems reasonable to suppose that amnesic patients (as well as normal subjects) know more about remote events than they are able to demonstrate in a single test session. In the limiting case, if a sufficient number of testing occasions were provided, one could suppose that amnesic patients might eventually produce as much information about remote events as normal subjects (Cermak and

O'Connor, 1983). This possibility has been tested by administering the same remote memory tests on multiple occasions during a 3-year period (Squire *et al.*, 1989b). On each test occasion, it was found that some information could usually be recalled that had not been recalled on previous tests. However, the amount of new information that amnesic patients could add at each test session eventually became quite small, and their cumulative performance score leveled off to an asymptote well before their recall performance reached normal levels. This result indicates that retrograde amnesia is not a problem in assessing memory that can be overcome with sufficient retrieval opportunity. On the contrary, it appears that amnesic patients simply possess less usable knowledge about past events than normal subjects, and retrograde amnesia is a stable feature of their memory impairment.

Recently, this view was questioned by a report that retrograde amnesia could be attenuated by altering the manner in which remote memory questions are presented. Specifically, findings from a single case of post-encephalitic amnesia suggested that retrograde amnesia was severe and extensive when assessed with standard tests, but that it was not observed at all when remote memory tests were redesigned as semantic memory tests (Warrington and McCarthy, 1988). Rather than assessing associative memory, the new remote memory tests assessed simple familiarity for famous names or name-completion ability. Yet, it seemed possible that such tests were simply too easy to detect a difference between normal and abnormal performance, i.e., impaired performance might have been obscured by a ceiling effect.

To explore this issue, we constructed similar tests but made them difficult enough that subjects did not achieve perfect performance (Squire *et al.*, 1990b). Two amnesic patients were tested with radiologically confirmed lesions that included the hippocampal formation bilaterally [patient Boswell (Damasio *et al.*, 1985) and patient WI (Squire *et al.*, 1990a)]. Both patients had severe and extensive retrograde amnesia as assessed by standard recognition tests of remote memory, i.e., they performed more poorly than the patients whose data appear in Fig. 1. [Note that the standard tests of remote memory are sometimes not very sensitive to retrograde amnesia when they are given in a recognition format (see Fig. 1, right panels). Accordingly, only severely impaired patients have room to improve on such tests, and only severely impaired patients can provide a test of the idea that performance will improve when the nature of the remote memory test is altered.] The first test (familiarity) asked subjects to select the famous name from a group of nonfamous names (e.g., Arthur Elliot, David Conner, Richard Daly). The second test asked subjects to complete a fragment to form a famous name (e.g., Adlai Stev___). The correct answers for both tests were taken from a standard test of remote memory for famous faces and spanned the time period 1940–1985.

On the redesigned tests, the amnesic patients did perform better than on more conventionally designed tests (e.g., "select from a group of famous names the one that matches a photograph"). However, the normal subjects also performed better on the redesigned tests, and they retained their substantial advantage over the amnesic patients. Indeed, the two amnesic patients scored outside the range of the scores obtained by normal subjects, and they were more than two standard deviations below the normal mean. These findings provide no basis for supposing that retrograde amnesia can be mitigated by simple changes in test procedure. Retrograde amnesia reflects a stable impairment in accessing past facts and events.

F. Temporally Graded Retrograde Amnesia

The data just reviewed show that retrograde amnesia is a typical feature of memory impairment. In most cases, retrograde amnesia is temporally graded and affects recent memory more than remote memory. Its severity and extent are related to the severity of anterograde amnesia and determined by the extent of damage within the medial temporal lobe and midline diencephalon. When damage is more extensive and includes, for example, lateral temporal neocortex, remote memory impairment can be severe and ungraded, perhaps because there is direct damage to memory storage sites. In these cases, the link between anterograde and retrograde amnesia is less clear.

Because very remote memories are typically preserved in amnesic patients, the site of permanent memory storage cannot be the hippocampal formation or any of the other damaged structures. For this reason, it has long been supposed that the hippocampus and related structures must have only a temporary role in memory storage. There are two fundamentally different ways to understand this idea. One possibility is that the structures damaged in amnesia are necessary for the storage and retrieval of memory, but especially the storage and retrieval of those components of memory that tend to be forgotten quickly. A complete memory for any single event, e.g., dinner with a friend, is assumed to consist of many component memories, which have different qualities and varying lifetimes. Details, context, and other incidental features, e.g., what the friend was wearing, will on average be forgotten quickly after the event and will be rare in very long-term memory. The more generic and central features of the event, e.g., that dinner with a friend did take place, will be remembered longer. If the structures damaged in amnesia are necessary for storing and retrieving the short-lasting components of memory, then it follows that amnesia will always appear to affect recent memory more than remote memory. By this scenario, temporally graded retrograde amnesia occurs simply because these components are more abundant in recent memory than in remote memory. There is no transformation or consolidation of information across time. There is simply differential attrition of memory by type. The structures damaged in amnesia have a temporary role in memory because the kind of memory served by these structures is present only temporarily.

A second possibility is that the structures damaged in amnesia have a temporary role because memories that initially depend on these structures become independent as time passes. That is, memories are reorganized or consolidated with the passage of time after learning. As time passes, memories gradually become independent of these structures.

These two possibilities can be distinguished experimentally by determining the precise shape of the performance curves in retrograde amnesia. Consider the two sets of hypothetical data shown in Fig. 4. In the left panel, the score for any particular time period is never lower than the score for a more remote time period. These data can be explained by supposing that memories for the very remote past that have survived

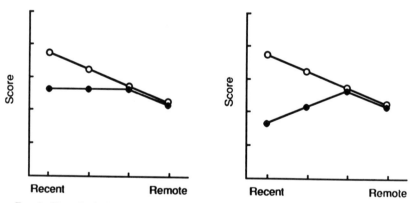

FIG. 4. Hypothetical data derived from an optimal remote memory test that can sample equivalently across time periods, i.e., the material from each time period was initially learned to the same level and then forgotten at the same rate. Only the data in the right panel require that memory is actively reorganized or consolidated as time passes after learning. The key feature of the data in the right panel is that memory for remote time periods is better than memory for more recent periods. (O) Normal subjects; (●) amnesic patients.

for many years never depended on the structures damaged in amnesia, even when they were first acquired. Only the more quickly forgotten memories depend on these structures. In this view, the ability to recall the recent past can never be poorer than the ability to recall the remote past. In the right panel, scores for recent time periods are actually lower than scores for more remote time periods. These data cannot be accounted for by supposing that amnesia especially impairs rapidly decaying memories. One must explain why, in amnesia, older memories could be remembered better than recent memories.

It has been difficult to decide between these two alternatives. The difficulty is that the precise shape of the temporal gradient of retrograde amnesia cannot be determined with certainty using the tests that are available to assess remote memory retrospectively in humans. Nevertheless, gradients of retrograde amnesia have been obtained in which the remote past was remembered better than the recent past. In one case, psychiatric patients prescribed electroconvulsive theory (ECT) were tested both before and after treatment using a test that was specially constructed to permit equivalent sampling of past time periods (Squire et al., 1975). After treatment, the patients had difficulty remembering events that had occurred 1 to 3 years previously, whereas more remote events were remembered normally. In a second case, mice were trained in a one-trial learning task and then given electroconvulsive shock (ECS) at different times after learning (Squire and Spanis, 1984). Memory for the training was impaired when the training occurred 1 to 3 weeks prior to ECS but not when it occurred at earlier times. These findings show (in agreement with the alternative illustrated in the right panel of Fig. 4) that long-term memory is dynamic and that memory must change as time passes after learning. However, treatments such as ECT and ECS cannot be usefully related to neuroanatomy.

Recently, a direct test of the alternatives in Fig. 4 was arranged by studying memory prospectively in monkeys with bilateral lesions of the hippocampal formation (the H+ lesion) (Zola-Morgan and Squire, 1990a). Monkeys were trained preoperatively on five different sets of 20 two-choice object discrimination pairs (for a total of 100 object pairs). Training on each 20-pair set began approximately 16, 12, 8, 4, and 2 weeks prior to surgery. For training, each object pair was presented for 14 trials, and during training performance improved from 55% correct on the first trial (chance = 50%) to 88% correct on the fourteenth trial (averaged across all 100 object pairs). One of the two objects was always rewarded, and the left–right location of the correct object varied randomly. The learning curves were numerically quite similar for the five training episodes (Fig. 5, top).

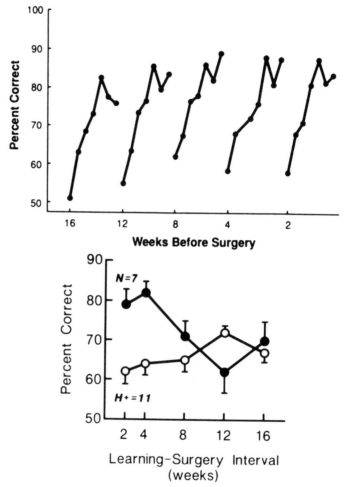

FIG. 5. Top: acquisition of 100 object discrimination problems (20 pairs/ time period) prior to surgery. Bottom: retention of the 100 object pairs as a function of learning–surgery interval. Monkeys with bilateral lesions of the hippocampal formation and parahippocampal gyrus (H +) exhibited temporally graded retrograde amnesia. Normal monkeys ($N = 7$) exhibited forgetting (from Zola-Morgan and Squire, 1990a) (Copyright 1990, © AAAS.)

Two weeks after surgery, memory was assessed by presenting a single trial for each of the 100 pairs in a mixed order. Figure 5 (bottom) shows the mean retention scores as a function of learning–surgery interval. Unoperated monkeys ($N = 7$) exhibited forgetting, ranging from 79% correct for objects learned recently to less than 70% correct for objects learned in the most remote time periods. The H + group (N = 11) exhibited temporally graded retrograde amnesia. Specifically, the operated monkeys performed more poorly than the normal monkeys on object pairs that had been learned 2–4 weeks before surgery ($p < 0.01$). The two groups did not differ at any other time periods. The key finding was that the operated monkeys remembered objects learned long before surgery significantly better than objects learned recently. In addition, the retrograde amnesia gradient was monotonic from 2 to 12 weeks (62, 64, 65, and 72%), and there was a significant linear trend ($p < 0.01$) across this portion of the performance curve. Indeed, of the 11 H + monkeys, only one remembered the objects learned 2 weeks before surgery better than the objects learned 12 weeks before surgery. For the 7 normal monkeys, the opposite was true: only one monkey remembered the 12-week-old objects better than the 2-week-old objects.

One would expect that, if all relevant time periods had been fully sampled, the performance curve of operated animals should approximate an inverted U. In other words, if the memory scores of operated monkeys do increase significantly as one moves from a recent to a more remote time period, at some point in very remote time periods the scores of operated monkeys would be expected to join the forgetting curve of normal monkeys.

These results provide evidence for a gradual process of consolidation or reorganization in memory as time passes after learning. Similar results have also been reported for mice and rats given hippocampal formation lesions, although in this case the gradients of retrograde amnesia covered a somewhat shorter time (Winocur, 1990; Cho et al., 1993; Kim and Fanselow, 1992). Thus, the hippocampal formation is essential for memory storage for only a limited period of time. A temporary memory is established in the hippocampal formation at the time of learning [in the form of a simple memory, a conjunction, or an index (Halgren, 1984; Marr, 1971; McNaughton, 1989; McNaughton and Nadel, 1990; Milner, 1989; Rolls, 1990; Squire et al., 1989b; Teyler and Discenna, 1986)]. The role of the hippocampal formation then gradually diminishes, and a more permanent memory is established elsewhere that is independent of this region.

These ideas about the significance of retrograde amnesia and the reorganization of memory over time are ideas specifically about declarative memory. Medial temporal lobe lesions in monkeys did not affect previously learned motor skills (Salmon et al., 1987). In addition, patients who were amnesic following a prescribed course of electroconvulsive therapy retained a mirror-reading skill that they had acquired prior to treatment, despite forgetting the words they had read as well as the training sessions (Squire et al., 1984b).

G. Retrograde Amnesia: A Summary

The facts of retrograde amnesia, as they are now understood, require a gradual process of reorganization or consolidation within declarative memory, whereby the contribution of the hippocampus and related structures gradually diminishes and the neocortex alone gradually becomes capable of supporting usable, permanent memory. This reorganization could depend on the development of effective cortico-cortical connections between the separate sites in neocortex, which together constitute a whole memory, or reorganization could require the development of new representations. In either case, it would seem that slow changes in synaptic connectivity must be involved. A theme of this essay is that consolidation is a part of the biologic process of forgetting, and that the connections between some elements of representations are lost over time while other connections grow stronger (for a computational approach to consolidation, see Alvarez and Squire, 1994).

Temporally graded retrograde amnesia has now been observed in mice, rats, monkeys, and humans. The length of the retrograde amnesic gradient was short in mice and rats (from a few days to 4 weeks), intermediate in monkeys (2–12 weeks), and longer in humans (1–3 years). The length of the gradient can be expected to vary depending on the extent of damage to the medial temporal lobe memory system and on the course of normal forgetting for the material being tested. It is also likely that more recently evolved, higher vertebrates have more slowly developing memory consolidation processes compared to simpler vertebrates. Indeed, the time required for neuroplasticity to develop may generally be slower in more complex nervous systems. For example, an independent, secondary epileptic focus (mirror focus) in the hemisphere contralateral to the site of an artifically induced primary epileptic lesion develops more slowly in cats and monkeys than in frogs, rats, and rabbits (Wilder, 1972).

More than 100 years have passed since Ribot first pointed out the lawfulness of memory loss for past events and the relative preservation of remote memory. Prospective studies involving experimental animals show how this observation should be interpreted. Sparing of remote memory in amnesia is not based on the greater rehearsal and repetition of remote events compared to recent events, because sparing of remote memory can occur in amnesia even when the remote material is remembered less well than recently learned material by normal subjects. In addition, sparing of remote memory does not reflect the survival of particular components of memory that did not depend at any time after learning on the structures damaged in amnesia. Rather, the phenomenon results from the fact that the damaged structures have only a temporary role in memory.

The concept of consolidation was originally advanced to explain retroactive interference (Muller and Pilzecker, 1900) but found its strongest support in the phenomenon of retrograde amnesia (Burnham, 1903). Subsequently, a large body of experimental work illustrated convincingly the utility of the concept of consolidation for understanding the phenomenon of retrograde amnesia (McGaugh and Gold, 1976; McGaugh and Herz, 1972). More recent work with experimental animals shows that consolidation can continue for a long period and suggests how the hippocampal formation is involved in the process. The hippocampal formation must initially participate in establishing representations, if memory is to be established in a usable way. Gradual reorganization of memory storage occurs such that storage and retrieval are eventually possible without the participation of the hippocampus or related structures.

The facts of retrograde amnesia can be summarized as follows:

1. When damage is limited to the CA1 region of human hippocampus, retrograde amnesia is limited to a period of a year or two at the most.

2. In patients with more complete damage to the hippocampal formation, retrograde amnesia can be extensive and temporally graded across a decade or more, with sparing of very old memories.

3. Hippocampal damage causes retrograde amnesia for both factual information and autobiographical, event-specific information.

4. The retrograde amnesia represents a loss of usable knowledge, not a loss of accessibility that can be overcome by multiple retrieval opportunities.

5. Retrograde amnesia is a retrieval deficit in the sense that lost memories return following transient amnesic episodes. However, memory for the time period just prior to the onset of amnesia is permanently lost. Moreover, it cannot be assumed that past memories would recover to the same extent if the period of amnesia lasted longer than it typically does in transient amnesia. Some clinical observations on this point (see Squire *et al.*, 1984a) raise the possibility that memory becomes progressively disorganized so long as the medial temporal lobe memory system remains dysfunctional. Thus, when the system regains its normal function quickly, as in transient global amnesia, past memories are once again available. However, if the system were to remain dysfunctional for many weeks or longer, memory might not recover so fully. These considerations suggest that, rather than describing retrograde amnesia as a retrieval deficit, it is more accurate to describe it as a loss of memory, the nature of which is determined by the status of memory in storage when amnesia occurs.

6. Retrograde amnesia is revealed in tests that require associative memory as well as in tests that require simple recognition based on familiarity. To date, there have been no convincing demonstrations that retrograde amnesia can be mitigated by changing test procedures (except in the theoretically uninteresting case in which two different tests have similar effects on both normal subjects and amnesic patients, e.g., administering a test of recognition memory instead of a test of recall).

7. Work with experimental animals provides direct evidence for gradual consolidation of memory during the period of normal forgetting and for the involvement of the hippocampus and related structures in this process. These structures are required initially for the storage and retrieval of memory, but not after sufficient time has passed.

IV. Conclusions

Coordinated neural activity in neocortex is thought to underlie perception and the capacity for immediate (short-term) memory (Damasio, 1989; Mishkin, 1982; Squire, 1987; Singer, 1990). If this neural activity is to cohere into a stable declarative memory, then convergent activity must occur within anatomical projections from these regions into the medial temporal lobe memory system.

In this view, simultaneous and coordinated activity in neocortex is sufficient for the task of perception and short-term memory. So long as a visual object is in view or in mind, its representation remains coherent. However, a distinct problem arises when attention shifts to a new scene or a new thought, and one then attempts at a later time to recover the visual object from memory. In the present account, the possibility of later retrieval is provided by the medial temporal lobe memory system because it has "bound together" the relevant cortical sites. A partial cue that is later processed through this system is able to reactivate all of the sites and thereby accomplish retrieval of the whole memory.

This state of affairs is only temporary. As the result of gradual processes that are still poorly understood, the organization of memory storage is slowly transformed as time passes after learning. This transformation could involve rehearsal, additional retrieval opportunities, or acquisition of related material; or it could be largely endogenous. In any case, with time, the role of medial temporal lobe structures diminishes until they are no longer necessary for either the maintenance of memory in storage or its retrieval. Concurrently, the sites of storage in neocortex undergo two, possibly related, kinds of changes. First, forgetting occurs, because of the establishment of new connections, which interfere with the coherence of already established networks, and because of actual weakening or loss of existing connections within established networks. Second, the distributed networks that together constitute a whole memory develop greater coherence, perhaps by developing functional cortico-cortical connections or by rerepresenting information in a more efficient form. As a result of these gradual changes, remembering becomes possible without the participation of the medial temporal lobe memory system.

References

Albert, M. S., Butters, N., and Levin, J. (1979). Temporal gradients in the retrograde amnesia of patients with alcoholic Korsakoff's disease. *Arch. Neurol. (Chicago)* **36,** 211–216.

Albert, M. S., Butters, N., and Brandt, J. (1981). Patterns of remote memory in amnesic and demented patients. *Arch. Neurol. (Chicago)* **38,** 495–500.

Alvarez, P., and Squire, L. R. (1994). Memory consolidation and the medial temporal lobe: A simple network model. *Proc. Natl. Acad. Sci. U.S.A.,* in press.

Bailey, C. H., and Chen, M. (1989). Time course of structural changes at identified sensory neuron synapses during long-term sensitization in *Aplysia. J. Neurosci.* **9,** 175–180.

Barr, W. B., Goldberg, E., Wasserstein, J., and Novelly, R. A. (1990). Retrograde amnesia following unilateral temporal lobectomy. *Neuropsychologia* **28,** 243–256.

Beatty, W. W., Salmon, D. P., Bernstein, N., and Butters, N. (1987). Remote memories in a patient with amnesia due to hypoxia. *Psychol. Med.* **17,** 657–665.

Beatty, W. W., Salmon, D. P., Butters, N., Heindel, W. C., and Granholm, E. A. (1988). Retrograde amnesia in patients with Alzheimer's disease or Huntington's disease. *Neurobiol. Aging* **9,** 181–186.

Brunham, W. H. (1903). Retroactive amnesia: Illustrative cases and a tentative explanation. *Am. J. Psychol.* **14,** 382–396.

Butters, N., and Cermak, L. S. (1986). A case study of the forgetting of autobiographical knowledge: Implications for the study of retrograde amnesia. *In* "Autobiographical Memory" (D. Ruben, ed.), pp. 253–272. Cambridge Univ. Press, New York.

Butters, N., and Stuss, D. T. (1989). Diencephalic amnesia. *In* "Handbook of Neuropsychology" (F. Boller and J. Grafman, eds.), Vol. 3. Elsevier, Amsterdam.

Cermak, L. S., and O'Connor, M. (1983). The anterograde and retrograde retrieval ability of a patient with amnesia due to encephalitis. *Neuropsychologia* **19,** 213–224.

Cermak, L. S., Talbot, N., Chandler, K., and Wolbarst, L. R. (1985). The perceptual priming phenomenon in amnesia. *Neuropsychologia* **23,** 615–622.

Cho, Y. H., Beracochea, D., and Jaffard, R. (1993). Temporally graded retrograde and anterograde amnesia following ibotenic entorhinal cortex lesion in mice. *J. Neurosci.* **13,** 1759–1766.

Cohen, N. J., and Squire, L. R. (1981). Retrograde amnesia and remote memory impairment. *Neuropsychologia* **119,** 337–356.

Corkin, S. (1984). Lasting consequences of bilateral medial temporal lobectomy: Clinical course and experimental findings in H. M. *Semin. Neurol.* **4,** 249–259.

Crovitz, H. F., and Schiffman, H. (1974). Frequency of episodic memories as a function of their age. *Bull. Psychon. Soc.* **4,** 517–518.

Damasio, A. R. (1989). Time-locked multiregional retroactivation: A systems-level proposal for the neural substrates of recall and recognition. *Cognition* **33,** 25–62.

Damasio, A. R., Graff-Radford, N. R., Eslinger, P. J., Damasio, H., and Kassell, N. (1985). Amnesia following basal forebrain lesions. *Arch. Neurol. (Chicago)* **42,** 263–271.

Daum, I., Channon, S., and Canavar, A. (1989). Classical conditioning in patients with severe memory problems. *J. Neurol. Neurosurg. Psychiatry* **52,** 47–51.

Gabrieli, J. D. E., Cohen, N. J., and Corkin, S. (1988). The impaired learning of semantic knowledge following medial temporal-lobe resection. *Brain Cognition* **7,** 157–177.

Galton, F. (1879). Psychometric experiments. *Brain* **2,** 149–162.

Goodman, C. S., and Shatz, C. J. (1993). Developmental mechanisms that generate precise patterns of neuronal connectivity. *Cell (Cambridge, Mass.)* **72,** 77–98.

Graf, P., Squire, L. R., and Mandler, G. (1984). The information that amnesic patients do not forget. *J. Exp. Psychol. Learn. Mem. Cognition* **10,** 164–178.

Graf, P., Shimamura, A. P., and Squire, L. R. (1985). Priming across modalities and priming across category levels: Extending the domain of preserved function in amnesia. *J. Exp. Psychol. Learn. Mem., Cognition* **11,** 386–396.

Graff-Radford, N. R., Tranel, D., Van Hoesen, G. W., and Brandt, J. (1990). Diencephalic amnesia. *Brain* **113,** 1–25.

Haist, F., Musen, G., and Squire, L. R. (1991). Intact priming of words and nonwords in amnesia. *Psychobiology* **19,** 275–285.

Halgren, E. (1984). Human hippocampal and amygdala recording and stimulation: Evidence for a neural model of recent memory. *In* "The Neuropsychology of Memory" (L. R. Squire and N. Butters, eds.), pp. 165–182. Guilford Press, New York.

Johnson, M. K., Kim, J. K., and Risse, G. (1985). Do alcoholic Korsakoff's syndrome patients acquire affective reactions? *J. Exp. Psychol. Learn. Mem., Cognition* **11,** 22–36.

Kim, J. J., and Fanselow, M. S. (1992). Modality-specific retrograde amnesia of fear. *Science* **256,** 675–677.

Knowlton, B. J., Ramus, S. J., and Squire, L. R. (1992). Intact artificial grammar learning in amnesia: Dissociation of category-level knowledge and explicit memory for specific instances. *Pscyhol. Sci.* **3,** 172–179.

Kopelman, M. D. (1989). Remote and autobiographical memory, temporal context memory and frontal atrophy in Korsakoff and Alzheimer patients. *Neuropsychologia* **27,** 437–460.

Kritchevsky, M., and Squire, L. R. (1989). Transient global amnesia: Evidence for extensive, temporally-graded retrograde amnesia. *Neurology* **39,** 213–218.

Kirtchevsky, M., Squire, L. R., and Zouzounis, J. A. (1988). Transient global amnesia: Characterization of anterograde and retrograde amnesia. *Neurology* **38,** 213–219.

MacKinnon, D., and Squire, L. R. (1989). Autobiographical memory in amnesia. *Psychobiology* **17,** 247–256.

Mahut, H., and Moss, M. (1984). Consolidation of memory: The hippocampus revisited. *In* "The Neuropsychology of Memory" (L. R. Squire and N. Butters, eds.), pp. 297–315. Guildord Press, New York.

Marr, D. (1971). Simple memory: A theory for archicortex. *Philos. Trans. R. Soc. London, Ser. B* **262,** 23–81.

Marslen-Wilson, W. D., and Teuber, H. L. (1975). Memory for remote events in anterograde amnesia: Recognition of public figures from news photographs. *Neuropsychologia* **13,** 353–364.

McGaugh, J. L., and Gold, P. E. (1976). Modulation of memory by electrical stimulation of the brain. *In* "Neural Mechanisms of Learning and Memory" (M. R. Rosenzweig and E. L. Bennett, eds.), pp. 549–560. MIT Press, Cambridge, MA.

McGaugh, J. L., and Herz, M. J., eds. (1972). "Memory Consolidation." Albion, San Francisco.

McNaughton, B. L. (1989). Neuronal mechanism for spatial computation and information storage. *In* "Neural Connection, Mental Computations" (L. Nadel, L. A. Cooper, P. Culicover, and R. M. Harnish, eds.), pp. 285–350. MIT Press, Cambridge, MA.

McNaughton, B. L., and Nadel, L. (1990). Hebb–Marr networks and the neurobiological representation of action in space. *In* "Neuroscience and Connectionist Theory" (M. Gluck and D. Rumelhart, eds.), pp. 1–63. Erlbaum, Hillsdale, NJ.

Meudell, P. R., Northern, B., Snowden, J. S., and Neary, D. (1980). Long-term memory for famous voices in amnesia and normal subjects. *Neuropsychologia* **18**, 133–139.

Milner, B., Corkin, S., and Teuber, H. L. (1968). Further analysis of the hippocampal amnesic syndrome: 14 year follow-up study of H.M. *Neuropsychologia* **6**, 215–234.

Milner, P. (1989). A cell assembly theory of hippocampal amnesia. *Neuropsychologia* **27**, 23–30.

Mishkin, M. (1982). A memory system in the monkey. *Philos. Trans. R. Soc. London, Ser. B* **298**, 85–92.

Muller, G. E., and Pilzecker, A. (1900). Experimentelle beitrage zur lehre von gedachlniss. *Z. Psychol. Suppl.* **1**.

Musen, G., and Squire, L. R. (1991). Normal acquisition of novel verbal information in amnesia. *J. Exp. Psychol. Learn. Mem. Cognition* **17**, 1095–1104.

Musen, G., and Squire, L. R. (1993). On the implicit learning of novel associations by amnesic patients and normal subjects. *Neuropsychology* **7**, 119–135.

Musen, G., Shimamura, A. P., and Squire, L. R. (1990). Intact text-specific reading skill in amnesia. *J. Exp. Psychol. Learn. Mem. Cognition* **16**, 1068–1076.

Nissen, M. J., and Bullemer, P. (1987). Attentional requirements of learning: Evidence from performance measures. *Cognit. Psychol.* **19**, 1–32.

Ostergaard, A. L. (1987). Episodic, semantic, and procedural memory in a case of amnesia at an early age. *Neuropsychologia* **25**, 341–357.

Ostergaard, A. L., and Squire, L. R. (1990). Childhood amnesia and distinctions between forms of memory: A comment on Wood, Brown, and Felton. *Brain Cognition* **14**, 127–133.

Press, G. A., Amaral, D. G., and Squire, L. R. (1989). Hippocampal abnormalities in amnesic patients revealed by high-resolution magnetic resonance imaging. *Nature (London)* **341**, 54–57.

Purves, D. (1988). "Body and Brain." Harvard Univ. Press, Cambridge, MA.

Purves, D., and Lichtman, J. W. (1980). Elimination of synapses in the developing nervous system. *Science* **210**, 153–157.

Ribot, T. (1881). "Les Maladies de la Mémoire." Germer Baillière, Paris.

Ribot, T. (1882). "Diseases of Memory" (Engl. Transl.). Appleton-Century-Crofts, New York.

Rolls, E. (1990). Principles underlying the representation and storage of information in neuronal networks in the primate hippocampus and cerebral cortex. *In* "An Introduction to Neural and Electronic Networks" (S. F. Zornetzer, J. L. Davis, and C. Lau, eds.), pp. 73–90. Academic Press, San Diego.

Sagar, H. H., Cohen, N. J., Corkin, S., and Growdon, J. M. (1985). Dissociations among processes in remote memory. *Ann. N. Y. Acad. Sci.* **444**, 533–535.

Sagar, H. H., Cohen, N. J., Sullivan, E. V., Crokin, S. and Growdon, J. M. (1988). Remote memory function in Alzheimer's disease and Parkinson's disease. *Brain* **111**, 185–206.

Salmon, D. P., Zola-Morgan, S., and Squire, L. R. (1987). Retrograde amnesia following combined hippocampus–amygdala lesions in monkeys. *Psychobiology* **15**, 37–47.

Sanders, H. I., and Warrington, E. K. (1971). Memory for remote events in amnesic patients. *Brain* **94**, 661–668.

Schacter, D. L., Cooper, L. A., Tharan, M., and Rubens, A. B. (1991). Preserved priming of novel objects in patients with memory disorders. *J. Cognit. Neurosci.* **3**, 117–130.

Scoville, W. B., and Milner, B. (1957). Loss of recent memory after bilateral hippocampal lesions. *J. Neurol., Neurosurg. Psychiatry* **20**, 11–21.

Shatz, C., and Sretavan, D. W. (1986). Interactions between retinal ganglion cells during the developemnt of the mammalian visual system. *Annu. Rev. Neurosci.* **9**, 171–207.

Singer, W. (1990). Search for coherence: A basic principle of cortical self-organization. *Concepts Neurosci.* **1**, 1–26.

Squire, L. R. (1987). "Memory and Brain." Oxford Univ. Press, New York.

Squire, L. R., and McKee, R. (1992). The influence of prior events on cognitive judgments in amnesia. *J. Exp. Psychol.: Learn. Mem. Cognition* **18**, 106–115.

Squire, L. R., and Spanis, C. W. (1984). Long gradient of retrograde amnesia in mice: Continuity with the findings in humans. *Behav. Neurosci.* **98**, 345–348.

Squire, L. R., and Zola-Morgan, S. (1983). The neurology of memory: The case for correspondence between the findings for human and non-human primate. *In* "The Physiological Basis of Memory" (J. A. Deutsch, ed.), pp. 199–268. Academic Press, New York.

Squire, L. R., and Zola-Morgan, S. (1991). The medial temporal lobe memory system. *Science* **253**, 1380–1386.

Squire, L. R., Slater, P. C., and Chace, P. M. (1975). Retrograde amnesia: Temporal gradient in very long-term memory following electroconvulsive theory. *Science* **187**, 77–79.

Squire, L. R., Cohen, N. J., and Nadel, L. (1984a). The medial temporal region and memory consolidation: A new hypothesis. *In* "Memory Consolidation" (H. Weingartner and E. Parker, eds.), pp. 185–210. Hillsdale, NJ. Erlbaum.

Squire, L. R., Cohen, N. J., and Zouzounis, J. A. (1984b). Preserved memory in retrograde amnesia: Sparing of a recently acquired skill. *Neuropsychologia* **22**, 145–152.

Squire, L. R., Haist, F., and Shimamura, A. P. (1989a). The neurology of memory: Quantitative assessment of retrograde amnesia in two groups of amnesic patients. *J. Neurosci.* **9**, 828–839.

Squire, L. R., Shimamura, A. P., and Amaral, D. G. (1989b). Memory and the hippocampus. *In* "Neural Models of Plasticity" (J. Byrne and W. Berry, eds.), pp. 208–239. Academic Press, San Diego.

Squire, L. R., Amaral, D. G., and Press, G. A. (1990a). Magnetic resonance measurements of hippocampal formation and mammillary nuclei distinguish medial temporal lobe and diencephalic amnesia. *J. Neurosci.* **10**, 3106–3117.

Squire, L. R., Zola-Morgan, S., Cave, C. B., Haist, F., Musen, G., and Suzuki, W. (1990b). Memory: Organization of brain systems and cognition. *Cold Spring Harbor Symp. Quant. Biol.* **55**, 1007–1023.

Squire, L. R., Knowlton, B., and Musen, G. (1993). The structure and organization of memory. *Annu. Rev. Psychol.* **44**, 453–495.

Stuss, D. T., Guberman, A., Nelson, R., and Larochelle, S. (1988). The neuropsychology of paramedian thalamic infarction. *Brain Cognition* **8**, 348–378.

Teyler, T. J., and Discenna, P. (1986). The hippocampal memory indexing theory. *Behav. Neurosci.* **100**, 147.

Tulving, E., and Schacter, D. L. (1990). Priming and human memory systems. *Science* **247**, 301–396.

Tulving, E., Schacter, D. L., McLachlan, D., and Moscovitch, M. (1988). Priming of semantic autobiographical knowledge: A case study of retrograde amnesia. *Brain Cognition* **8**, 3–20.

Warrington, E. K., and McCarthy, R. A. (1988). The fractionation of retrograde amnesia. *Brain Cognition* **7**, 184–200.

Weiskrantz, L., and Warrington, E. K. (1979). Conditioning in amnesic patients. *Neuropsychologia* **17**, 187–194.

Wilder, B. J. (1972). Projection phenomena and secondary epileptogenesis—Mirror foci. *In* "Experimental Models of Epilepsy" (D. Purpura, J. Penry, D. Tower, D. Woodbury, and R. Walter, eds.), pp. 85–111. Raven Press, New York.

Wilson, R. S., Kaszniak, A. W., and Fox, J. H. (1981). Remote memory in senile dementia. *Cortex* **17**, 41–48.

Winocur, G. (1990). Anterograde and retrograde amnesia in rats with dorsal hippocampal or dorsomedial thalamic lesions. *Behav. Brain Res.* **38**, 145–154.

Zola-Morgan, S., and Squire, L. R. (1990a). The primate hippocampal formation: Evidence for a time-limited role in memory storage. *Science* **250**, 288–290.

Zola-Morgan, S., and Squire, L. R. (1990b). Neuropsychological investigations of memory and amnesia: Findings from humans and nonhuman primates. *In* "The Development and Neural Basis of Higher Cognitive Function" (A. Diamond, ed.), pp. 434–456. N. Y. Acad. Sci., New York.

Zola-Morgan, S., Squire, L. R., and Amaral, D. G. (1986). Human amnesia and the medial temporal region: Enduring memory impairment following a bilateral lesion limited to field CA1 of the hippocampus. *J. Neurosci.* **6**, 2950–2967.

IMPLICIT KNOWLEDGE: NEW PERSPECTIVES ON UNCONSCIOUS PROCESSES*

Daniel L. Schacter

Department of Psychology
Harvard University
Cambridge, Massachusetts 02138

I. Introduction

Recent evidence from cognitive science and neuroscience indicates that brain-damaged patients and normal subjects can exhibit nonconscious or implicit knowledge of stimuli that they fail to recollect consciously or perceive explicitly. Dissociations between implicit and explicit knowledge, which have been observed across a variety of domains, tasks, and materials, raise fundamental questions about the nature of perception, memory, and consciousness. This article provides a selective review of relevant evidence and considers phenomena such as priming and implicit memory in amnesic patients and normal subjects, perception without awareness and "blindsight" in patients with damage to visual cortex, and nonconscious recognition of familiar faces in patients with facial-recognition deficits (prosopagnosia). A variety of theoretical approaches to implicit/explicit dissociations are considered. One view is that all of the various dissociations can be attributed to disruption or disconnection of a common mechanism underlying conscious experience; an alternative possibility is that each dissociation requires a separate explanation in terms of domain-specific processes and systems. More generally, it is concluded that rather than reflecting the operation of affectively charged unconscious processes of the kind invoked by psychodynamic or Freudian theorists, dissociations between implicit and explicit

* This article has been reprinted from PNAS (1992). **89**, 11113–11117.

271

knowledge are a natural consequence of the ordinary computations of the brain.

Consider the following two clinical scenarios. In the first, a patient with memory problems is shown a list of familiar words and several minutes later is unable to remember any of the list items when asked to recollect them; indeed, he denies that a list of words had been presented. But when he is required to perform an incidental test that does not require conscious recollection of the list, the patient's performance indicates perfectly normal retention of the previously studied words. In the second scenario, a patient with perceptual problems is exposed to a bright visual stimulus and claims to see nothing. Yet when asked to "guess" in which of two locations the stimulus appeared, the patient performs well above the chance level, indicating that she has in some sense "seen"—despite the absence of conscious experience—the target stimulus.

The foregoing scenarios may seem surprising and even bizarre: How can a patient exhibit memory without remembering or perception without perceiving? It is tempting to suggest that the patients suffer from psychiatric problems or, perhaps, are engaging in outright deception of the examiner. On the contrary, however, these two scenarios represent examples of what have become almost commonplace observations in the neuropsychological laboratory and are often referred to as dissociations between explicit and implicit knowledge (1). *Explicit* knowledge refers to knowledge that is expressed as conscious experience and that people are aware that they possess; the everyday uses of such terms as "seeing" and "remembering" refer to explicit knowledge. *Implicit* knowledge, by contrast, refers to knowledge that is revealed in task performance without any corresponding phenomenal awareness; implicit knowledge is often expressed unintentionally and tapped indirectly. Far from reflecting psychiatric symptoms or dissimulation, dissociations between explicit and implicit knowledge are providing important new insights into the fundamental nature of perception, memory, and conscious experience.

The terms explicit and implicit knowledge are quite similar in meaning to conscious and unconscious knowledge, and the two sets of terms can be used interchangeably. However, traditional conceptions of unconscious knowledge have been tied closely to Freudian and other psychodynamic constructs such as repression, drive, conflict, and the like. As this article should make evident, these concepts have little relevance to the kinds of phenomena that have been the subject of recent neuropsychological and cognitive studies. Because the classical notion of the "unconscious" is so closely linked to psychodynamic ideas, it seems prudent to use terminology that is not similarly burdened [for more extended discussion, see Greenwald (2)].

The article provides a selective overview of research that has documented and explored dissociations between explicit and implicit knowledge. It will focus primarily on explicit/implicit dissociations in patients with memory disorders and perceptual disorders, although similar phenomena that have been documented in other patient populations will also be noted. In addition, some attention will be paid to analogous dissociations that have been produced in cognitive studies of normal, non-brain-damaged subjects. The article will conclude by surveying theoretical accounts of the various dissociations and by considering whether these diverse phenomena depend on similar underlying mechanisms. Taken together, the neuropsychological and cognitive evidence suggests that, rather than reflecting the operation of affectively charged psychodynamic processes, many implicit or unconscious expressions of knowledge occur as a relatively routine consequence of the ordinary computations of the brain.

II. Memory Disorders

The most extensively studied neurological disorder of memory is known as the *amnesic syndrome*, which occurs as a consequence of various kinds of pathological conditions (e.g., stroke, encephalitis, anoxia) that produce damage to medial temporal and diencephalic brain regions (3,4). Amnesic patients are characterized by a marked inability to remember recent experiences together with normal perception and intelligence. Their memory disorders are evident on a variety of explicit memory tests, including free recall, wherein patients attempt to retrieve recently presented items without the aid of experimenter-provided cues; cued recall, wherein various cues or hints are provided to assist recollection; and recognition, wherein previously studied items are presented together with new items, and subjects indicate which item they recollect from the study list.

Despite their severe impairments in explicitly remembering recently presented information, it has been established beyond dispute that amnesic patients can show intact implicit memory for aspects of the same information. One of the most intensively studied implicit memory phenomena in amnesia is known as repetition or direct *priming*: the facilitated ability to identify, or make judgments about, target stimuli as a consequence of a recent exposure to them (5). In a typical priming experiment, subjects are shown a list of familiar words and are later given an apparently unrelated test that does not require explicit memory for the study list. For example, on a stem completion test, subjects would be given three-letter word beginnings (e.g., T-A-B--) and asked to complete them with the first word that comes to mind. Half of the stems could be completed with words that had appeared previously on the study list (e.g., TABLE), and the other half could not be completed with words from the study list. Priming is said to occur when subjects provide the target completion more frequently to stems that represent studied words than to stems that represent nonstudied words. Early studies by Warrington and Weiskrantz (6) indicated that amnesic patients show what we would now call normal priming effects on the stem-completion task despite poor explicit memory, although Warrington and Weiskrantz did not refer to the phenomenon as priming. Subsequent experiments confirmed and extended the finding of normal stem-completion priming in amnesia and also revealed that amnesics exhibit normal priming effects on a variety of other implicit memory tasks [7–12; for review, see Shimamura (13)].

Recent research has extended further the boundaries of the priming phenomenon. In early experiments, the target items presented for study were well-learned materials, such as familiar words, that exist in memory before the experiment. Thus, it was possible to argue that priming effects in amnesic patients reflect the temporary activation of preexisting memory representations (7,14). However, it has now been established that amnesic patients can show intact priming for novel information that does not have a preexisting memory representation, including pseudowords (e.g., "numdy") 15,16) and nonverbal materials, such as novel objects or patterns (17–20). It has also been shown that priming effects in amnesia can be quite long-lived, lasting across retention intervals of days, weeks, or months (21–23).

Research on priming effects in amnesic patients has been complemented by a large and ever-increasing literature on normal subjects, indicating that priming can be dissociated sharply from explicit memory (24–26). One particularly important finding is that priming effects on various implicit memory tests are relatively unaffected by manipulations of how subjects encode target materials during study-list presentation. For example, when subjects are induced to process the semantic attributes of words at the time of study (e.g., make judgments about a word's meaning), their recollection of the word on subsequent explicit memory tests is generally much higher than when they are induced to process nonsemantic physical features of the target words (e.g., count the number of vowels in a word). But the magnitude of priming effects is similar following the two kinds of study tasks (20,27,28). Moreover, the priming effect appears to be modality specific: it is reduced by study-to-test changes in visual or auditory modality of presentation (28,29). Under certain circumstances, priming is even reduced by study-to-test changes in the particular type font or case in which a word appears (30,31) or the voice in which a word is spoken (32). These kinds of observations, taken together with the amnesia data, have led to a vigorous debate concerning the psychological and neurophysiological processes and systems that subserve priming and explicit memory, respectively (3,25,33).

Priming is not, however, the only example of preserved implicit memory in amnesic patients. It has been known since the classic studies of Milner and Corkin and their colleagues (34) that amnesic patients can acquire new motor skills across numerous training sessions, and it is now clear that they can gradually acquire perceptual and cognitive skills as well (35–37). Amnesics have also exhibited normal implicit learning of the rules of an artificial grammar (38) and a complex spatio-temporal sequence (39) and have proved capable of acquiring classically conditioned responses (40,41). Severely amnesic patients have even been able to learn (although not at a normal rate) the complex knowledge and skills needed to operate and program a computer and have exhibited robust retention of such knowledge over delays of 5–9 months (42,43)—despite little or no explicit memory for their learning experiences.

Some of this work on implicit memory for complex knowledge and skills has a parallel in—and, in fact, was inspired by—studies of normal subjects. For example, Reber has reported a series of studies over the past 25 years (44,45) that have provided evidence for implicit learning of grammatical rules: after exposure to a list of consonant strings that are ordered according to the complex rules of an artificial grammar, subjects can later distinguish novel grammatical strings from novel non-grammatical strings, even though the subjects are unable to articulate the nature of the rule [for a critique, see Dulaney et al.(46)]. Similarly, Lewicki and colleagues (47) have provided evidence that subjects can learn complex patterns and contingencies despite poor explicit knowledge of them.

Taken together, the data from amnesic patients and normal subjects indicate clearly that memory for various kinds of experiences can be expressed independently from, and in the absence of, conscious recollection of those experiences.

III. Perceptual Disorders

At about the same time that early evidence was accumulating on implicit memory in amnesic patients, there were reports of a puzzling

and, in some respects, analogous phenomenon in patients with disturbances of visual perception. Initially documented by Poppel, Held, and
Frost (48), the phenomenon was referred to as "blindsight" by Weiskrantz
and colleagues (49), in reference to the seemingly paradoxical nature of
the visual behavior exhibited by certain patients with lesions to primary
(striate) visual cortex. Such patients appeared to be "blind" in the sense
that they denied seeing a stimulus presented in certain parts of the visual
field. But when asked to guess about the location or other attributes of
the same stimulus, the patients exhibited "sight" in the sense that their
guessing performance was well above chance and sometimes nearly
perfect.

The experimental paradigm used most frequently to demonstrate
blindsight involves requiring patients to localize a stimulus presented in
the blind field, either by pointing to or reaching toward the target location
or by making a verbal response. Blindsight can also be exhibited when
patients are asked to make visual discriminations about other kinds of
targets by guessing, including simple figures (e.g., X vs. O) and line
orientations (e.g., horizontal vs. vertical). However, Perenin and
Jeannerod (50) failed to find evidence for pattern discrimination, and
Weiskrantz (51) has suggested that orientation discrimination is more
fully preserved than form discrimination in blindsight patients. Finally,
blindsight has also been demonstrated by using experimental paradigms
in which information presented in the blind field influences patients'
perceptions of, and responses to, information presented in the sighted
field (52).

One of the most intriguing questions about blindsight concerns exactly what patients experience when they respond accurately to stimuli
presented in the blind field and how these "perceptions" differ from
those of conscious visual experience. Although it is most often reported
that patients claim to see nothing and are merely guessing, it has also
been reported that some patients occasionally describe a rather primitive
visual awareness of a target. For example, a patient studied by Weiskrantz
(51) claimed to sense "a definite pinpoint of light" but when probed
further insisted that it did not "actually look like a light [but]...nothing
at all" (51, p. 378). It has also been reported that with extensive practice
and training, patients can develop a heightened awareness of stimuli in
their blind fields (51,53). In view of this evidence, some critics have
suggested that rather than representing implicit or nonconscious perception of target stimuli, blindsight can be attributed to cautious responding
on the basis of degraded (but conscious) vision that is produced by
scattered light (54). However, such explanations have difficulty accom-
modating various kinds of evidence (1,55).

Recent research has revealed implicit perceptual knowledge in other kinds of brain-damaged patients that is, in some respects, similar to that observed in blindsight. One particularly striking example comes from the study of *visual form agnosia*, a disorder in which patients have difficulty perceiving and recognizing virtually all kinds of visual objects. Goodale, *et al.* (56) described a patient who was severely impaired in making judgments about the width of three-dimensional objects but made entirely normal motor adjustments of hand position as she reached toward a target object; the positioning of her finger–thumb grip varied directly as a function of the object's width despite her impairment of conscious perception.

There has also been a good deal of recent research on implicit knowledge in patients with *prosopagnosia*—the impaired ability to recognize familiar faces, usually because of bilateral lesions to occipito-temporal cortex. Although such patients typically deny any familiarity with faces that ordinarily would be well known to them (e.g., a spouse or relative), there is now considerable evidence that they possess implicit knowledge of those faces. Early evidence was provided in a psychophysiological study by Bauer (57), in which a prosopagnosic patient viewed a familiar face and at the same time listened to the experimenter read a series of names; one belonged to the face and the others did not. Despite failing to recognize the face explicitly, the patient showed a maximal skin conductance response to the correct name. Tranel and Damasio (58) replicated and extended this phenomenon using a different paradigm for eliciting the skin-conductance responses to familiar faces that their patient failed to recognize explicitly.

Young and De Haan and their colleagues have provided a systematic series of studies using behavioral measures to demonstrate and explore implicit facial familiarity in prosopagnosic patients (59). For example, they reported the case of a patient who performed at chance levels when required to choose which of two faces (one famous, one unknown) was familiar. However, when given a matching task in which subjects judged whether two simultaneously exposed faces were the same or different, the patient—just like normal control subjects—responded more quickly when the two faces were famous than when they were unknown. Similarly, they also found that the patient was slower to learn a name–face pairing when a familiar face was paired with an incorrect name than when it was paired with a correct name, even though he claimed that none of the faces were familiar; and presentation of a famous face that was unfamiliar to the patient speeded up his ability to make judgments about verbal information associated with the face (e.g., seeing a photo of Prince Charles facilitated his response to the name Princess Diana).

Interestingly, Young and colleagues have reported another case in which the patient failed to show evidence for implicit knowledge of unrecognized faces [see also Humphreys *et al.* (60)].

The data from blindsight, visual form agnosia, and prosopagnosia indicate clearly that conditions exist in which some patients can show implicit knowledge of visual stimuli that they fail either to perceive or to recognize explicitly. Cognitive research with normal, non-brain-damaged subjects has long been concerned with the possible existence of "perception without awareness" or "subliminal perception." Early research in this area was fraught with methodological difficulties and marked by controversy (2,61). Although some of the confusion still persists in contemporary work, a number of findings and ideas have emerged during the past decade that have helped to clarify the sense in which, and extent to which, perception without awareness can be said to exist.

In a typical paradigm for studying perception without awareness, two kinds of evidence are provided: (1) explicit or direct measures that are used to document subjects' failure to perceive a stimulus consciously and (2) implicit or indirect measures that reveal an impact of the undetected stimulus on some aspect of performance. For example, in a semantic priming paradigm, the subject may claim that he or she fails to detect the presence of the word chair when it is flashed briefly and obscured by a visual mask; but the subject will nevertheless be faster to identify or make a judgment about the related word table when it is presented immediately after the word chair than when it is presented after a semantically unrelated word (62). The existence of a semantic priming effect suggests that subjects have, indeed, registered some features of the target stimulus despite the apparent absence of conscious perception.

Why has research of this kind been dogged by controversy? As Merikle (63, p. 792) has stated, the controversy "has centered on the issue, What constitutes an adequate behavioral measure of conscious perceptual experience? Depending upon one's answer to this question, the evidence for perception without awareness is either overwhelming or nonexistent." Cheesman and Merikle (64) proposed a useful distinction between *subjective* and *objective* measures of conscious perception. Subjective measures typically involve a person's verbal statement that he or she does not detect the presence of a target stimulus, as in the foregoing example. Objective measures, by contrast, typically involve tasks such as forced-choice judgment in which subjects must choose between the presented stimulus and a nonpresented alternative, even when they feel that they are just guessing. As Merikle (63) points out, if one accepts as valid subjective measures of conscious perception, then the evidence for perception without awareness is strong (e.g., there is evidence for semantic priming from stimuli that subjects claim that they do not see); if one insists on an objective measure, however, then the evidence is weak or nonexistent (e.g., there is little evidence of semantic priming from stimuli about which subjects are unable to make accurate forced-choice discriminations).

Although the intricacies of this debate are beyond the purview of the present article, it is worth noting that the distinction between objective and subjective measures of conscious perception has implications for our understanding of neuropsychological phenomena, such as blindsight. In the blindsight literature, failures of conscious perception are typically inferred from subjective measures; patients claim that they do not see a target stimulus. Moreover, evidence for *implicit knowledge* or *nonconscious* perception is frequently inferred from above-chance performance on a forced-choice test in which the patient claims to be guessing—precisely the kind of test that some would refer to as an objective measure of *conscious* perception! To make matters even more complex, chance-level performance on forced-choice tests has been taken as evidence for an absence of conscious perception in some studies of implicit or covert recognition in prosopagnosia (59). Merikle (63) has delineated several reasons why it probably makes sense to accept data from subjective measures as evidence for failure of conscious perception. Nevertheless, it seems clear that careful attention must be paid to possible differences in underlying mechanisms when implicit knowledge is inferred from failures on subjective or objective measure of conscious perception, respectively.

IV. Additional Neuropsychological Evidence for Implicit Knowledge

Although most of the work on implicit knowledge in neuropsychological syndromes has involved disorders of memory and perception, similar kinds of evidence have been gleaned from patients with a variety of neuropsychological deficits. Milberg and Blumstein (65) and their colleagues, for example, have studied aphasic patients who exhibit severe deficits on explicit tests of language comprehension and yet show robust semantic priming effects for words that they fail to understand explicitly. Tyler (66) has described other kinds of aphasic patients who are unable to make explicit judgments about the meaning and grammaticality of sentences. But the performance of these patients on a target-monitoring task was disrupted by semantic and grammatical violations, and the pattern of disruption was similar to that observed in normal control subjects.

Evidence for implicit knowledge has also been seen in studies of patients with reading disorders, who appear able to make judgments about properties of words that they cannot identify consciously (67). And observations suggestive of implicit knowledge have been reported in patients who exhibit spatial neglect, associative agnosia, and unawareness of deficit (1).

V. Theories and Mechanisms

The seemingly ubiquitous evidence for preserved implicit knowledge despite impaired explicit knowledge across a variety of patient groups, experimental tasks, and knowledge domains is compelling. Moreover, the converging evidence in several instances from studies of non-brain-damaged subjects indicates that the basic phenomenon is characteristic of normal cognitive function and is not some sort of exotic curiosity that occurs only in pathological conditions. What are we to make of these striking and counterintuitive phenomena? Although current theoretical understanding of them is rather modest, several different approaches can be distinguished.

The "family resemblance" among the various implicit/explicit dissociations across a variety of conditions has suggested to some that it is appropriate to seek a common explanation for them. For instance, Schacter *et al.* (1), speculated that a common mechanism may underlie conscious experiences of perceiving, knowing, and remembering—a high-level system that takes as its input the extensively processed output of perceptual and semantic representation systems and that must be activated for phenomenal awareness in different domains (68). They suggested further that this mechanism can become selectively disconnected from individual brain modules that process and represent particular kinds of information. If such modules continue to function relatively normally, then the information on which they operate could affect performance and behavior implicitly, without any corresponding phenomenal awareness. A disconnection account of this kind seems to fit well with the neuropsychological data because patients do not suffer from generalized impairments of conscious experience; their problems with explicit knowledge are domain specific (55). One difficulty with this approach, however, is that it implies the existence of a "consciousness module" despite the paucity of experimental evidence for such a model. Another approach to a common explanation for a variety of implicit/explicit dissociations has been put forward by Edelman (69), who suggested that they may be attributable to selective dysfunctions of *reentrant loops*—connections among brain regions that, when activated, are ordinarily responsible for particular kinds of conscious experiences of perceiving, knowing, and remembering. This approach represents a parsimonious attempt to accommodate numerous implicit/explicit dissociations without postulating a consciousness module, but there is, as yet, no direct empirical support for it.

In contrast to these attempts to develop a single account for a variety of phenomena, other researchers have focused on individual implicit/explicit dissociations. For example, a number of investigators have suggested that priming, skill learning, and other manifestations of implicit memory reflect the activity of memory systems that are spared in amnesic patients. These systems can function independently of the memory system that ordinarily supports explicit memory, depends on the integrity of the hippocampus and related structures, and is impaired in amnesia (3,4,35,70). To illustrate, it has been suggested that priming depends on changes in early-stage perceptual representation systems that preserve information about the form and structure, but not the meaning and associated properties, of words and objects (5,33,70,71). Neuropsychological and neuroimaging evidence indicates that such systems depend on posterior cortical structures (33,72), which is consistent with the proposal that they can function normally in amnesic patients. Although experience-induced changes in perceptual representation systems can provide a basis for facilitated identification of degraded words and objects, they do not provide access to the kind of contextual and associative information that is important for conscious recollection and that appears to depend on the hippocampus and related structures. Thus, by this view priming and explicit remembering depend on different underlying memory systems.

An important observation supporting this kind of multiple memory systems account is that amnesic patients typically exhibit *normal* levels of implicit memory despite severely impaired explicit memory; accordingly, it makes sense to postulate that independent brain systems support the two forms of memory. By contrast, in the other neuropsychological syndromes discussed in this article, patients typically do not exhibit entirely normal performance on tasks that tap implicit knowledge, so it is more difficult to argue that independent brain systems underlie explicit and implicit knowledge [for discussion of the "multiple visual systems" approach to blindsight, see Weiskrantz (55), Goodale *et al.* (56), and Cowey and Stoerig (73)]. For example, Wallace and Farah (74) have suggested that, in some cases of prosopagnosia, residual implicit knowledge may be a natural consequence of impairment to the facial processing system that normally supports explicit knowledge. They noted that in simulations of prosopagnosia with a neural network, when "lesions" are made to a part of the network that supports facial recognition, the network still shows some residual ability to "perform" tasks analogous to those used to demonstrate implicit facial knowledge in prosopagnosic patients. This kind of observation is consistent with the idea that when patients exhibit some, but not normal, levels of implicit knowledge, the effect may be attributable to the impaired functioning of a damaged system that normally supports explicit knowledge.

Because research in this area is still in its infancy, it is too early to state confidently whether a unified theoretical account of different implicit/explicit dissociations will be possible or whether it will be necessary to construct separate domain-specific theories for each particular kind of dissociation. Current evidence does suggest, however, that demonstrations of fully intact implicit memory in amnesic patients probably demand a different kind of explanation compared to explanations of demonstrations of residual (but not normal) implicit knowledge in blindsight, prosopagnosia, and other syndromes.

Whatever the ultimate theoretical account of implicit/explicit dissociations, the fact that these phenomena can be observed in normal subjects as well as neurological populations indicates that they are not exotic or unusual symptoms that represent pathological consequences of brain damage. Nor are these dissociations intimately intertwined with emotional conflicts or psychodynamic processes (e.g., repression) that were crucial to postulation of the Freudian unconscious (75). Rather, dissociations between implicit and explicit knowledge seem to arise as a natural consequence of the functional architecture of the brain and reflect the activity of computations that are routinely performed during the course of perceiving, recognizing, and remembering. A major challenge for future research is to understand more deeply the properties of the architecture and the nature of the computations responsible for dissociations between implicit and explicit knowledge.

References

1. Schacter, D. L., McAndrews, M. P., and Moscovitch, M. (1988). In "Thought Without Language" (L. Weiskrantz, ed.), pp. 242–278. Clarendon, Oxford.
2. Greenwald, A. G. (1992). Am. Psychol. **47,** 766–779.
3. Squire, L. R. (1992). Psychol. Rev. **99,** 195–231.
4. Weiskrantz, L. (1985). In "Memory Systems of the Human Brain: Animal and Human Cognitive Processes" (N. M. Weinberger, J. L. McGaugh, and G. Lynch, eds.), pp. 380–415. Guilford Press, New York.

5. Tulving, E., and Schacter, D. L. (1990). *Science* **247**, 301–306.
6. Warrington, E. K., and Weiskrantz, L. (1974). *Neuropsychologia* **12**, 419–428.
7. Graf, P., Squire, L. R., and Mandler, G. (1984). *J. Exp. Psychol.: Learn., Mem., Cognition* **10**, 164–178.
8. Cermak, L. S., Talbot, N., Chandler, K., and Wolbarst, L. R. (1985). *Neuropsychologia* **23**, 615–622.
9. Jacoby, L. L., and Witherspoon, D. (1982). *Can. J. Psychol.* **36**, 300–324.
10. Moscovitch, M. (1982). *In* "Human Memory and Amnesia" (L. S. Cermak, ed.), pp. 337–370. Erlbaum, Hillsdale, NJ.
11. Shimamura, A. P., and Squire, L. R. (1984). *J. Exp. Psychol., Gen.* **113**, 556–570.
12. Schacter, D. L. (1985). *Ann. N.Y. Acad. Sci.* **444**, 44–53.
13. Shimamura, A. P. (1986). *Q. J. Exp. Psychol.* **38A**, 619–644.
14. Rozin, P. (1976). *In* "Neural Mechanisms of Learning and Memory" (M. R. Rosenzweig and E. L. Bennet, eds.), pp. 3–48. MIT Press, Cambridge, MA.
15. Cermak, L. S., Bleich, R. P., and Blackford, M. (1988). *Brain Cognition* **7**, 145–156.
16. Haist, F., Musen, G. and Squire, L. R. (1991). *Psychobiology* **19**, 275–285.
17. Gabrieli, J. D. E., Milberg, W., Keane, M. M., and Corkin, S. (1990). *Neuropsychologia* **28**, 417–428.
18. Musen, G., and Squire, L. R. (1992). *Mem. Cognition* **20**, 441–448.
19. Schacter, D. L., Cooper, L. A., Tharan, M., and Rubens, A. B. (1991). *J. Cognit. Neurosci.* **3**, 118–131.
20. Bowers, J. S., and Schacter, D. L. (1994). *In* "Implicit Memory: New Directions in Cognition, Neuropsychology, and Development" (P. Graf and M. E. J. Masson, eds.). Academic Press, San Diego (in press).
21. Cave, C. B., and Squire, L. R. (1992). *J. Exp. Psychol.: Learn., Mem., Cognition* **18**, 509–520.
22. MacAndrews, M. P., Glisky, E. L., and Schacter, D. L. (1987). *Neuropsychologia* **25**, 497–506.
23. Tulving, E., Hayman, C. A. G., and MacDonald, C. (1991). *J. Exp. Psychol.: Learn., Mem., Cognition* **17**, 595–617.
24. Richardson-Klavehn, A., and Bjork, R. A. (1988). *Annu. Rev. Psychol.* **36**, 475–543.
25. Roediger, H. L., III (1990). *Am. Psychol.* **45**, 1043–1056.
26. Schacter, D. L. (1987). *J. Exp. Psychol.: Learn., Mem., Cognition* **13**, 501–518.
27. Graf, P., Mandler, G., and Haden, P. (1982). *Science* **218**, 1243–1244.
28. Jacoby, L. L., and Dallas, M. (1981). *J. Exp. Psychol., Gen.* **110**, 306–340.
29. Roediger, H. L., III, and Blaxton, T. A. (1987). *Mem. Cognition* **15**, 379–388.
30. Graf, P., and Ryan, L. (1990). *J. Exp. Psychol.: Learn., Mem., Cognition* **16**, 978–992.
31. Marsolek, C. J., Kosslyn, S. M., and Squire, L. R. (1992). *J. Exp. Psychol.: Learn., Mem., Cognition* **18**, 492–508.
32. Schacter, D. L., and Church, B. (1992). *J. Exp. Psychol.: Learn., Mem., Cognition* **18**, 915–930.
33. Schacter, D. L. (1992). *Am. Psychol.* **47**, 559–569.
34. Milner, B., Corkin, S., and Teuber, H. L. (1968). *Neuropsychologia* **6**, 215–234.
35. Cohen, N. J., and Squire, L. R. (1980). *Science* **210**, 207–210.
36. Saint-Cyr, J. A., Taylor, A. E., and Lang, A. E. (1988). *Brain* **111**, 94–959.
37. Squire, L. R., and Frambach, M. (1990). *Psychobiology* **18**, 109–117.
38. Knowlton, B. J., Ramus, S. J., and Squire, L. R. (1992). *Psychol. Sci.* **3**, 172–179.
39. Nissen, M. J., and Bullemer, P. (1987). *Cognit. Psychol.* **19**, 1–32.
40. Daum, I., Channon, S., and Canavar, A. (1989). *J. Neurol., Neurosurg. Psychiatry* **52**, 47–51.

41. Weiskrantz, L., and Warrington, E. K. (1979). *Neuropsychologia* **17**, 187–194.
42. Glisky, E. L., and Schacter, D. L. (1988). *Neuropsychologia* **26**, 173–178.
43. Glisky, E. L., and Schacter, D. L. (1989). *Neuropsychologia* **27**, 107–120.
44. Reber, A. S. (1967). *J. Verbal Learn. Verbal Behav.* **6**, 855–863.
45. Reber, A. S. (1989). *J. Exp. Psychol., Gen.* **118**, 219–235.
46. Dulaney, D. E., Carlson, R. A., and Dewey, G. I. (1984). *J. Exp. Psychol., Gen.* **113**, 541–555.
47. Lewicki, P., Hill, T., and Czyzewska, M. (1992). *Am. Psychol.* **47**, 796–801.
48. Poppel, E., Held, R., and Frost, D. (1973). *Nature (London)* **243**, 2295–2296.
49. Weiskrantz, L., Warrington, E. K., Sanders, M. D., and Marshall, J. (1974). *Brain* **97**, 709–728.
50. Perenin, M. T., and Jeannerod, M. (1978). *Neuropsychologia* **16**, 1–13.
51. Weiskrantz, L. (1980). *Q. J. Exp. Psychol.* **32**, 365–386.
52. Torjussen, T. (1978). *Neuropsychologia* **16**, 15–21.
53. Zihl, J. (1980). *Neuropsychologia* **18**, 71–77.
54. Campion, J., Latto, R., and Smith, Y. M. (1983). *Behav. Brain Sci.* **6**, 423–486.
55. Weiskrantz, L. (1986). "Blindsight." Clarendon, Oxford.
56. Goodale, M. A., Milner, A. D., Jakobson, L. S., and Carey, D. P. (1991). *Nature (London)* **349**, 154–156.
57. Bauer, R. M. (1984). *Neuropsychologia* **22**, 457–469.
58. Tranel, D., and Damasio, A. R. (1985). *Science* **228**, 1453–1454.
59. Young, A. W., and De Haan, E. H. F. (1992). *In* "The Neuropsychology of Consciousness" (A. D. Milner and M. D. Rugg, eds.), pp. 69–90. Academic Press, San Diego.
60. Humphreys, G. W., Troscianko, T., Riddoch, M. J., Boucart, M., Donnelly, N., and Harding, G. F. A. (1992). *In* "The Neuropsychology of Consciousness" (A. D. Milner and M. D. Rugg, eds.), pp. 39–68. Academic Press, San Diego.
61. Holender, D. (1986). *Behav. Brain Sci.* **9**, 1–23.
62. Marcel, A. J. (1983). *Cognit. Psychol.* **15**, 197–237.
63. Merikle, P. M. (1992). *Am. Psychol.* **47**, 792–795.
64. Cheesman, J., and Merikle, P. M. (1986). *Can. J. Psychol.* **40**, 343–367.
65. Milberg, W., and Blumstein, S. E. (1981). *Brain Lang.* **14**, 371–385.
66. Tyler, L. K. (1992). *In* "The Neuropsychology of Consciousness" (A. D. Milner and M. D. Rugg, eds.), pp. 159–178. Academic Press, San Diego.
67. Shallice, T., and Saffran, E. M. (1986). *Cognit. Neuropsychol.* **3**, 429–458.
68. Schacter, D. L. (1989). *In* "Varieties of Memory and Consciousness" (H. L. Roediger, III and F. I. M. Craik, eds.), pp. 355–389. Erlbaum, Hillsdale, NJ.
69. Edelman, G. (1991). "Bright Air, Brilliant Fire: On the Matter of the Mind." Basic Books, New York.
70. Schacter, D. L. (1992). *J. Cognit. Neurosci.* **4**, 244–256.
71. Schacter, D. L. (1990). *Ann. N.Y. Acad. Sci.* **608**, 543–571.
72. Squire, L. R., Ojemann, J. G., Miezin, F. M., Petersen, S. E., Videen, T. O., and Raichle, M. E. (1992). *Proc. Natl. Acad. Sci. U.S.A.* **89**, 1837–1841.
73. Cowey, A., and Stoerig, P. (1992). *In* "The Neuropsychology of Consciousness" (A. D. Milner and M. D. Rugg, eds.), pp. 11–37. Academic Press, San Diego.
74. Wallace, M. A., and Farah, M. J. (1992). *J. Cognit. Neurosci.* **4**, 150–154.
75. Kihlström, J. (1987). *Science* **237**, 1445–1452.

SECTION IV
DISCUSSION

Virtually no other aspect of brain function has attracted as much attention from psychologists and neuroscientists as the nature of memory. By the same token, no other neuroscientific problem has fueled so much fierce debate, often placing the opponents in ideological camps with names such as "holism" or "localizationism." Everyone agrees that memory involves some kind of structural change ("storage") somewhere in the brain; however, opinions differ widely on what is stored where, and for how long, or how the stored traces are accessed. Can selectionism offer a new and fresh perspective?

There is an important connection between memory and categorization. The way animals or humans categorize stimuli in their environments has a deep impact on the way memory is stored and accessed in their nervous systems. How are categories structured and how are they represented in the brain? Solutions to this problem have been cast in both localizationist or antilocalizationist terms. A protagonist of the localizationist position would claim that the sensory information about a stimulus item, after going through distinct processing stages, comes together in a particular part of the nervous system. In an extreme case, every stimulus (or stimulus class) would excite its particular dedicated part of the nervous system. The activation of that part (ultimately the infamous "grandmother cell") would then signal the presence of a stimulus item of a particular class. Most localizationist theories are also hierarchical; processing of the sensory input occurs sequentially in defined and largely autonomous stages, each of which in turn occupies a circumscribed area of the brain. Localizationism also implies that memory is based on sets of distinct, independently accessible and generally nonisomorphic traces. This view of memory may be called replicative memory, and it faces a number of theoretical problems that are closely linked to the ones facing single-cell theories of perception (discussed in more detail in Section III). Opposing this view, a distributionist would claim that the perception of a stimulus does not, in general, involve the activation of a stimulus-specific (or class-specific) part of the brain. Instead, many parts of the brain subserve perceptual tasks in an overlapping manner, and the activity patterns in response to stimuli are distributed throughout these parts. Distributionist theories are often (but not always) heterarchical and put less emphasis on the distinctness of levels in sensory processing. Some distributionist theories still assume replicative memory: recall works by addressing distinct but distributed traces that are laid down or stored at multiple places in the nervous system. Nonreplicative theories of memory are always distributionist, because they always assume that memory involves the activation of large sets of neurons. Nonreplicative memory theories stress the interrelationships between stored items, their preservation in the representational structure, and the continuity (in fact indistriminability) of storage and recall processes. In the context of categorization, nonreplicative memory stresses the procedural character of memory; it refers to the enhanced ability of the animal to categorize stimuli in its environment. Memory, in short, is recategorization, not exact replication.

On the basis of this view of memory, we may attempt to sketch out some basic properties of the proposed neural "representational" structure of categories in the nervous system. (Differing from its use in cognitive science, the term "representation" simply refers to that part of the nervous system that responds when presented with stimulus items belonging to a particular category.) Neural representations of natural categories are *nonsymbolic* (there is no message-passing between neurons along labeled lines), *distributed* (across functionally differentiated brain regions, with integration, generalization, and association achieved by reentrant links), *gradually emerging* (depending on synaptic changes accumulating during perceptual experience), *dynamic* (due to inherent temporal dynamics and ongoing synaptic changes leading to constant reorganization and readjustment), and *polymorphic* and *degenerate* (due to the "family resemblance" structure of perceptual categories).

This last point deserves a brief comment. There is a relationship between polymorphism (in the internal structure of categories) and degeneracy (of the responding elements in the nervous system). Degeneracy is one of the key properties of the basic units in a selective system. It allows these units to respond over a wide range of stimuli. In a selective categorizing system, the responding elements that have been selected to comprise a neural representation of a given category will tend to respond to a subset of members of this category, but some will continue also to respond to nonmembers. This degeneracy of responses across category boundaries is important for the maintenance of variability to allow further selective events to take place, as well as the creation of superordinate categories within the framework of an overall taxonomical order. In addition, the degenerate structure of neural representations naturally preserves individual characteristics of sensory stimuli, while at the same time permitting classification due to their family resemblance structure.

The synthetic neural models discussed by George Reeke (designed along the lines of known neuroanatomy and neurophysiology) shed an interesting light on the nature of memory and are consistent with recategorical memory: whereas the models are able to increase their performance in various learning paradigms, it is often not easy to say precisely where the "memory trace" is located in their modeled nervous systems. Changes in synaptic weights occur in many different places, but generally it is difficult if not impossible to attribute a specific memorial function to any particular synapse or cell. The model's memory is a system property, is expressed as increased behavioral performance, e.g., the increased ability to recategorize the surrounding world of stimulus objects; it is not replicative or localized in a precise fashion. Behavioral performance (i.e., the measurable effect of "memory") can be degraded in various ways and to various extents by "lesions" in different parts of the model (some of them far removed from locales of synaptic change). This may not sound surprising: neural network models have often been used to show the distributed nature of memory. However, in the case of Reeke's models, memory is not just the delocalized property of a single network, but is distributed among several functionally distinct "brain areas." In addition, because of the incorporation of actual behavioral output, memory becomes directly measurable as increased or decreased levels of performance.

Squire's review illuminates the differential involvement of different brain regions in different aspects of memory, from the initial construction of a mental scene to short-term memory, long-term consolidation, and recall. Implicit/explicit dissociations, though not directly dealing with processes related to memory formation, also highlight the distributed nature of memory function. An obvious question concerns the neurobiological basis for the segregation of different aspects of memory and the interaction between them. Here it is useful to reconsider the key concept of reentry introduced and elaborated in Section III. The anatomical basis for integrating multiple centers of the brain involved in memory might be the reciprocal connectivity linking different brain areas. It is an open question whether the "transfer" of stored memories from the medial temporal lobe system to neocortex is mediated by reentrant interactions between these two systems and whether the eventual storage within or between neocortical areas is accomplished by the formation of functional (e.g., strengthened) cortico-cortical connections. Similarly, the dissociation between implicit and explicit memory could be due to functional or anatomical disconnection of brain areas involved in these two aspects of memory. (This does not necessarily imply a precise localization of these aspects in segregated areas.) Reentrant interactions are becoming more accessible to experimental study and manipulation, particularly with the advent of powerful techniques in multielectrode recording and functional neuroimaging. Perhaps modeling studies of the kind reviewed by Reeke could help in formulating specific hypotheses concerning the function of reentrant pathways in memory.

An important, even essential, aspect of memory within a selectional framework is its historical and unique character, an aspect of higher brain function that is discussed in some more detail in Section V. Again, to understand better how this uniqueness relates to selective principles, it is useful to consider some results from work in categorization. A major obstacle to elucidating the representational structure of even the simplest categories is the frequent inability to decompose stimuli into "meaningful" features that are the basic elements of this representational structure. Stated simply, can we really tell what are the defining elementary features of a chair, or a motorboat, or a running shoe? Though it is easy to come up with an answer that will fit most examples, it is virtually impossible to come up with one that fits all. The featural dimensions of almost any given stimulus category are basically inaccessible. How, then, does an organism select the relevant features when faced with the task of categorizing its environment? According to the selectionist paradigm, relevant stimulus attributes are constructed by the organism's sensorimotor apparatus while interacting with the world; they are the product of developmental and experiential selection. Therefore stimulus attributes will, in general, correspond to those features that are most typical, but they may also correspond to disjunctive criteria that are logically hard to grasp, but are naturally acquired through adequate sensory sampling. This is somewhat reminiscent of the individuality expressed by Thelen's infants as they acquire motor skills; whereas some global convergence exists, the "movement attributes" (e.g., the basic components of synergies) can differ from infant to infant. From a selectionist perspective, memory is the result of developmentally and historically determined interactions of an individual with its world. Thus, inevitably, each individual's memory is truly his own.

SECTION V

PSYCHOPHYSICS, PSYCHOANALYSIS, AND NEUROPSYCHOLOGY

This final section contains three papers that, in different ways, indicate how a selectionist perspective can be applied, with surprising and illuminating results, to what would normally be considered as "high-level" aspects of human neural activity—clinical syndromes and complex psychological experience.

Vilayanur Ramachandran discusses two clinical syndromes, phantom limbs and somatophrenic delusions, and attempts to elucidate their relationship to normal and abnormal cortical function. His main focus is on the perceptual correlates of cortical reorganization. Several lines of research over the last decade have shown that the representation of the body surface in the somatosensory cortex changes in response to changes in peripheral input, after amputation or deafferentation as well as after overstimulation. These experiments have played a key role in supporting selectionist notions as illustrated by the work of Merzenich and others. Ramachandran finds that within weeks or months of an amputation or severe peripheral nerve damage patients report "referred sensations," i.e. sensory stimulation of a still existing part of their body surface (e.g., the face) will result in perceived sensations in the no longer existing limb (e.g., the arm or hand). So-called phantom limbs (referring to the continued sensory presence of a limb that no longer exists) have been studied in clinical medicine for quite some time. Ramachandran postulates that phantom limbs are the result of a remapping of the body surface representation in response to injury; he offers some speculations as to the mechanistic basis of the phenomenon. Ramachandran also considers somatophrenic delusions, in which patients deny the existence of their own paralyzed limb after suffering brain damage involving the right hemisphere. He creates a link between this delusional syndrome and Freudian repression of "unpleasant" memories.

The next chapter, by Arnold Modell, takes us from psychophysics to the domain of psychoanalytic theory and practice. Modell argues that both psychic development and the therapeutic setting can be interpreted in terms of the selectionist concept of memory as recategorization, which is related to Freud's early view of memory as *Nachträglichkeit*, or retranscription. Modell's thesis is that a failure of recategorization is at the origin of many intrapsychic conflicts. The therapeutic setting can be seen as a situation in which such retranscription or recategorization is actuated in the presence of the analyst. Modell also discusses the need to replace Freud's instinct theory, which he considers to be devoid of solid biological foundations, with Edelman's concept of value as it applies to selectionist systems.

The final chapter in the book is by a neurologist, Oliver Sacks. In his clinical practice, Sacks has been able to collect and examine in detail many neurological and neuropsychological case histories, histories of individuals that shed a new light on the interpretation of neurological syndromes, and that present a serious challenge to classical viewpoints. Sacks, who has written extensively about these subjects, was at first frustrated in his attempts to achieve a general framework for understanding them. Over the last few years, however, he has come to the conclusion that the theory of neuronal group selection may constitute precisely such a framework. It is a global theory, and it is a selectionist one. In his chapter, Oliver Sacks summarizes several aspects of this theory as they relate to and illuminate the clinical observations that are the object of his studies.

PHANTOM LIMBS, NEGLECT SYNDROMES, REPRESSED MEMORIES, AND FREUDIAN PSYCHOLOGY

V. S. Ramachandran

Brain and Perception Laboratory, Psychology Department and Neurosciences Program, University of California, San Diego, La Jolla, California 92093-0109

I. Introduction

In this essay I would like to consider two of the most fascinating syndromes in clinical medicine: phantom limbs and somatoparaphrenic delusions. In the case of phantom limbs, the patient continues to experience a limb that has long ceased to exist, whereas in somatophrenia he insists that his paralyzed limb does not belong to him. He may even attribute his limb to his spouse or to his physician. These two syndromes have long been regarded as enigmatic clinical curiosities. My goal, however, will be to bring them into the respectable arena of modern neuroscience and to point out that they illustrate certain important principles concerning the functional organization of the normal human brain.

II. Phantom Limbs as a Perceptual Marker for Somatosensory Plasticity

When I began my career as a medical student nearly 15 years ago, I was taught that no new neural connections can be formed in the adult mammalian brain. Once connections have been laid down in fetal life, or in early infancy, it was assumed that they hardly change later in life. It is this stability of connections in the adult brain, in fact, that is often used to explain why there is usually very little functional recovery after damage to the nervous system and why neurological diseases are so notoriously difficult to treat. In this article I will present some evidence suggesting that we may need to revise these views radically.

It is known that a complete somatotopic map of the entire body surface exists in the somatosensory cortex of primates (Mountcastle, 1957; Merzenich *et al.*, 1983; Kaas *et al.*, 1981; Jones, 1982). In a series of pioneering experiments, Merzenich *et al.* (1984) amputated the middle finger of adult primates and found that within 2 months the area in the cortex corresponding to this digit starts to respond to touch stimuli delivered to the adjacent digits, i.e., this area is "taken over" by sensory input from adjacent digits. If more than one finger was amputated, however, there was no take over beyond about 1 mm of cortex. Merzenich and co-workers concluded from this that the expansion is probably mediated by arborizations of thalamo-cortical axons that typically do not extend beyond 1 mm.

This figure—1 mm—was often cited as the fixed upper limit of reorganization of sensory pathways in adult animals (Calford, 1991). A remarkable experiment performed by Pons *et al.* (1991), however, suggests that this view might be incorrect. They found that after long-term (12 years) deafferentation of one upper limb, the cortical area originally corresponding to the hand gets taken over by sensory input from the face. The cells in the "hand area" now start responding to stimuli applied to the lower face region! Because this patch of cortex is over 1 cm in width, we may conclude that sensory reorganization can occur over at least this distance—an order of magnitude greater than the original 1-mm "limit."

A. PERCEPTUAL CORRELATES OF PLASTICITY IN HUMANS

Despite the wealth of physiological experiments demonstrating striking plasticity in the primary sensory areas of primates, there has been almost no attempt to look directly for the behavioral consequences of this reorganization. The observation by Pons *et al.* (1991), for example, makes the curious prediction that if one were to touch a monkey's face after long-term deafferentation, the monkey should experience the sensations as arising from the hand as well as from the face. To test this prediction, we studied the localization of sensations in several adult human subjects who had undergone amputation of an upper limb. Two of these subjects (VQ and WK) have been described in detail elsewhere (Ramachandran *et al.*, 1992a,b, 1993; Ramachandran, 1993). In this essay, I will briefly summarize our findings for these two patients and will also describe some preliminary results from new patients (FA and DS).

1. Patient VQ

Patient VQ was an intelligent, alert 17-year-old male whose left arm was amputated 6 cm above the elbow about 4 weeks prior to our testing him. He experienced a vivid phantom hand that was "telescoped," i.e., it felt like it was attached just a few centimeters below his stump and was pronated. We studied localization of touch (and light pressure) in this patient using a cotton swab that was brushed at various randomly selected points on his skin surface. His eyes were shut during the entire procedure and he was simply asked to describe any sensations that he felt and to report the perceived location of these sensations. Using this procedure, we found that even stimuli applied to points remote from the amputation line were often systematically mislocalized to the phatom arm (Fig. 1). Furthermore, the distribution of these points was not random (Ramachandran *et al.*, 1992b). There appeared to be two clusters of points, with one cluster being represented on the lower part of the face ipsilateral to the amputation. There was a systematic one-to-one mapping between specific regions on the face and individual digits (e.g., from the cheek to the thumb, from the philtrum to the index finger, and from the chin to the fifth finger). Typically, the patient reported that he simultaneously felt the cotton swab touching his face and a "tingling" sensation in an individual digit. By repeatedly brushing the swab on his face, we were even able to plot "receptive fields" (or "reference fields") for individual digits of the (phamtom) left hand on his face surface (Fig. 1). The margins of these fields were remarkably sharp and stable over successive trials. Stimuli applied to other parts of the body such as the

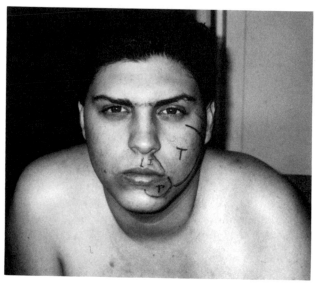

FIG. 1. Regions on the left side of the face of patient VQ, which elicited precisely localized referred sensations in the phantom digits. Reference fields, regions that evoke referred sensations, were plotted by brushing a cotton swab repeatedly on the face. The region labeled T always evoked sensations in the phantom thumb; P denotes the "pinkie" (fifth finger); I, the index finger; and B, the ball of the thumb. This patient was tested 4 weeks after amputation.

tongue, neck, shoulders, trunk, and axilla were never mislocalized to the phatom hand and no referred sensations were ever felt in the other (normal) hand. There was, however, one specific point on the contralateral cheek that always elicited a tingling sensation in the phantom elbow.

The second cluster of points that evoked referred sensations was found about 7 cm above the amputation line. Again there was a systematic one-to-one mapping, with the thumb being represented medially on the anterior surface of the arm and the fifth finger laterally, as if to mimic the pronated position of the phantom hand.

We repeated the whole procedure again after 1 week and found a very similar distribution of points. We conclude, therefore, that these one-to-one correspondences are stable over time—at least over the 1-week period that separated our two testing sessions (but see below).

2. Patient WK

In testing the second patient (WK) we found a very similar pattern of results, although there were some interesting differences as well. This patient had a right forequarter disarticulation, i.e., his entire right arm and right scapula were removed. We tested him exactly 1 year after amputation.

We had WK close his eyes and we firmly rubbed the skin of his right lower jaw and cheek with one of our fingers or the tip of a ballpoint pen. A representation of the entire phantom arm was found on the ipsilateral face, with the hand being represented on the anterior lower jaw, the elbow on the angle of the jaw, and the shoulder on the temporo-mandibular joint. Again, as in patient VQ, there appeared to be a precise and stable point-to-point correspondence between points on the lower jaw and individual digits.

A second cluster of reference fields representing the hand was found just below the axilla. Because this region is close to the line of amputation, it may be analogous to the cluster of points we found on the upper arm of VQ. In this region, even a cotton swab was effective in eliciting referred sensations in the thumb, forefinger, fifth finger, or palm. And last, there was also a third cluster of points near the right nipple, and the arrangement of these points also showed some hint of topography. Thus it would appear that there is a tendency toward the spontaneous emergence of multiple somatotopically organized maps even in regions remote from the line of amputation. The exact mechanism by which such maps are formed remains an interesting question for future research.

We have now studied nine patients after upper limb amputation and found that sensations were referred from the face to the phantom arm in only four of them. The cluster(s) of points just proximal to the line of amputation, however, was seen in eight patients. We shall discuss the reason for this variability in a later section.

3. Patient FA

FA lost his right arm as a result of an accident on a fishing boat in 1982. His arm had been amputated about 8 cm below the elbow crease. He experienced a very vivid phantom hand that was usually telescoped, i.e., the hand felt like it was directly attached to the stump with no intervening forearm. He could, however, voluntarily extend his hand so that it acquired a subjectively normal length and indeed he could even attempt to grasp objects, fend off blows, or break a fall with his phantom.

FA was one of the subjects we examined who did not initially have a map on his face. As in the other patients, however, he had points near the amputation line that elicited referred sensations. After carefully mapping these points, we established that there were two distinct somatotopic representations that were almost completely identical to each other (Fig. 2). One of these extended from the amputation line to about 3 cm below the elbow, whereas the second one extended from about 6 cm

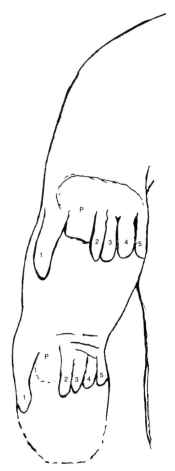

FIG. 2. Somatotopic maps of referred sensations in patient FA. Notice that there are two distinct maps, one close to the line of amputation and a second one 6 cm above the elbow crease. The maps are almost identical except for the absence of fingertips in the upper map. When patient FA imagined he was pronating his phantom, the entire upper map shifted in the same direction by about 1.5 cm (see text). 1, Thumb; 2, index finger; 3, middle finger; 4, right finger; 5, fifth finger. These reference fields usually elicited sensation in the glabrous portions of these digits. The dorsal surface of the hand was represented on the dorsolateral part of the upper arm lateral to the palm (P) and thumb representations. No referred sensations in the phantom could be elicited by stimulating the skin region in between these two maps.

above the crease to about 14 cm. Stimuli applied to points in between these two maps were completely ineffective in producing referred sensations, even though skin sensitivity was normal in this region. Note that the two maps are very similar except for the absence of fingertips in the second map.

4. Patient DS

Patient DS had a brachial avulsion following a motorcycle accident, and his arm was amputated a year after the accident. He experienced a vivid phantom that felt "paralyzed"—as if to mimic the paralysis that preceded the amputation. We mapped the distribution of reference fields in this patient extensively on three separate occasions, the first two separated by 24 hours and the third one after 6 months. The arrangement of reference fields is shown in Fig. 3a. Notice the topographic arrangement of digits on the face (e.g., digits 1 to 4 are neatly laid out on the zygoma). The thumb receptive field was especially large, as in some of our other patients. Curiously, there was also a second map of sorts on the mandible, with the digits following approximately the same sequence as on the zygoma. (Stimulating the buccal region in between these two maps elicited diffuse tingling on the palm.) Thus, each digit appeared to be represented twice, but the reference field on the zygoma usually corresponded to the distal interphalangeal joint, whereas the one on the mandible elicited sensations from the base of the digit.

The map remained stable during the first two testing sessions, but when we saw the patient again after 6 months, there had been some small but noticeable changes (Fig. 3b). In particular, the thumb region appeared to have expanded to stretch across the entire mandible—the base of the thumb near the ramus and the tip near the symphysis menti. It was unclear why the map had changed in this manner, but it may have occurred as a result of changing patterns of sensory input (and spontaneous activity) from the face and from the stump. It might be interesting to test this hypothesis by actually stimulating a specific region of the map (e.g., the index finger reference field) for a few days to see if this increases the size of that reference field (see also Section III,E). A second map was found in the region of the deltoid muscle and this, too, was topographically organized. Unlike the face map, however, it remained stable across all three testing sessions (Fig. 3c).

An especially convincing way of demonstrating topography in patient DS was as follows. When the cotton swab was moved continuously from the angle of the mandible to the symphysis menti, the referred sensation also felt like "it was moving from the ball of the thumb to the tip in an arclike motion." This observation was replicated several times. Also, if

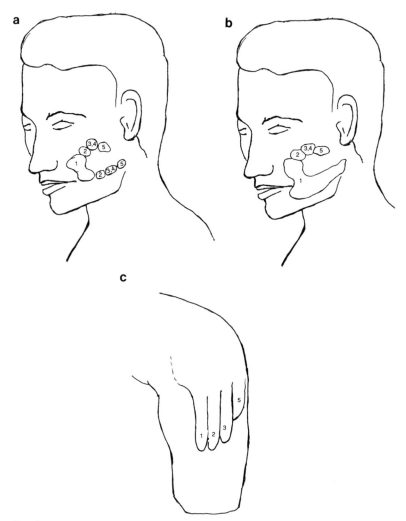

FIG. 3. (a) Distribution of reference fields in patient DS. Notice the prominent representation of the thumb (1), which we have seen in several patients, and the roughly topographic arrangement of digits 2, 3, 4, and 5 on the face. This pattern was nearly identical 24 hours later, but after 6 months the representations of some of the digits had changed noticeably (b). This may occur as a result of sensory input and spontaneous activity from the face (and stump) continuously remodeling neural connections in S1. If this interpretation is correct, then phantom limbs might provide a valuable preparation for studying the manner in which sensory maps emerge and change in the adult nervous system. (c) The second map in the region of the deltoid muscle. Patient DS's arm always felt completely extended and paralyzed; it was never telescoped into the stump.

a short excursion was made on the jaw, the excursion on the hand was correspondingly short. Curiously, however, if the direction of motion of the cotton swab was reversed, DS reported a diffuse tingling in the thumb; there was no reversal of the direction of motion on the thumb. Thus, distance and velocity were accurately referred but direction was not.

A similar effect could also be evoked by moving the cotton swab across the digits' reference fields on the deltoid muscle, and in this case reversing the direction of the cotton swab also reversed the direction of motion on the phantom hand.

Finally, it was our general impression that in patient DS as well as in other patients, the topography was usually much more precise in the map proximal to the stump than on the face. The reason for this difference is not clear.

B. MODALITY-SPECIFIC EFFECTS

The neural pathways that mediate the sensations of pain, warmth, and cold are quite different from those that carry information about touch from the skin surface to the brain (Kenshalo et al., 1971; Landgren, 1960; Kreisman and Zimmerman, 1971). We wondered whether the remapping effect reported by Pons and his collaborators occurs separately in each of these pathways or only in the touch pathways. To find out, we tried placing a drop of warm water on VQ's face. He felt the warm water on his face, of course, but remarkably he reported (without any prompting) that his phatom hand also felt distinctly warm.[1] On one occasion when the water accidentally trickled down his face, he exclaimed, with surprise, that he could actually feel the warm water trickling down the length of his phantom arm! We have now seen this effect in three patients, two patients after upper limb amputation and one after an avulsion of the brachial plexus. The latter patient was better able to use his normal hand to trace out the exact path of the illusory trickle along his paralyzed arm as a drop of cold water flowed down his face. (The distance traversed by this illusory trickle was about five times the

---

[1] Modality-specific referral from the stump (but not the face) was also noticed by William James (1887) and Wier Mitchell (1871). This finding, however, is open to multiple interpretations, e.g., due to reinnervation of the stump by severed axons (which may also be modality specific) or due to the fact that phantom is often "telescoped" so that its phenomenal location is superimpsoed on the stump.

distance on the face, as one might expect from the obvious differences in cortical magnification for the face and arm representations.) Finally, in patient DS, a vibrator placed on the jaw evoked a compelling sensation of vibration in the phantom hand.

How does the point-to-point referral of temperature sensations compare with that of touch? To explore this, we tried applying a drop of warm (or cold) water on different parts of the face of patient DS and found that the heat or cold was usually referred to individual fingers so that there was a sort of crude map of referred temperature that was roughly superimposed on the touch map (e.g., touching the thumb reference field on the face with warm water evoked warmth in the thumb alone, whereas touching the fifth finger part of the map evoked a warm sensation confined to that finger). To make sure that these effects were not simply due to simultaneous activation of touch receptors, we also tried touching the thumb reference field on the face with warm water while simultaneously applying tepid water to the fifth finger region of the map. The patient then reported that he could feel the touch in both digits—as expected—but that the warmth was felt only in the thumb. Reversing the stimulation on the face produced corresponding reversal in the phantom. If these preliminary results are confirmed, they would imply that there are independent modality-specific reference fields for touch, heat, and cold on the face and that these reference fields are usually in approximate spatial registration.

C. COMBINING REFERRED SENSATIONS

These observations raise an interesting question. What would happen if dissimilar stimuli were applied to the thumb reference field on the face versus the corresponding reference field on the upper arm? For example, one could put hot water on the thumb region of the face and ice-cold water on the thumb region of the arm. Would the sensation in the phantom thumb then be an average of the two, so that it felt neutral? How would the brain resolve the conflict? The result was clear. On every occasion that we tried the test, the patient reported a clear alternation of the sensations "a flash of heat followed by a flash of cold, followed once again by the heat," etc. It would be interesting to see what would happen if the two temperature sensations were closer in degree, e.g., tepid and very warm (rather than cold and hot). This might lead to an averaging or blending of the sensations rather than to an alternation.

D. "Learned" Paralysis of Phantom Limbs

Another puzzling observation we made also deserves mention. Most patients who have lost a limb experience a very compelling phantom arm or leg that they can "move" voluntarily. (As we shall see later, we have also studied a patient who was congenitally missing both arms, but nevertheless experienced vivid phantom arms.) Yet, we noticed that if the patient had a preexisting paralysis of the arm caused by a peripheral nerve lesion (e.g., a brachial plexus avulsion or infiltration by carcinoma), then the patient usually complained that although he experienced a phantom arm, he could not voluntarily move the phantom—it felt paralyzed and always assumed the same position and length as that of the paralyzed arm before amputation (e.g., neither patient DS nor patient WK could move his phantom voluntarily, whereas FA and VQ had no difficulty). This raises an interesting question. Why does the mere fact that a limb was paralyzed (say) a few months before amputation cause the phantom to be paralyzed, whereas patients who have lost the whole limb, and therefore never moved it for many years, can still imagine voluntary movement? How can a phantom be paralyzed?

The answer is surely that in the former case the patient has learned that the limb is paralyzed, i.e., every time he tried to move his limb there was both visual feedback and proprioceptive feedback from the limb muscles informing him that the limb was not following the command; the brain was receiving evidence that the limb was paralyzed. In the amputees, on the other hand, when the subject tried to move the limb, there was simply no feedback from the limb that either confirmed or contradicted the command signals. Thus, it looks as though the contradictory signals that were sent to the brain during the months preceding the amputation were somehow "wired" into the brain so that there was a permanent memory trace of the paralysis left in place.

E. Relevance to Stroke Rehabilitation: The Virtual Reality Box

If the phantom is paralyzed because the patient's brain has learned that it is paralyzed, then would it be possible to "unlearn" the paralysis so that the limb starts moving once again? Liz Franz and I realized that one way to achieve this might be to encourage the patient simply to perform a mirror-symmetric movement with his other normal hand because this might facilitate the corresponding neural circuits in equivalent locations in the other hemisphere (some phantom limb patients do, in fact, spontaneously report that movement of the phantom can be facilitated by making a corresponding movement with the other hand; e.g., patient FA could not ordinarily flex and extend his phantom hand but could do so if his normal hand performed a similar movement at the same time).

A cleverer method might be to use a "Virtual Reality Box" to trick the patient into thinking that his phantom was moving (Ramachandran, 1994). A mirror is placed vertically on a table in front of the patient. (Imagine a book on the table; if you opened the front cover so that it stood vertically, you would be mimicking the position and orientation of the mirror.) The patient is then asked to view the reflection of his normal hand in the mirror in order to create the illusion that he now has two hands. He would have to move his normal hand until its mirror reflection was superimposed on the felt position of his phantom hand. If he now attempts to execute mirror-symmetric movement with both of his hands, he will see his phantom come to life and move as if it was obeying his commands! Would this revive the lifeless phantom so that it no longer felt paralyzed?

I recently tried this experiment on patient DS and the result was quite astonishing. Just a few seconds after he had tried the "mirror therapy," he exclaimed, with considerable surprise, that he could vividly feel (and not just see) his phantom arm moving as though it was under his voluntary control again! "Mind-boggling," he said. "My arm is plugged in again; it's as if I am back in the past. I can actually *feel* my arm moving, doctor. It no longer feels like it's lying lifeless in a sling." I then removed the mirror and verified that, as before, he could no longer feel his phantom moving even if he closed his eyes and tried mirror-symmetric movements. ("It feels frozen again," he said, "as though in a plaster cast.") Patient DS also tried moving his index finger and thumb alone while looking in the mirror but, this time, the phantom thumb and index finger remained paralyzed—they were not revived. (This is an important observation, for it rules out the possibility that the previous result was simply a confabulation in response to unusual task demands.) After a dozen such 15-minute sessions of "mirror therapy" (distributed over three weeks), he found, to his amazement, that for the first time in nine years, his hand became telescoped permanently into his stump with his phantom fingers dangling from his shoulder!

The concept of "learned paralysis" may have important implications for rehabilitation from stroke. One ordinarily thinks of the hemiplegia that arises from stroke as being the result of permanent irreversible neural damage. There is undoubtedly some truth to this view, but is it conceivable that at least some of the paralysis that these patients experience is "learned"? For example, even if there is some degree of recovery—as a result of "remapping"—the patient may not use his arm because his brain has learned during the acute stages that his limb is paralyzed. If so, mirror therapy may eventually prove useful in accelerating recovery of function in at least a subset of stroke victims.

F. DISCUSSION

The occurrence of referred sensations in the phantom limb is not new. It has been noticed by many researchers (Mitchell, 1871; Cronholm, 1951) that stimulating points on the stump often elicits sensations from missing fingers, and the great American psychologist William James (1887) once wrote, "A breeze on the stump is felt as a breeze on the phantom." Unfortunately, because the results of Pons and his collaborators were not available at that time, such findings were often attributed to direct reinnervation of the stump by the severed axons. Even when points remote from the stump were found to be effective in producing referred sensations, the phenomenon was often attributed to "diffuse" connections in the nervous system (Melzack, 1992). I would argue, instead, that the effects I have observed are a direct consequence of the remapping observed by Pons *et al.* (1991), which in turn is constrained by proximity of maps in the brain. The reason that there are two clusters of points—for example, one on the face and one near the upper arm— is that the hand area in the Penfield homunculus is flanked on one side by the face and on the other side by the upper arm, shoulder, and axilla (Fig. 4). If the sensory input from the face and from around the stump were to "invade" the cortical territory of the hand, one would expect precisely this sort of clustering (Ramachandran *et al.*, 1992b) of points. In the rest of this essay I shall refer to this view as the "remapping hypothesis" of referred sensations (Ramachandran *et al.*, 1992b). I would emphasize, especially, the topographic arrangement of points on the face, the referral of complex sensations such as "trickling" from the face to the phantom, and the extreme rapidity with which the referred sensations emerge. (Our study was carried out after 4 weeks rather than 12 years.)

This rapidity might suggest that the reorganization is based on the unmasking of silent synapses (e.g., through disinhibition) rather than on anatomical sprouting. Whatever the interpretation, however, these findings represent the first clear demonstration that highly organized, modality-specific "rewiring" of the adult mammalian brain can occur in

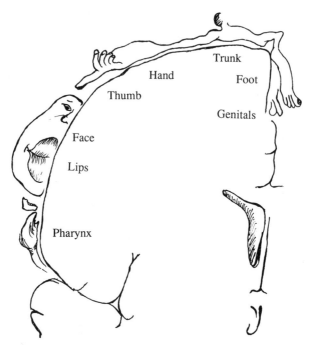

FIG. 4. The Penfield homunculus. Notice that the sensory hand area is flanked below by the face and above by the upper arm and shoulder—the two regions where we usually find reference fields in arm amputees. Also, note that the area representing the genitals is just below the foot representation, a face that might explain the frequent occurrence of certain foot fetishes even among normal individuals.

as little as 4 weeks and that this rewiring can be functionally effective. It remains to be seen, of course, whether this latent capacity can be exploited for therapeutic purposes.

1. *Sprouting or Unmasking?*

What is the actual neural mechanism underlying the expanded hand representation in the Silver Spring monkeys and in our patients? We need to consider two theories:

1. When a patch of sensory neurons (e.g., in the "hand area") is deprived of sensory input, it might begin to secrete some neurotrophic factors that provide sprouting of new axon terminals from neurons supplying anatomically adjacent cortical areas. These same trophic factors might subsequently "attract" these terminals to the denervated zone.

2. Perhaps even in normal individuals any given point on the skin projects simultaneously to several locations, e.g., the sensory input from the face projects simultaneously to both the face and the hand neurons in the cortex (or thalamus). The unwanted input to the hand area, however, might be subject to tonic presynaptic inhibiton (e.g., via an inhibitory interneuron) by the "correct" axons that arrive there from the hand. If the arm is amputated, on the other hand, this occult input is unmasked through disinhibition and this would lead to mislocalized sensations.

There is at present no strong reason for favoring one hypothesis over the other. The elegant work of Wall (1971) provided the first clear evidence that rapid "unmasking" of synapses can indeed occur in the somatosensory system (see also Calford and Tweedale, 1990; Rasmusson and Turnbull, 1983; Kelahan and Doetsch, 1981). Such short-term changes, however, usually result in an enlargement of receptive field size, and there is no strong evidence that topography can be altered. Furthermore, the unmasking idea is rendered somewhat unlikely by the fact that neither the arborization of a thalamo-cortical axon terminals nor cortico-cortical connections have been found spanning more than a few millimeters of the cortex (Calford, 1991; Pons, 1992).

Even if the sprouting hypothesis turns out to be correct, however, one would still have to account for the emergence of topography and modality specificity, i.e., the sprouting would have to be organized and the new axon terminals would have to find their appropriate targets. The guidance of such new terminals to appropriate targets would, if it occurred at all, have to depend on poorly understood mechanisms such as chemoaffinity.

III. Some Potential Problems

A. INTERSUBJECT VARIABILITY

How general are the findings we have reported here? Of the nine patients we have seen so far, the map on the face was seen in four. The second cluster of points near the line of amputation, on the other hand, was seen in eight patients.

Why do some patients not have a cluster of points on the face? There are at least five possibilities that are not mutually exclusive. First, the brain maps might vary slightly from patient to patient, and this, in turn, might influence the degree of remapping. Second, some patients may eventually "learn" to ignore the referred sensations from the face by using visual feedback. Third, even without visual feedback the plasticity exhibited by the afferent pathways may be propagated further along the pathways to perception so that the input gets correctly interpreted as originating from the face alone [i.e., the peripheral organ might "specify" the central connections, as suggested by Weiss (1939)]. Fourth, the aberrant connections that are formed may get deleted by the same genetic mechanism that causes their elimination in the embyro. And fifth, if the patient uses the stump constantly, the skin corresponding to it may "regain" the territory that was initially lost to the face.[2] Obviously, more extensive testing of a large number of patients is needed before we can distinguish between these possibilities.

Halligan and Marshall (1993) have recently studied a patient whose arm had been amputated at the shoulder level. They were able to replicate and significantly extend our basic observation—the occurrence of a map on the ipsilateral lower face. Curiously, they found that although the map was nearly complete and was in many ways quite similar to the one we had observed, it lacked an index finger and thumb. Careful questioning of the patient revealed that she had completely lost sensations in her thumb and index finger for over a year preceding the amputation (she had suffered from carpal tunnel syndrome). It was as though this sensory loss had been carried over into her phantom!

B. MULTIPLE MAPS

The "remapping" hypothesis predicts that after arm amputation two clusters of points should be seen—one near the face and one near the line of amputation. As we have seen, this is generally true (e.g., one hardly ever sees points on the ipsilateral leg, contralateral chest, contralateral leg, and abdomen). However, in two of our patients there was more

---

[2] If this argument is correct, then the face map should be seen much more consistently in patients with brachial plexus avulsion than in amputees, and we have some evidence that this is indeed true. The reason for this difference is that in amputees the nerves that supply the arm can reinnervate the stump, after an initial period of retrograde degeneration, whereas in the avulsion cases, the roots degenerate permanently and there is no possibility of reinnervation. It was our impression, also, that patients who referred sensations from the face to the phantom either had a preexisting long-standing pathology in that arm (e.g., a brachial avulsion, infiltration by carcinoma) or were seen soon (e.g., 4 weeks) after amputation. Patients who were seen several years after a "clean" amputation (with no preexisting pathology) tended not to have a map on the face. Clearly, additional experiments are needed to see if this distinction holds up.

than one map near the line of amputation and we have no simple explanation for this. For example, WK (whose arm had been disarticulated at
the shoulder) had at least two maps proximal to the amputation line—one
below the axilla and a second less distinct one near the ipsilateral nipple.
Likewise, patient FA, described above, had two distinct maps—one that
was 3 cm below the elbow crease and the second map (identical to the
first) 6 cm above the crease, with nothing in-between! There are, of
course, multiple representations of the body surface in both the thalamus
and in S1, and one wonders whether the multiple maps that we observed
reflect remapping occurring separately in each of these brain areas.

In some patients, we have also occasionally seen similar dual representation of the hand on the face (e.g., sensations in the phantom index
finger could be evoked by stimuli on either of two separate points on
the face—one on the lower jaw and one on the upper cheek). One
possible explanation for such dual reference fields comes from the recent
physiological work of Lund *et al.* (1994), who found that the "hand area"
of the cortex is actually flanked by two separate maps of the face within
S1. It is conceivable, therefore, that after upper limb deafferentation,
the sensory input from the thumb destined for the hand area of S1 now
projects additionally to separate parts of the two flanking face maps,
e.g., to the "cheek" region of one map and the "jaw" region of the other.
The outcome of such remapping would be two separate thumb reference
fields on the patient's face.

C. Contralateral Points

Points on the normal skin surface that elicited referred sensations in
the phantom were usually clustered around regions proximal to the
line of amputation and around the ipsilateral face as predicted by the
remapping hypothesis, although the details of the maps varied considerably from patient to patient (e.g., in two patients the maps were on the
lower jaw but in a third patient they were mainly clustered on and around
the temporomandibular joint and pinna).

These observations are, on the whole, consistent with the remapping
hypothesis, but mention must be made of the occasional presence of
small maps in the contralateral limb at locations that were approximately
mirror-symmetrical with the line of amputation. In one patient (RW),
for example, in addition to the two clusters that are usually found (i.e.,
on the face and near the amputation line), a small (2-cm diameter) well-
circumscribed region of skin near the contralateral elbow was found that
elicited referred sensations in the phantom hand. Moving a pencil in

this region produced a vivid sensation of movement in an equivalent direction in the phantom and scratching it was effective in eliminating itch sensations in the phantom! (Other regions on the normal arm were completely ineffective in producing these effects.) In the second patient (FA) we found a clearly organized map on the normal arm that was an exact mirror image of the map that was above the line of amputation. The curious thing about this map, however, was that the sensation was referred to the finger of the normal limb. Again, no other areas of skin surface on the normal arm were effective in evoking referred sensations.

These contralateral effects are difficult to account for in terms of the remapping hypothesis as it currently stands, but they might be explicable in terms of the transcallosal effects reported by Calford and Tweedale (1990). These authors found that digital nerve block in flying foxes and primates produces the expected immediate expansion of receptive fields in the contralateral hemisphere, but there were also striking changes in the mirror-symmetric locations of the ipsilateral hemisphere corresponding to the normal hand—changes that took less than 20 minutes to emerge. It is not known how long the changes last, but it is conceivable that remapping effects of the kind observed by Merzenich *et al.* (1983, 1984) and Pons *et al.* (1991) may also induce analogous long-term changes in the other hemisphere. If such changes were to occur, they would explain the maps we saw in the normal arms of our two patients.

D. ROLE OF THE CORPUS CALLOSUM

In this section, I will describe a novel perceptual effect that we observed in a 23-year-old patient who fell off a train and lost his left arm 19 days prior to our testing him. The effect provides additional evidence for strengthening or reactivation of preexisting connections. After verifying first that our patient was neurologically intact, we blindfolded him and applied sensory stimuli to various parts of his body and asked him to report where he felt the sensations. Like some of our other patients, he referred sensations from his lower ipsilateral face to his phantom fingers, but there were no clearly defined reference fields—possibly because not enough time had elapsed after the amputation. An especially intriguing effect was observed, however, when we touched the normal hand. For example, when we touched an individual finger of the right hand, he felt he was also being touched simultaneously on the corresponding finger of the phantom hand. Remarkably, even the subjective quality of the sensation was carried over vividly into the phantom, e.g., when his right index finger was scraped with a knee hammer, he experienced his phantom index finger also being "scraped." When we held his fifth finger or index finger and passively dipped either finger into a glass of hot or ice-cold water, he felt the corresponding finger on the phantom also "dipping into water," although, curiously, the warmth or cold was felt only in the right hand—it was not referred to the phantom. This rules out confabulation, for if the patient were confabulating, why should he refer only the "dipping" sensation and not the temperature? We conclude, therefore, that we are dealing with a genuine sensory phenomenon. No referral of sensations occurred from any other part of the body and the effects remained stable across two successive testing sessions separated by 24 hours. (The patient could not be followed up subsequently because he left the country.)

The phenomenon bears a suggestive resemblance to allesthesia, which is seen in neurological patients with right parietal lobe disease. In this condition, the patient detects a stimulus applied to his left arm but attributes it to his normal (right) arm. It has been suggested that the illusion arises because the patient neglects the left side of his body and therefore tends to assimilate sensations from the contralesional (left) side into his "surviving cognitive scheme" or body image associated with the left hemisphere (Brain and Walton, 1969).

What causes allesthesia? We suggest that in parietal lobe syndrome as well as in phantom limbs, the phenomenon arises from activation of preexisting transcallosal connections. There is physiological evidence suggesting that even in normal individuals, touching a finger on (say) the right hand activates not only the "finger" area of the left hemisphere but also the mirror-symmetric location in the right hemisphere (Calford and Tweedale, 1990). One reason normal individuals do not experience allesthesia might be that they ordinarily have countermanding signals from the left hand informing the brain of the absence of touch signals. If the left hand is amputated, however, there is no contradictory information and the brain simply accepts the null hypothesis that both hands are being touched. The fact that temperature is not referred argues against a cognitive explanation and suggests that there are no transcallosal fibers concerned with this modality.

A second possibility is that the callosal input from the right hand to the right hemisphere is ordinarily subliminal, i.e., too weak to activate the neurons in area 3b that get a much stronger input from the left hand. After amputation of the left hand, however, this weak input from the right hand gradually "takes over" these neurons and becomes strong enough to activate them, thereby leading to referred sensations. [This would be analogous to shifts in ocular dominance or eye preference observed in young monkeys after monocular deprivation (Wiesel and

Hubel, 1965).] This interpretation is different from unmasking, of course, but it does imply a strengthening of preexisting connections rather than a sprouting of new axons across the corpus callosum!

1. Nonspecific Effects

In addition to the clearly defined reference fields described so far, we also observed that sensations could occasionally be evoked in the phantom using very nonspecific stimuli applied to the normal skin surface. These nonspecific effects could be distinguished from reference fields by using the following criteria: (1) The sensations evoked in the phantom tended to be diffuse and not localized to specific points on the phantom limb. They were also usually less intense. (2) Unlike sensations produced by stimulation of reference fields, the nonspecific referred sensations were usually highly variable in their occurrence and distribution, e.g., stimulating the same point would evoke sensations in very different locations in the phantom on different trials. (3) The distribution of the points that evoked these highly variable sensations was usually quite random, i.e., there was no clearly discernible pattern such as the clustering of reference fields on the lower jaw and around the amputation line. Occasionally, even points on the contralateral torso, neck, shoulder, etc. were effective in producing such nonspecific sensations.

The mechanisms underlying these nonspecific effects are obscure but they may have more in common with diffuse "arousal" than with the remapping that we have considered so far (e.g., the barrage of spontaneous activity from neuromas may be normally gated, but nonspecific arousal might make the cortex more sensitive to such impulses). Some support for the arousal interpretation comes from the recent physiological work of Dykes et al. (1994), who found two classes of novel responses in the deafferented hand area of the cortex (S1) of cats. First, there were cells with clearly defined receptive fields of the kind observed by Pons et al. (1991) in monkeys. A second class of responses, however, could be obtained by touching almost any part of the animal, i.e., there were no clearly defined receptive fields. Dykes et al. suggest that these responses are not "truly sensory in character" and that they may be mediated by brainstem arousal mechanisms. This second category of responses usually appeared very soon after deafferentation and may account for some of the nonspecific referred sensations that we observed in our patients. (The prediction would be that such sensations should also emerge earlier after amputation than specific, organized reference fields.)

2. Stability of Maps over Time

In patients WK, VQ, and FA the overall features of the map were remarkably stable with repeated testing across weekly intervals (For 4 weeks). In patient FA, however, we made a very intriguing observation suggesting that the fine details of the map may be dynamically maintained.

Recall that FA lost his arm 10 years ago when the beam of a sailboat landed on his arm and crushed it. His arm was subsequently amputated 8 cm below the elbow crease. On careful questioning, we discovered that FA's phantom hand usually occupied a position halfway between pronation and supination with the fingers slightly flexed as though he was holding an imaginary vertical staff. We were also struck by the fact that the topography of points on the upper arm seemed to approximately mimic the position of the phantom fingers—a tendency that we had also previously noticed in other patients. Out of curiosity, we asked him to pronate his phantom hand all the way and we remapped the points on the upper arm while his hand was still pronated. To our astonishment, we found that the entire map had shifted systematically leftward by about 1 cm as if to follow the pronation partially (Ramachandran, 1993). Because the arm below the elbow was clamped, this shift in the map could not be attributed to accidental upper arm movements. Also, when he returned the phantom to its resting position, the map also shifted rightward and returned to its original location. A particularly convincing way of demonstrating this effect was to place a constant stimulus such as a small drop of water on (say) the fifth finger region of the map. When he was then asked to pronate his phantom, he reported that he very distinctly felt the drop of water moving from the fifth finger to the ring finger.

To explore this effect further, we also tried placing a drop of hot water on the index finger reference field and, as expected, this produced a referral of both the touch (tingling) and the warmth sensations to the phantom index finger when the hand was in its normal position. When he pronated his hand, the touch sensation was felt to move to his thumb, as one would expect from the previous experiment, but to our surprise (and to the patient's!) the warmth sensation did *not* move; it remained confined to the index finger. This experiment was repeated several times and on two consecutive days, with identical results. The results have at least four interesting implications. First, the referral of warmth does not depend on the simultaneous coactivation of touch receptors. Even though the touch was referred to a new digit, temperature was confined to the original digit. Second, the shift in the reference fields that occurs during pronation of the phantom cannot be confabulatory, for if it were, why should only touch be referred to a new digit and not temperature? Third, there must be separate maps of reference fields for different modalities such as temperature and touch, and these maps must be in approximate registration (although, of course, they may vary in resolution). Fourth, the dynamic shifts in the sensory map, based, presumably, on the motor commands sent to the hand, occur only for the touch map, but not for the temperature map. One reason for this might be that touch is represented cortically in a topographically organized manner, whereas the response to temperature might be primarily thalamic rather than cortical.

Changes in reference fields were also observed in patient FA when he simply clenched and unclenched his phantom fingers. When he made a fist, for example, touch sensations from the original thumb reference field moved to the palm, but when he unclenched his fingers, the sensation was referred once again to the thumb. (This was true for other digits as well.)

Finally, modulation of referred sensations was also observed, albeit on a smaller scale, on the face map in patient FA. No actual shift was observed, but when he clenched and unclenched his fist, the thumb reference field disappeared and reappeared. (Again, this effect was repeatable across testing sessions.)

These observations are quite remarkable: although their functional significance is not obvious, they suggest that the fine details of the map may be dynamically maintained and that either the map in S1 or in subsequent read-out can be profoundly modified by reafference signals from motor commands sent to the hand. We are currently exploring such effects using magnetoencephalography (MEG) and, obviously, it would also be interesting to study cortical maps in awake, behaving monkeys while they were actually moving their hands.

E. Long-Term Changes in Maps of Referred Sensations: Neural Darwinism?

With regard to the stability of maps, two additional observations were made in patient FA that deserve comment. First, we noticed that during the first three testing sessions there were no reference fields on the face at all. Yet when we repeatedly prodded his face for obtaining MEG recordings (Yang *et al.*, 1993, 1994), he reported, with some surprise, that he had started to notice some sensations in his phantom hand! These referred sensations were more noticeable the following day when he was shaving, than during the actual MEG recording session. It was as though the repeated mechanical stimulation had somehow revived dormant connections that had always been there. (Alternately, the sensations might have emerged spontaneously even without the prodding. This needs to be explored in additional patients.) Interestingly such sensations were now evoked for both sides of the face, although less reliably from the contralateral side than from the ipsilateral side.

The short-term and long-term changes may be based on very different mechanisms, but whatever the explanation might be, they are sure to have important implications for our understanding of brain function. They provide the first behavioral evidence for the views of Merzenich *et al.* (1983) and Edelman (1989), that even in the adult brain, neural connections are being modified all the time.

F. A Theory of Phantom Limbs

The remapping hypothesis not only explains referred sensations but may also provide a novel explanation for the very existence of phantom limbs. The old clinical explanation of phantom limbs is that the illusion arises from irritation of severed axon terminals in the stump by the presence of scar tissue and neuromas. Unfortunately, as emphasized out by Melzack (1992), this explanation is quite inadequate, because injecting local anesthetic into the stump or even removing the neuromas surgically often fails to abolish the phantom or to eliminate phantom limb pain. Indeed, as early as 1836, it was pointed out by Valentin that central factors must be invoked to account for the phenomenology of phantom limbs (Valentin, 1836).

We suggest that the phantom limb experience arises because tactile and proprioceptive inputs from the face and tissues proximal to the stump take over the hand region not only in area 3b as shown by Pons *et al.* (1991), but possibly also in "proprioceptive" maps. Consequently, spontaneous discharges from these tissues would be misinterpreted as arising from the missing limb and might therefore be felt as a phantom (Ramachandran *et al.*, 1992a,b). This hypothesis is different from, although not incompatible with, the view that phantom limbs arise from the persistence of a "neurosignature" in a diffuse neural matrix (Melzack, 1992). We would argue, however, that the effect arises from mechanisms of a more specific nature, such as remapping.

The remapping hypothesis does not, however, explain all aspects of the phantom limb experience. Consider, for example, the observation that phantom limbs are occasionally seen in patients who have congenital absence of limbs. We have recently studied one such patient (DB), a 20-year-old lady whose arms had both been missing from birth. All she had on each side was the upper end of the humerus—there were no hand bones and no radius or ulna. Yet she claimed to experience very vivid phantom limbs that often gesticulated during conversation! It is unlikely that these experiences are due to confabulation or wishful thinking, for two reasons. First, she claimed that her arms were "shorter" than they should be by about a foot. (She knew this because her hand did not fit into the prosthesis like a hand in a glove "the way it was supposed to".) Second, her phantom arms did not feel like they were swinging normally as she walked—they felt rigid! These observations suggest that her phantom limbs did not originate simply from her desire to be "normal." It is also difficult to see how the remapping hypothesis, in its simple form, can explain the vivid gesticulation and other spontaneous movements that both DB and other patients experience. We would suggest, instead, that the sensations arise from reafference signals derived from the motor commands sent to the phantom. What is remarkable, however, is that the neural circuitry generating these gesticulatory movements was hardwired and had actually survived intact for 20 years in the absence of any visual or kinesthetic reinforcement.

Based on these observations, we suggest that the phantom limb experience probably depends on integrating information from three different sources: first, from the spontaneous activity of tissues in the face and tissues proximal to the amputation, i.e., the "remapped" zones; second, from reafference signals that accompany motor commands sent to the muscles of the phantom limb; and third, to some extent even from the neuromas—as taught by the old textbooks. Information from these three sources is probably combined in the parietal cortex to create a vivid dynamic image of the limb—an image that persists even when the limb is removed. Indeed, there is at least one case on record of a patient actually *losing* his phantom (Head and Holmes, 1911) as a result of a stroke affecting his right parietal cortex, just as one might expect from our hypothesis.

IV. Conclusions on the Remapping Hypothesis

After 100 years of meticulous neurology, it would have been quite remarkable if no one had noticed referred sensation in phantom limbs, and indeed such effects have been reported several times (see Mitchell, 1871; James, 1887; Cronholm, 1951). In a monograph published in 1951, Cronholm noted clearly that points remote from the stump could sometimes evoke sensations in the phantom. What these researchers did not recognize, however, was that there was something special about the face or that there was a specific pattern of distribution of points yielding referred sensations—one set of points on the ipsilateral lower face and one on the upper arm. Nor did they suggest that this clustering of points can be explained in terms of Penfield's map, an explanation that we refer to as the "remapping hypothesis." Notice, especially, that this hypothesis dissociates proximity in the brain from proximity on the body surface (because of certain peculiarities of the brain map such as proximity of face to hand and genitals to feet).

With regard to our empirical results, what is new may be summarized as follows:

1. There were well-defined reference fields on the body surface remote from the stump. Also, the reference fields were not distributed randomly; there were two clusters, one on the lower face region and one near the amputation.

2. Reorganization is relatively rapid; the study was carried out after 4 weeks rather than 12 years. This rapidity might suggest that the reorganization is based on the unmasking of silent synapses (e.g., through disinhibition) rather than on anatomical sprouting. This claim receives further support from the recent studies of Aglioti et al. (1994a), who reports emergence of referred sensation in 5 days after radical mastectomy.

3. The possible existence of topography[3] on the face, e.g., in one patient, when we moved the cotton swab from the temporomandibular joint along the mandible toward the symphysis menti, he experienced an equivalent movement of referred sensation on his phantom arm.

4. The referral of complex sensations from regions remote from the line of amputation, e.g., warm water trickling down the face was felt as a sensation of warm water trickling down the phantom hand.

5. The induction of permanent telescoping using a virtual reality box.

6. The "rivalry" of warmth and cold sensations following simultaneous stimulation of two maps.

7. The shifting map proximal to the stump when the phantom hand is pronated, supinated, or flexed. (This occurred whether the phantom was telescoped or not.)

8. The long-term changes in maps observed in patient FA. It remains to be seen whether this was a consequence of the repeated facial stimulation that occurred during the EMG recording sessions.

In the older neurological literature, there are several examples of vague suggestions to the effect that phantom limbs have a central rather

---

[3] The presence of topography on the stump (but not on the face) was also noted by Cronholm (1951), but he attributed this (incorrectly, in my view) to the fact that the phantom was telescoped onto the stump.

than peripheral origin. Yet surprisingly, no attempt was made to formulate a precise, testable hypothesis. (One reason for this may be simply
that the work on primates was not available at that time.) What we call
the remapping hypothesis, on the other hand, makes the following simple
predictions: (1) Sensations should be referred from the face to this hand
after upper limb amputation and a second cluster of points should be
seen just proximal to the stump. As we have seen, this is true at least in
some patients. (2) There should be topography or both on the face and
proximal to the stump. Again, this appears to be true in many patients,
although for some reason, the topography is usually clearer near the
stump. (3) Sensations should be referred from the genitals to feet after
lower limb amputation, and we have seen this in at least two patients
(Ramachandran, 1993). There have also been previous reports of defeca-
tion and micturition causing referred sensations in the phantom (see
Sunderland, 1959, for a review), but no attempt was made to relate this
to the Penfield map. Our observations on the link between genitals and
feet have now been confirmed and significantly extended by Aglioti
et al. (1994b). (4) The hypothesis might also explain the widespread
prevalence of foot fetishes and the relative scarcity of (say) hand or nose
fetishes (e.g., there might be a slight "error" in mapping during fetal
development). We prefer this neurological explanation to Freud's psychodynamic interpretation, which postulates a visual resemblance between the foot and the penis. (5) Sensations should be referred from
foot to penis after penis amputation (e.g., for carcinoma) and from hand
to face after trigeminal ganglion section. The latter prediction would be
especially easy to test. (6) To determine whether the remapping is cortical
or subcortical, it would be interesting to look for referred sensations in
neurological patients who have sustained damage to the sensory thalamo-
cortical fibers in the internal capsule. A subset of these patients have
complete sensory loss on the contralateral side of the body, but a sparing of the face. Would these patients also refer sensations from the face
to hand? If so, one could conclude that the remapping was cortical.
(7) Finally, because the "magnification factor" has increased for the face,
one might also expect to see an actual improvement in sensory discrimination thresholds on the face.[4]

---

[4] Haber (1958) and Teuber *et al.* (1949) noticed an improvement in two-point thresholds
on the stump, and suggested, with considerable foresight, that this improvement may
occur as a result of "recruitment" of adjacent brain areas. The improvement, however,
could also be attributed other nonspecific "practice" effects, because patients tend to use
their stumps a great deal. To rule out this possibility it would be especially interesting to
look for improvement in touch thresholds, point localization, and two-point discrimination
on the face following amputation.

Thus, although the remapping hypothesis may eventually turn out to be wrong in detail, it leads to several testable predictions and may point to some new directions of research. As noted by Charles Darwin: "False facts are highly injurious to the progress of science, for they often endure long; but false views, if supported by some evidence, do little harm, for everyone takes a salutary pleasure in proving their falseness."

V. Neurology, Freud, and the Inner Ear

The social scientists have a long way to go to catch up, but they may be up to the most important scientific business of all, if and when they finally get to the right questions. Our behavior toward each other is the strangest, most unpredictable, and almost entirely unaccountable of all the phenomena with which we are obliged to live. (Lewis Thomas)

A. Neglect, Denial of Illness (Anosagnosia), and Somatoparaphrenic Delusions

We will now consider what might be loosely regarded as the converse of the phantom limb experience, namely, the syndrome of somatoparaphrenic delusions associated with right hemisphere stroke. Whereas in the case of phantom limbs the patient vividly experiences an arm that he knows to be missing, in somatoparaphrenia he asserts that his own paralyzed limb does not belong to him. "This is your arm, doctor," he might say, pointing to his own left arm!

Right hemisphere stroke usually results in a paralysis of the left side of the body (hemiplegia) and somatoparaphrenia is seen only in a small subset of these patients, usually those who have associated right parietal lobe damage. Curiously, left parietal disease does *not* result in denial of the right arm. A much more common manifestation of right parietal disease, however, is not an actual delusion that the arm belongs to someone else, but simply a denial of paralysis. [For insightful discussions on these topics, see Edelman (1991), Prigatano and Schacter (1991), and Weinstein and Kahn (1950).] Such a denial of paralysis was first recognized by Babinski, who coined the term "anosagnosia" to describe the condition. I became interested in this condition for two reasons. First, I believe that this disease provides an experimental approach to certain hitherto mysterious aspects of human nature such as the denial or repression of unpleasant memories or unpleasant facts about oneself. These phenomena are normally relegated to the realm of Freudian psychology, but I believe they can be brought into the realm of experimental neurology. Second, as we shall soon see, denial and neglect have considerable relevance to the problem of rehabilitation of neural function.

Consider, first, the relevance to rehabilitation from stroke. We usually think of neglect and denial as manifestations of injury or lesions in the right parietal cortex. But if this is true then how does one explain the fact that parietal lobe syndrome is one of those few neurological disorders that show a very high rate of spontaneous remissions within a few weeks? One argument might be that, as in the case of phantom limbs, some other part of the cortex (e.g., the other hemisphere) might take over some of these functions, but a remarkable discovery made by Bisiach and co-workers (1991) suggests an alternative, more exciting possibility. Bisiach *et al.* studied a patient who had sustained a right hemisphere stroke and was suffering from the delusion that his left arm belonged to someone else. They found, to their surprise, that when they simply poured cold water in the patient's left ear canal, there was a complete disappearance of symptoms! Unfortuantely, a few hours after the caloric stimulation had worn off, the symptoms returned and the patient once again started denying ownerhsip of his arm. Even so, Bisiach's discovery has two important far-reaching implications. First, it may pave the way toward a therapy for neglect and denial and other manifestations of parietal lobe disease. (Would repeated caloric stimulation accelerate recovery? Can a more pleasant substitute be found for vestibular stimulation?) Second, the result implies that many of the so-called syndromes of clinical neurology, which we ordinarily think of as irreversible hardware damage, may in fact represent deranged software (although, admittedly, the distinction between hardware and software is somewhat poorly defined for a biological system such as the brain). If this conclusion is correct, than the relevance of these findings for all kinds of therapy and rehabilitation becomes obvious.

B. How Deep Is the "Denial" of Anosagnosia?

Since Babinski's original description of this disease, there have been remarkably few studies on the question of *why* patients with right parietal disease deny their paralysis. With most neurological syndromes, the patient loses some specific mental capacity (e.g., syntax in Broca's aphasia and face recognition in prosopagnosia), but the integrity of the person remains largely intact. What is especially fascinating about anosognosia, on the other hand, is that the very notion of a "person" or self" is called into question (Galin, 1992).

To emphasize this further I will briefly describe a patient I saw recently after she was admitted to our hospital following a right hemisphere stroke. This patient (BM) was a 76-year-old lady who had complete paralysis of the left side of her body as a result of her stroke, but she persistently denied the paralysis even on repeated questioning. The following conversation[5] was typical:

VSR: *Mrs. M, when were you admitted to the hospital?*

BM: *I was admitted on April 7th because my daughter felt there was something wrong with me.*

VSR: *What day is it today and what time?*

BM: *It is sometime late in the afternoon on Tuesday. [This was an accurate response.]*

VSR: *Mrs. M., can you use your arms?*

BM: *Yes.*

VSR: *Can you use both hands?*

BM: *Yes, of course.*

VSR: *Can you use your right hand?*

BM: *Yes.*

VSR: *Can you use your left hand?*

BM: *Yes*

VSR: *Are both hands equally strong?*

BM: *Yes, they are equally strong.*

VSR: *Mrs. M, point to my student with your right hand. [Patient points.]*

VSR: *Mrs. M, point to my student with your left hand. [Patient remains silent.]*

VSR: *Mrs. M, why are you not pointing?*

BM: *Because I didn't want to.*

The same sequence of questions was repeated the next day with identical answers, except that toward the end of the session the patient looked at me and asked:

BM: *Doctor, whose hand is this [pointing to her own left hand]?*

VSR: *Whose hand do you think it is?*

BM: *Well, it certainly isn't yours!*

VSR: *Then whose is it?*

BM: *It isn't mine either.*

VSR: *Whose hand do you think it is?*

BM: *It is my son's hand, Doctor.*

---

[5] Patient BM was of Hispanic origin and a Spanish-speaking interpreter had to be used both during the testing and for subsequent analysis of the videotaped sessions.

Notice how the patient begins with rather simple denial of paralysis, but when her paralysis becomes increasingly obvious to her with repeated questioning, she is pushed into a corner and the only way she can rationalize the failure of her arm to perform is to progress into the even more full-blown delusion that the arm belongs to her son! (This is analogous to what Freud might call projection.) What we are seeing here on a compressed time scale, is an amplified version of the same kinds of delusions and rationalizations that all of us engage in some time or the other (Ramachandran, 1994).

A second, less psychodynamic interpretation of the same findings is also possible. One could argue, for instance, that she denies her arm because her body image is damaged in such a way that she "loses" half the image. (Even if this were true, however, one would still have to account for the subsequent bizarre rationalization that her arm belongs to her son.) What is puzzling about these cases, however, is the extreme lengths to which the patients will take the process, even though their intelligence, clarity of thought, and mentation are relatively unaffected in every other domain *except* for matters concerning the left hand! The patient I just described, for example, refused a box of candy, saying, "I am diabetic, Doctor—I can't eat candy. You should know that!" Thus, her anosagnosia included her limb but did not extend to her diabetes.

How does one go about studying anosagnosia in the laboratory? And to what extent does it affect prospects for effective rehabilitation? For if the patient is in a state of denial, what possible motivation could she have for engaging in rehabilitative therapy? These are difficult questions but we have recently begun a series of experiments that might help provide some answers. One interesting question, for example, concerns the depth of the patient's denial. Is the denial of paralysis mainly at the semantic/verbal level or does it run deeper? If it is mainly semantic, then is it possible that the patient is subconsciously aware that he/she is in fact paralyzed? We devised four novel tests to try and answer these questions (Ramachandran, 1994).

1. Test 1

We used our virtual reality box to trick the patient into thinking that her left hand was moving in response to her command. This was achieved by simply placing an 18" by 18" mirror vertically on the table so that it was perpendicular to the table as well as to the patient's chest (e.g., imagine opening a book so that the front cover stands upright; the front cover would then be the mirror). The mirror was concealed in a large wooden box and the patient simply inserted her two hands through circular windows cut into the face of the box, so that they lay on either side of the mirror, palm down on the floor of the box. The top of the box was opaque on the left so that the patient could not directly see her left hand, but the box was clear on the right so that she could see both her right hand and the reflected image of her right hand in the mirror. Because the hands were placed parallel and close to each other on either side of the mirror, the mirror image of the right hand was exactly superimposed on the "felt" position of the left hand. The result was that the patient was tricked into thinking that she was seeing her own two hands. When instructed to move both hands up and down, she obviously saw her right hand obey her command but she also saw her lifeless left hand suddenly coming to life, moving as though it was following her command! Our question was, would the patient register surprise, especially if she knew at some subconscious level that her left arm was paralyzed? Or would she fail to find it surprising because she believed that both her hands were functioning normally? Surprise was measured using two techniques—a galvanic skin response (GSR) and changes in expression, such as raised eyebrows. (The entire session was videotaped for subsequent analysis.)

2. Test 2

In the second test, the patient was given a choice between performing two tasks: a simple bimanual task (e.g., tying a shoelace into a bow knot or cutting a circular disk out of a sheet of cardboard) versus a unimanual task (e.g., threading a bolt). She was told, also, that she would be given a large box of candy if she successfully completed the first task and a small box of candy for the second task. (She was, of course, not explicitly told that the tasks were unimanual and bimanual.) Our question was, would the patient show a spontaneous preference for the unimanual task, despite the smaller reward, even though she denied the paralysis of her left arm? In other words, can a dissociation between "procedural" and "declarative" knowledge be observed in anosagnosia?

3. Test 3

The patient was asked to reach out and grab a tray with glasses on it. Would her right hand automatically reach for the handle on the right side or would it go straight for the middle of the tray?

4. Test 4

In the fourth task, the suject simply viewed herself in a large full-length mirror while being instructed to perform simple movements with her left or right hand alternately. Ordinarily, the patient will refuse to acknowledge her failure of performance by saying, "I didn't want to move it that time," or, "I'm not usually very ambidextrous" (as one patient once told us). Would seeing her failure in a mirror or videtape, however, enable her to adopt a more "abstract" attitude, i.e., enable her to distance herself from her own body image and thereby allow her to acknowledge her paralysis?

We have, so far, tried some of these experiments on two patients (BM and LR)[6] and the preliminary results were most intriguing (Ramachandran, 1994). The patients (LR) clearly did *not* show "subconscious knowledge" of paralysis on any of the tasks, suggesting that the denial must be very deep indeed; it cannot simply be the inverse of hysterical paralysis (or of malingering). On the unimanual versus bimanual task, for example, patient LR consistently chose the bimanual task (e.g., tying a shoelace). This was true even when the test was prefaced with the question "Mrs. LR, how many hands would you need to tie a bow knot or a shoelace? And how many hands do you need to thread the bolt?" She answered both questions correctly, but went straight for the shoelace task and kept trying to tie a bow knot with one hand! Patient BM, however, chose the nut/bolt unimanual task on one occasion. When asked why she preferred this task even though a larger reward had been offered for tying a shoelace, she replied, "The other task might be too difficult for me" "Why is it more difficult?" I asked, to which she replied, "I don't know why. It just seems like it might be." Computerized tomograpy scans revealed right parietal lesions in both patients, but one wonders whether there were subtle differences to the extent of lesion that might account for the differences in depth of anosagnosia.

C. Repressed Memories

An even more remarkable piece of evidence for subconscious knowledge comes from another experiment we did on patient BM. The reader

---

[6] Patient LR was a 79-year-old, right-handed lady who was admitted for left-sided weakness; she was seen by us for 4 weeks after her admission. A CT scan revealed an infarct in the region supplied by the right middle cerebral artery. Neurological examination revealed a residual left hemiplegia affecting the left upper extremity quite severely, a left-sided neglect (line crossing and line bisection tests), and a mild dysarthria. She was quite alert and attentive and her memory, both short and long term, was intact. She had no obvious dementia or aphasia.

Patient BM was a 76-year-old Hispanic woman who was admitted for sudden-onset left-sided hemiplegia and was seen by us 2 weeks later. She had clear neurological signs of left hemiplegia and neglect (e.g., extreme right gaze preference), was accurate but somewhat sluggish in responding to questions or commands, and was able to communicate clearly with the examiner. An MRI revealed a right parieto-occipital lesion along with slight involvement of the right thalamus and head of the caudate nucleus.

will recall that this patient denied her paralysis even on repeated questioning, and she finally asserted that the arm belonged to her son. Having been inspired by the experiments of Bisiach *et al.* (1991), I decided to try a caloric test on this patient. After she had repeated several times that she was not paralyzed and her arm belonged to her son, I administered 10 ml of ice-cold water into her left ear and waited until nystagmus appeared. My main interest was not only in replicating Bisiach's observation, but also in specifically asking her questions about her memory, an issue that had never been studied directly before on a systematic basis.

VSR:	*Do you feel okay?*
BM:	*My ear is very cold but other than that I am fine.*
VSR:	*Can you use your hands?*
BM:	*I can use my right arm but not my left arm. I want to move it but it doesn't move.*
VSR:	*[holding the arm in front of the patient] Whose arm is this?*
BM:	*It is my hand, of course.*
VSR:	*Can you use it?*
BM:	*No, it is paralyzed.*
VSR:	*Mrs. M, how long has your arm been paralyzed? Did it start now or earlier?*
BM:	*It has been paralyzed continuously for several days now.*

After the caloric effect had worn off completely, I waited for $\frac{1}{2}$ hour and asked:

VSR:	*Mrs. M, can you use your arm?*
BM:	*No, my left arm doesn't work.*

Finally, the same set of questions was repeated to the patient 8 hours later by one of our colleagues.

EX:	*Mrs. M, can you walk?*
BM:	*Yes.*
EX:	*Can you use both your arms?*
BM:	*Yes.*
EX:	*Can you use your left arm?*
BM:	*Yes.*
EX:	*This morning, two doctors did something to you. Do you remember?*
BM:	*Yes. They put water in my ear; it was very cold.*
EX:	*Do you remember they asked some questions about your arms, and you gave them an answer? Do you remember what you said?*

BM: *No, what did I say?*
EX: *What do you think you said. Try and remember.*
BM: *I said my arms were okay.*

These observations have several remarkable implications. First, they confirm the observation of Bisiach *et al.* about remission from anosagnosia and delusion following caloric stimulation. Second, they also allow us to draw certain important new inferences about denial and memory repression. Specifically, her admission that she had been paralyzed for *several days* suggests that even though she had been continuously denying her paralysis, the information about the paralysis was being continuously laid down[7] in her brain, i.e., the denial did not prevent memory consolidation (Ramachandran, 1994). Again, we may conclude that at some deeper level she does indeed have knoweldge about the paralysis. (Also, the insight gained during the caloric stimulus seemed to last at least for $\frac{1}{2}$ hour after the stimulation had ceased!) Finally, when tested 8 hours later, she not only reverted to denial, but also "repressed" the admission of paralysis that she had made during her stimulation. The remarkable theoretical implication of these observations is that memories can indeed be selectively repressed although, it is unclear whether this repression occurs during consolidation or during the subsequent split second recollection.

Seeing patient BM also convinced me, for the first time, of the reality of the repression phenomena that form the cornerstone of classical psychoanalytical theory. Selective memory repression was also seen in patient LR, whom we tested three times at weekly intervals, and she denied each time that her left arm was paralyzed. Furthermore, she always chose the bimanual task, instead of the unimanual one, and continued to do so with no sign of frustration despite her repeated failures. Finally, after her last try on the third week, I asked her to point to my student with her left hand. She tried to do so and then admitted for the first time in 3 weeks that she could not use her left hand. (And 10 minutes later when asked to point again, she spontaneously admitted her paralysis.) A week later, when my student questioned LR again in my absence, she admitted to remembering me as, "The nice Indian doctor who asked

---

[7] Part of this, of course, could have been a confabulatory "gap-filling," i.e., she sees now that she is paralyzed and she knew that she was admitted for stroke several weeks ago and therefore makes the obvious inference (whether consciously or not) that she must have been paralyzed for that entire period. Her use of the phrases "several days" and "continuously paralyzed" suggests, however, that this was not the case. Mrs. BM's apparent lack of surprise when she admitted paralysis (during caloric stimulation) is also noteworthy, because it implies that she was also repressing the denial that she had been engaging in just a few minutes earlier!

me to tie shoelaces," and then went on to add, "He asked me to tie the laces on a small shoe. I was able to do so *using both my hands*." But when my student queried her specifically about pointing, she admitted at once, "Yes, he asked me to point with my left hand. I was unable to do so."

Thus, she had selectively repressed her failure to tie laces (perhaps because her failure was never explicitly pointed out to her), but had not repressed her inability to point! Doing so might have required her to stretch the truth to a degree that she was simply not capable of, given, especially, that she was probably already in partial remission 8 weeks after the stroke.

It would be premature to draw any firm conclusions from these very preliminary observations, but clearly the findings are sufficiently provocative that they warrant a systematic large-scale effort to understand these phenomena. Perhaps the reason Mrs. BM repressed her previous admission of paralysis was that there was no way she could honestly deny her present paralysis and still acknowledge the insight she gained during caloric-stimulation—without falling apart. We may conclude, therefore, that remembering something, even from the recent past, entails a complete reordering of one's conscious experience to accommodate current demands.

D. A Darwinian Theory of Defense Mechanisms

In my view, the various defense mechanisms, rationalization, repression, etc., arise because the brain tries to arrive at the most probable and globally consistent interpretation of the evidence derived from multiple sources. By way of analogy, consider a military general trying to make a major strategic decision, e.g., whether to invade a particular city at a particular time. He would ordinarily collect evidence from a large number of scouts, weigh the evidence, and arrive at a firm decision. Now, if one scout were to provide information that was somewhat contradictory to the rest (e.g., he might indicate that the enemy had 10,000 soldiers rather than 5000), the general would be unlikely to change his strategy. He may ask the scout to be silent and to discard the evidence, or, for fear of mutiny, he may actually ask the scout to "march in tune" with the others, and if necessary, even lie to the other officers in the army. (The former would be analogous to denial and the latter to rationalization or confabulation.) A perpetually indecisive general, on the other hand, would be quite incapable of winning a war.

Oddly enough, something like this also seems to occur when the visual system tries to combine multiple sources of information about relative depth (e.g., perspective, stereo, occlusion, motion parallax, shading) to yield a vivid coherent impression of depth (Ramachandran, 1988). The rules that the visual system uses to combine multiple cues are poorly understood, but may involve two processes: (1) taking a weighted average (the weighing is important because, statistically speaking, some cues might be inherently more reliable than others, and this "wisdom" might be wired into the visual system during ontogeny and phylogeny) and (2) looking for consistency (e.g., if six cues yield random values and two yield identical values, then the visual system may "choose" the latter instead of averaging the values). This is because accidental inconsistencies are common in nature (due to noise) but accidental consistencies are rare.

Interestingly, once a global interpretation of depth has been reached, the system simply ignores or suppresses the conflicting information. The purpose of this might be to avoid going into a perpetually indecisive state, i.e., the rule might be that any firm decision is better than none at all. Now the remarkable thing is that the visual system may, on occasion, even hallucinate some of the required evidence in order to preserve consistency, i.e., there appears to be a tendency to actually impose coherence. It was as though the general had decided not only to ignore the advice of one of his scouts, but also insisted that the scout actually fabricate the evidence required in order to fit the "big picture."

A striking example of this can be observed with the illusory square (Fig. 5), which is created by simply aligning four disks from which pie-shaped sectors have been removed (Kanizsa, 1979). What people usually see when viewing this display is an opaque white square partially occlud-

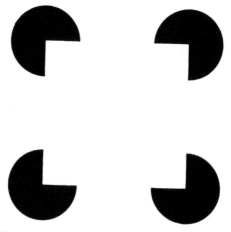

Fig. 5. An illusory square (after Kanizsa, 1979).

ing four back disks, rather than four disks that have been deceitfully aligned by the experimenter.

Now it should be obvious that when seeing a square in this display, the visual system has to discard the contrary evidence from the homogeneous paper surface about the absence of an edge (for such an edge would usually be associated with a change of luminance). But instead of discarding the perception of a square, the visual system seems to opt for actually hallucinating an illusory edge, which even has an illusory brightness change associated with it (an example of "Vector Completion"). So here is a clear example of the visual system "jury rigging" the evidence in order to impose a coherent interpretation.

Now in my view, the same sort of thing happens in the cognitive/emotional domain. We have a tremendous need to impose a sense of order and coherence in our lives—we need a "story." Of course, when most of the evidence favors one particular interpretation of the available data, we have no difficulty in simply accepting that interpretation. For example, even when a patient's arm is paralyzed, her motor cortex sends messages to her limb and there is a comparator in her brain that ordinarily monitors these feed-forward signals and informs her "self" that, "I am moving my limb." Therefore her conscious self tentatively accepts this story.[8] When the evidence is conflicting, however (e.g., if the patient's vision tells her that her arm is not obeying her commands), then instead of wasting time in conflict or oscillating between alternate decisions, her cognitive system simply picks one story and adheres to it. Again, in order to do this, it either ignores the conflicting evidence (denial) or actually fabricates new evidence (rationalization). The evolutionary purpose of such defense mechanisms might be that when limited time is available, *any* decision, however uncertain, is better than an indecisive vacillation—so long as it is the best interpretation of the current data. But to deal with a conflicting source of information that keeps nagging away at the central processor, the latter may actually insert the relevant evidence so that it can go about the rest of its business. What you end up with, therefore, is a rationalization or a denial.

And that brings me to my last point. The purpose of a rationalization, we have seen, is to eliminate discrepancy by creating fictitious evidence (or false beliefs). But clearly there must be limits to this process, for

---

[8] This is similar to the function of the "interpreter" in the left hemisphere that Gazzaniga (1992) has postulated, to account for the rationalization that one observes in split brain patients. What I have tried to do in this chapter, however, is to consider the biological role of such a mechanism. I also postulate a second mechanism in the right hemisphere that is required for monitoring the magnitude of discrepancy and for generating a paradigm shift.

otherwise defense mechanisms would soon become maladaptive and threaten the individual's survival. It may be a good thing to repress an extremely traumatic memory in order to avoid being paralyzed with fear. This *would* be adaptive. It would be maladaptive, however, to repress every memory that was unpleasant because that would defeat the very purpose of having aversive memories in the first place. I suggest, therefore, that there is a special-purpose mechanism in the right parietal lobe whose sole purpose is to periodically "challenge" the left hemisphere's story, detect discrepancies, and make sure that the discrepancy is not too large. (You can think of this, if you like, as a center for intellectual honesty or integrity.) Hence, I might be willing to engage in some minor rationalization, i.e., make some small false assumptions to get on with my life, but when the false beliefs become too far removed for reality, my discrepancy detector kicks in and makes me reevaluate the situation (e.g., if I was a general about to wage war, it would be quite appropriate, usually, to ignore contrary evidence from a single scout, but if he told me that the enemy was waving a white flag or had nuclear arms, I would be foolish to adhere to my original decision). I suggest, further, that the mechanism for imposing consistency (i.e., the small rationalizations and repressions) is located in the left hemisphere, whereas the global anomaly detector that monitors the level of discrepancy and reacts with the appropriate emotion is in the right hemisphere[9]. This would explain why right hemisphere patients are willing to engage in much more elaborate and fanciful rationalizations than normal individuals or individuals with left hemisphere damage. Conversely, left hemisphere stroke patients may not be able to manage even a minimal amount of denial, rationalization, or confabulatory gap-filling and consequently become profoundly depressed. This would be a new interpretation of the common clinical observation that depression is most often associated with left hemisphere stroke. (The more common interpretation is that the right hemisphere is the emotional hemisphere, so that the affect is inappropriate when it is damaged.)

This theory may also help explain another major psychological puzzle—the biological significance of laughter and humor. When the "discrepancy detector" in the right hemisphere questions and corrects the

---

[9] Another way to characterize the difference between the hemispheres would be to note that their manner of dealing with anomalies is different. When small local errors are detected, the left hemisphere tries to impose consistency by ignoring or suppressing the evidence, whereas when there are large, global anomalies, an interaction with the right hemisphere forces a change in world view—a paradigm shift. Until we have a clearer idea of the underlying neural mechanisms, such a metaphorical explanation will have to serve as a temporary substitute.

rationalization or tentative hypothesis of the left hemisphere, the net result can be a strong emotional response. The defenses crumble and force a revision of world view; composure must be given up in order to correct behavior (e.g., by fight or flight). But if the correction is only of relatively trivial consequence (e.g., the burglar turns out to be a neighbor's cat), then the tension that is built up is discharged by a convulsive laughter. (This hypothesis would predict that right hemisphere patients should lack a sense of humor but should, paradoxically, sound funny to the physician.)

E. FREUD AND THE INNER EAR: A NEUROLOGICAL APPROACH TO PSYCHOTHERAPY

Finally, let us consider the extent to which these defense mechanisms (such as denial and projection) are domain specific, i.e., do they apply only to the patient's paralyzed limb or to all of the patient's maladies? (The reader will recall that patient BM denied her paralysis but was concerned about her diabetes!) We propose to test this experimentally using our mirror test (Test 2 described earlier), except that the patient will be asked to view the left side of the mirror so that she sees the reflection of her paralyzed left hand superimposed on the felt position of her (hidden) right hand. If she is now asked to move her right hand, she will, of course, feel her movement, but the hand will appear not to move. With this sensory conflict, the question, is, will she now rationalize the disability by saying, "Oh, I did see the hand move" or "I wasn't *really* trying to move my hand," or will she express surprise just as you and I would in that situation? In other words, does her tendency to confabulate affect only her left arm or does it also affect her other arm?

Is it conceivable that there are mechanisms in the right hemisphere that are concerned with detecting not only a discrepancy involving the corporeal self but with detecting other types of discrepancies as well? According to classical psychoanalytical theory, many forms of neuroses arise because the patient's defense mechanisms have become so extreme that they have actually become maladaptive instead of being simply used as a coping strategy. Providing insight into these maladaptive defense mechanisms is, therefore, one of the goals of Freudian psychoanalysis, and this is usually achieved by several months or years of intensive psychotherapy. But if we are correct in arguing that that insight can be enhanced using caloric left ear stimulation in patients with parietal lesions, is it conceivable that such insight could also be induced in neurotic patients who are neurologically intact, in order to eliminate the maladaptive defenses that are said to produce the psychoneuroses? (Notice that the efficacy of this would not necessarily depend on whether the denial is encapsulated; all we have to assume is that caloric stimulation can also eliminate other types of anosagnosia and amnesia by activation of the right hemisphere—a proposition that can be tested experimentally.) After all, in patient BM, caloric stimulation not only eliminated denial but also allowed the repressed memory of the paralysis to be overcome. What I am suggesting, then, is that left ear caloric stimulation[10] may eventually be used actually to replace psychoanalysis as a device for reviving repressed memories and for producing insight. If so, a few dozen sessions of cold water stimulation of the left ear might prove just as effective as several months of costly and intensive psychotherapy. Obviously, these are highly speculative and tentative ideas, but at least they are testable and they may eventually suggest new ways to rehabilitate and reeducate the malfunctioning brain.

VI. Conclusions: Is There Reason for Optimism?

The main conclusion to emerge from our experiments [together with the important recent work of Aglioti et al. (1994a,b) and Halligan and Marshall (1993)] is that we must give up the notion that the human brain is composed of a fixed set of anatomical connections specified largely by the genome. Our results suggest, instead, that even the adult brain is a dynamic biological system in which new connections are being created all the time, partly in response to novel sensory inputs and partly as a result of self-organizing principles. Everyone recognizes, of course, that some changes must be possible even in the adult brain, for otherwise, it would not be possible to account for phenomena such as learning and memory. What our results imply, however, is that even the basic circuitry or hardware in the brain—such as the sensory maps—can be altered with surprising rapidity. No one would have suspected, for example, that the famous Penfield homunculus, which every medical student learns about, can be reorganized over a distance of 2 cm or more in less than 4 weeks. And remarkably, the remapping, at least in some cases,

---

[10] Why does caloric stimulation produce these apparently miraculous effects? One possibility is that vestibular stimulation generates "orientating" through cortical activation, as shown in animals (Fredrickson, 1964). A second more intriguing possibility is that the eye movements generated by the caloric stimulation directly derepress memories in the right hemisphere in a manner analogous to the derepression of memories that occurs during dreaming in rapid eye movement (REM) sleep.

is precise and orderly, for if it was not, one could not account for the emergence of a topographically organized, modality-specific reference field on the face or for the referral of complex sensations such as "trickle" from the face to the phantom. It is unclear, at present, how one could harness this latent ability of the brain to accelerate recovery from brain injury, but if our view of the brain is correct, then there is at least reason for optimism.

The second set of experiments, on patients with denial and neglect, also has obvious relevance to stroke rehabilitation. But more importantly, perhaps, these experiments may eventually turn out to have broader implications for understanding the biological origin of defense mechanisms. The results of our studies may, in fact, suggest an experimental approach to these enigmatic aspects of human nature and eventually may lead to new types of treatment for the many intractable psychological problems to which our species is notoriously prone.

Acknowledgments

We thank F. H. C. Crick, D. Galin, J. Bogen, P. Churchland, O. Sacks, L. Franz, P. Halligan, J. Marshall, A. Damasio, T. Sejnowski, H. Pashler, D. Rogers-Ramachandran, M. Stallcup, R. McKinney, and J. Ramachandran for stimulating discussions; M. Botte, L. Stone, and G. Arcilla for referring their patients to us; and L. Levi, who collaborated with me on the caloric stimulation experiment. P. Halligan and J. Marshall (personal communication) have also independently observed long-term changes in the map on the face in one of their patients. The research reported in this paper received partial support from the AFOSR and ONR. The work was carried out in the newly formed Center for Research on Brain and Cognition at the University of California, San Diego.

References

Aglioti, S., Cortese, F., and Franchini, C. (1994a). Rapid sensory remapping in the adult human brain as inferred from phantom breast perception. *Neuroreport* **5**, 473–476.

Aglioti, S., Bonazzi, A., and Cortese, F. (1994b). Phantom lower limbs as a perceptual marker of neural plasticity in the mature human brain. *Proc. Roy. Soc. Lond.* (in press).

Bisiach, E., Rusconi, M. L., and Vallar, G. (1991). Remission of somatophrenic delusion through vestibular stimulation. *Neuropsychologia* **29**, 1029–1031.

Brain, R., and Walton, J. W. (1969). "Brain's Diseases of the Nervous System." Oxford Univ. Press, London.

Calford, M. (1991). Neurobiology. Curious cortical change. *Nature (London)* **352**, 759–760.

Calford, M. B., and Tweedale, R. (1990). Interhemispheric transfer of plasticity in the cerebral cortex. *Science* **249**, 805–807.

Cronholm, B. (1951). Phantom limbs in amputees. A study of changes in the integration of centripetal impulses with special reference to referred sensations. *Acta Psychiatr. Neurol. Scand. Suppl.* **72**, 1–310.

Dykes, R., Avendano, C., and Leclere, S. (1994). Evolution of cortical responsiveness to peripheral nerve transection. *J. Comp. Neurol.* (in press).

Edelman, G. M. (1989). "The Remembered Present." Basic Books, New York.

Fredrickson, J., Kornhuber H, and Schwarz, D. W. (1974). *In* "Handbook of Sensory Physiology" (H. Kornhuber, ed.), Vol. 6, 565–583. Springer-Verlag, New York.

Galin, D. (1992). Theoretical reflections on awareness, monitoring and self in relation to anosagnosia. *Consciousness and Cognition* **1**, 152–162.

Gazzaniga, M. (1992). "Nature's Mind." Basic Books, New York.

Halligan, P., and Marshall, J. (1993). *Neuroreport* **4**, 233–236.

Haber W. B. (1958). Reactions to the loss of a limb. *Ann. N.Y. Acad. Sci.* **74**, 14–24.

Head H., and Holmes G. (1912). Sensory disturbances from cerebral lesions. *Lancet* **1**, 144–152.

James, W. (1887). The consciousness of lost limbs. *Proc. Am. Soc. Psychical Res.* **1**, 249–258.

Jones, E. (1982). Thalamic basis of place- and modality-specific columns in monkey somatosensory cortex: A correlative anatomical and physiological study. *J. Neurophysiol.* **48**, 546–568.

Kaas, J. H., Nelson, R. J., Sur, M., and Merzenich, M. M. (1981). "The Organization of the Cerebral Cortex," pp. 237–261. MIT Press, Cambridge, Massachusetts.

Kanizsa, G. (1979). "The Organization in Vision." Praeger, Santa Monica, CA.

Kelahan, A. M., and Doetsch, G. S. (1981). Short term changes in the functional organization of somatosensory cortex of adult racoons after digit amputation. *Soc. Neurosci. Abstr.* **7**, 540.

Kenshalo, D. R., Hensel, H., Graziade, I. P., and Fruhstorfer, H. (1971). *In* "Oral-facial Sensory and Motor Mechanisms" (R. Dubner and Y. Kawamura, eds.), pp. 23–45. Appleton-Crofts, New York.

Kreisman, N. R., and Zimmerman, I. D. (1971). Cortical unit responses to temperature stimulation of the skin. *Brain Res.* **25**, 184–187.

Landgren, S. (1960). Thalamic neurons responding to cooling of the cat's tongue. *Acta Physiol. Scand.* **48**, 255–267.

Lashley, K. (1950). In search of the Engram. *Soc. Exp. Biol. Symp. No. 4.* Cambridge Univ. Press, London and New York.

Lund, J. P., Gond, D. S. and Lamarre, Y. (1994). *Science* (submitted).

Melzack, R. (1992). Phantom limbs. *Sci. Am.* **266**, 90–96.

Merzenich, M. M., Kaas, J. H., Wall, J. T., Nelson, R. J., Sur, M., and Felleman, D. (1983). Topographic reorganization of somatosensory cortical areas 3b and 1 in adult monkeys following restricted deafferentation. *Neuroscience* **8**, 33–55.

Merzenich, M. M., Nelson, R. J., Stryker, M. S., Cynader M. S., Schoppmann, A., and Zook, J. M. (1984). Somatosensory cortical map changes following digit amputation in adult monkeys. *J. Comp. Neurol* **224**, 591–605.

Mitchell, S. W. (1871). Lippincott's *Mag. Popular Lit. Sci.* **8**, 563–569.

Mountcastle, V. B. (1957). Modality and topographic properties of single neurons in a cat's somatosensory cortex. *J. Neurophysiol.* **20**, 408–434.

Pons, T. (1992). Perceptual correlates of massive cortical reorganization. *Science* **258**, 1159–1160.

Pons, T. P., Preston, E., Garraghty, A. K., *et al.* (1991). Massive cortical reorganization after sensory deafferentation in adult macaques. *Science* **252**, 1857–1860.

Prigatano, G., and Schacter, D. (1991). "Awareness of Deficit after Brain Injury." Oxford Univ. Press, London.

Ramachandran, V. S. (1988). The perception of shape from shading. *Sci. Am.* **269,** 76–83.

Ramachandran, V. S. (1993). Behavioural and MEG correlates of neural plasticity in the adult human brain. *PNAS* **90,** 10413–10420.

Ramachandran, V. S. (1994). How deep is the denial (anosagnosia) of parietal lobe syndrome? *Soc. Neurosci Abstr.*

Ramachandran, V. S., Rogers-Ramachandran, D., and Stewart, M. (1992a). Perceptual correlates of massive cortical reorganization. *Science* **258,** 1159–1160.

Ramachandran, V. S., Stewart, M., and Rogers-Ramachandran, D. C. (1992b). Perceptual correlates of massive cortical reorganization. *NeuroReport* **3,** 583–586.

Ramachandran, V., Rogers-Ramachandran, D., and Grush, R. (1993). *Soc. Neurosci Abstr.* **19** (in press).

Rasmusson, D., and Turnbull, B. (1983). Immediate effects of digit amputation on S1 cortex in the raccoon: Unmasking inhibiting fields. *Brain Res.* **288,** 368–373.

Sunderland, S. (1959). "Nerves and Nerve Injuries." Saunders, Philadelphia, Pennsylvania.

Teuber, H. L., Krieger, H. P., and Bender M. B. (1949). Reorganization of sensory function in amputation stumps. *Fed. Proc.* **8,** 156.

Valentin, G. (1836). Uber die subjectiven gefule von personen. *Rep. Anat. Physiol.* **1,** 328–3371.

Wall, P. (1971). The presence of inaffective synapses and the circumstances which unmask them. *Phil. Trans. Roy. Soc. Lond. Ser. B* **278,** 361–372.

Weinstein, E. A., and Kahn, R. L. (1950). The syndrome of anosagnosia. *Arch. Neurol. Psych.* **64,** 772–791.

Weisel, T. N., and Hubel, D. H. (1965). Comparison of the effects of unilateral and bilateral eye disease on cortical unit responses in young kittens. *J. Neurophysiol.* **28,** 1029–1040.

Weiss, P. (1939). "Principles of Development." Holt, New York.

Yang, T., Gallen, C., Ramachandran, V. S., Cobb, S., and Bloom, F. (1993). *Soc. Neurosci. Abstr.*

Yang, T., Gallen, C., Schwartz, B., Bloom, F., Ramachandran, V. S., and Cobb, S. (1994). Sensory maps in the human brain. *Nature (London)* **368,** 592–593.

NEURAL DARWINISM AND A CONCEPTUAL CRISIS IN PSYCHOANALYSIS

Arnold H. Modell

Harvard University
Cambridge, Massachusetts 02138

My introduction to Edelman's theory of neuronal group selection (TNGS) was quite fortuitous, as it was purely by chance that I happened to read "Neural Darwinism" (1987). At that time I was preparing a book on the theory of psychoanalytic treatment and was excited to discover that Edelman's concept that memory as recategorization was very similar to a theory of memory that Freud had proposed in 1896. The similarity between Edelman's and Freud's theory of memory may be no coincidence in that Freud was also constructing a global theory of the brain. In the previous year, 1895, Freud wrote "The Project for A Scientific Psychology," his failed attempt to describe psychological phenomena as a neurophysiological process. His insight was as follows: memory, as Edelman also claims, is not isomorphic with experience; memory is not laid down once but several times over, at the boundary of successive developmental epochs (see Freud's letter to Fleiss, December 6 1896; Masson, 1985). At these boundaries a new transcription or translation takes place. Repression leads to psychopathology because of a failure of retranscription. I have retained Freud's term *Nachträglichkeit* to describe his theory of memory. *Nachträglichkeit* may be roughly translated as a retranscription or, more awkwardly, as subsequentiality. The etymological roots of this German word are of some interest because there is a connection with the verb "to carry" as well as the Greek verb *metaphorein*, "to transport," from which we derive the noun "metaphor."

The psychoanalyst has frequent opportunity to observe that affective memories are categorical. I use the term "affects" to describe what we ordinarily refer to as feelings. These categorical memories, encountered in the multileveled intersubjective relationship between analyst and patient, are the memories of experiences that remain unassimilated. A patient of mine reported the following incident (see Modell, 1990): Due to the fact that his airline went out on strike, my patient was stranded in a distant city and was unable to return home. He did everything possible to obtain passage on another airline: he cajoled and pleaded with the functionaries of other airlines, all to no avail. Although my patient was usually not unduly anxious and was in fact a highly experi-

335

enced traveler, who, in the past remained calm under circumstances that would frighten many people, in this particular situation he experienced an overwhelming and generalized panic. He felt as if the unyielding airline representatives were like Nazis and that the underground passages of the airline terminal resembled a concentration camp. The helplessness of not being able to return home, combined with the institutional intransigence of the authorities, evoked the following categorical memory. When this man was 3 years old he and his parents were residents of a central European country and, as Jews, were desperately attempting to escape from the Nazis. They did in fact manage to obtain an airline passage to freedom, but until that point the outcome was very much in doubt. Although my patient did not recall his affective state at that time, his parents reported that he seemed cheerful and unaffected by their great anxiety. In this example, his helpless inability to leave a foreign city triggered or evoked an unassimilated categorical memory from age 3 years. It is not unreasonable to infer that the specific events in current time, his inability to find an airline passage, triggered a conceptual match with a salient memory from age 3 years, the affects of which were then experienced in current time. The events were remembered but the affects associated with those events were repressed. It can be said that a translation had not occurred subsequently; a recategorization had not taken place.

The idea of memory as a retranscription is central to a theory of the therapeutic action of psychoanalysis (this topic is reviewed in Modell, 1990). Through the retranscription of memory, the present can alter the past. One of the means through which psychoanalysis alleviates psychic pain is the recreation of old traumatic experiences within the context of the new relationship with the analyst in current time. By this process, old affective memories of traumatic experiences are retranscribed. This recategorization is also consistent with a procedural aspect of TNGS in its emphasis on motor activity that seeks a match between past and present salient memory categories. Psychoanalysts have long observed a parallel process in that patients are unconsciously driven to test whether their perception of the analyst in current time corresponds to their memories of those persons in the past with whom they have had traumatic experiences. It is not uncommon for patients unconsciously to provoke the analyst to act a similar part as the person with whom they have had a traumatic experience. This familiar repetition within the transference, Freud attributed to the repetition compulsion, which he had mistakenly understood as a fundamental quality of instinct. According to TNGS, repetition is a fundamental quality, not of instinct but of memory.

Categorical memory is a potential memory awaiting activation. I find that this idea clarifies the seemingly incongruous notion of unconscious affects. Some authors have attempted to deal with this problem by distinguishing unconscious affects from conscious affects by referring to the latter as feeling (Sandler and Joffe, 1969). Psychoanalysts speak of psychic structure in many different contexts. In one such context, psychic structures are equivalent to the long-term memory of affective experiences. For example, a repeated traumatic interaction with a caretaker may be internalized as an identification in which subject and object are represented. That is to say, the traumatic relationship is memorialized so that the affective components of both self and other become part of the self. The affects associated with this experience can be said to be unconscious in that they exist only as a potential awaiting activation. The following clinical vignette may make this clear (reported in Modell, 1990).

One if my patients had a traumatic relationship with her father in that he was subject to unexpected, violent, and totally irrational rage reactions. When her father lost control of his temper, my patient, understandably, experienced herself as the innocent victim because she believed that her father's rage was totally unprovoked—it came totally out of the blue. My casual use of the words "out of the blue" triggered the following episode. During our session I experienced the patient to be very withdrawn and almost completely silent and yet she complained that I was not making any useful comments or interpretations. I replied, probably with a slight edge of irritation, that she wanted me to produce something "out of the blue." This comment resulted in a violent rage reaction, which I then experienced as unprovoked, as coming "out of the blue." This categorical memory of the attacker and the attacked was recreated in current time with a reversal of roles. I experienced the affects that I believe my patient experienced when being attacked by her father—I felt a sense of surprise, of bewilderment, and overall a sense of the unfairness of being attacked when I, as far as I knew, had done nothing wrong. *I* became the "innocent" victim. What is also of interest is that when we discussed this episode some days later, my patient was unaware that she was angry or provocative. Her rage was dissociated; it could be described as unconscious.

I wish now to consider a somewhat different subject, the possible relevance for psychoanalysis of the concept of value, and the theory of consciousness presented in "The Remembered Present" (Edelman, 1989). For those animals who posses a higher order consciousness, the adaptive function of consciousness is fairly explicit, in that consciousness enables the organism to have a coherent model of present, past, and future that frees it from the tyranny of current inputs. This higher order consciousness can be said to imply a concept of self in that current perceptual events are recategorized in accordance with past value category matches. I would speculate that in humans this process results in a sense of continuity and coherence. The fact that value will exercise a selective preference or bias on perception and consciousness requires a discrimination between self and non-self. To quote from "The Remembered Present" (p. 98): "Current perceptual events are recategorized in terms of past value-category matches. It is the *contrast* of the special linkage of value and past categories with currently arriving categories, and the *dominance* of the self-related special memory systems in this memorial linkage, that generate the self-referential aspect of consciousness." According to TNGS the organism is a *creator* of those criteria that lead to information. If I were to extend this theory to the psychology of the self, the self can be seen as creator of meaning. From the perspective of the self, meaning is created through the memories of salient affective experiences. I firmly believe that the need to maintain the sense of the continuity and coherence of the self is an evolutionary given [this point is discussed further in Modell (1993)]. It is a homeostatic function that occurs outside of consciousness in the same sense that we are not usually aware of our breathing except when it is imperilled.

It seems to me that it is necessary to include affects in the sequence between value, consciousness, and meaning, inasmuch as affects are the internal value-generated signals that ensure survival. Affects can be thought of as amplifiers of value [for a discussion of affects as amplifiers, see Tomkins (1988)]. Our motives are most directly influenced by our feelings. We are motivated by our feelings in both a positive and negative sense. Such feelings would include not only pleasurable and painful affects but also specific unlearned anxieties that provide the individual with an adaptive advantage. An obvious example is separation anxiety.

I believe that this linkage between value and affects is a necessary element for any future construction of a biology of meaning. This view encompasses ever-increasing levels of complexity. If one accepts the hypothesis that affects are internal value-related signals essential for survival, there is a clear progression between value as an evolutionary property, and affects and meaning in the psychological domain. It is affect that defines meaning as personal significance.

It is apparent that I have chosen one definition of meaning among many. The psychoanalyst spends his days asking patients: "What does this mean to you?" Meaning here is defined as personal significance or private meaning. There is a tautology, for what is of personal significance is to some extent invested with feeling. This definition of meaning as personal significance refers essentially to private meaning or meanings. If we define meaning as personal significance, it exists prior to language; gestures and thoughts are endowed with meaning prior to their communication through a shared language. Meaning as personal significance is not the subject that interests most philosophers of language, who study the communal aspect of meanings (for contrary views, see Lakoff, 1987; Johnson, 1987; Rommetveit, 1985).

What I am attempting to portray is a loop between value, affects, meaning, and a psychoanalytic conception of the self. I ask your indulgence, for the moment, to be able to move back and forth from the level of the brain to psychoanalytic observation without being troubled by the ever-present mind/brain problem. Meaning is generated through the scanning function of the self, where past (salient) categorical memories are matched with current perceptual inputs. This process presupposes a certain intactness or coherence of the self. When psychopathology interferes with this coherence, there will be a constriction in the extent to which events are endowed with meaning. There is a considerable body of clinical evidence that indicates that traumatic experiences may result in a dissociative split within the self (Fairbairn, 1952; Kernberg, 1976). What may remain dissociated and unconscious are the affects and/or the ideational contents of those traumatic experiences. This dissociation or splitting of the self prevents the recontextualization of memories that would normally occur, as Freud predicted. This splitting or dissociation of the self also entails an altered relation to time and an alteration of the self's historical dimension. As Freud indicated, there is a failure of translation of the memories from one developmental stage to the next. The failure of retranscription interferes with the experience of cyclic time, that is, with the capacity to create a coherent model of past, present, and future. I would describe the continuity and coherence of the self as *a value that generates further emergent interpersonal* motives, such as the need to maintain the privacy of the self.

When someone remains estranged from their affective core, there is a resultant sense of emptiness and futility—experiences become less meaningful and ultimately life may become meaningless. This profound sense of emptiness can be observed in its most extreme forms in the so-called narcissistic disorders. These personality disorders are different from depression, although in severe depression there is an analogous disturbance of the self, for in cases of depressive psychomotor retardation there is also an inability to generate meaning. There is ample clinical observation to suggest that in disturbances of the sense of self there is some interference in the capacity to generate meaning.

This loss of contact with the deeper structures of the self can be observed in its most severe form in the so-called borderline case, a very severe personality disturbance, on the border between neurosis and psychosis. When there is a profound dissociation from this inner, affective core of the self, this may be experienced as a form of psychic death.

Total dissociation from the deep structures of the self is an unparalleled psychic catastrophe, because one loses contact with this inner core of the self—there is an inability to attribute meaning to experience. Some borderline and schizophrenic patients describe this catastrophe as a "black hole." For defensive reasons the self has compressed itself into nonexistence. Like the astronomer's black hole, an implosion has occurred. The term *"black hole"* is an attempt to name the ineffable, to give a name to an absence that results in chaos, nothingness, and meaninglessness.

I have been attempting to demonstrate the congruence of TNGS with certain psychoanalytic observations. Some of my psychoanalytic colleagues would reject this application of a neurobiological model to psychoanalysis on the grounds that it is reductionistic. They would claim that the concepts and theories of any science or academic discipline are bound to the context of the particular methods employed in observation (for example, see Edelson, 1988). Therefore neurobiological concepts cannot have relevance for psychoanalytic observation. They might further argue that in a certain sense the human species, in its capacity for language and culture, is disjunctive with other animals so that a neurobiologic theory would not apply to what is a cultural or humanistic discipline.

There is within psychoanalysis today a complete absence of consensus regarding the relation of psychoanalysis to biology in general and to neuroscience in particular. Some view the mind and brain as a seamless web, whereas others believe that a psychology of the mind is an autonomous, free-standing science such as economics, or possibly no science at all.

It can be said of contemporary psychoanalytic theory that it has lost its central organizing principle; in Kuhn's sense it has lost its paradigm. There is little agreement regarding basic assumptions and accordingly psychoanalysts have segregated within a variety of schools. It is evident that Freud's theoretical edifice has lost its conceptual glue. I would suggest that one of the root causes of this conceptual anarchy is that psychoanalysis has lost its tie to biology. Freud had no doubt that psychoanalysis needed to borrow certain crucial concepts, such as instinct, from evolutionary biology. But, unfortunately, for psychoanalysis, he backed the wrong horse. For, as you know, the concept of instinct has virtually disappeared from biology. To consider distinct instinctual entities or categories, in my opinion, is a vestige of thinking of Platonic essences, which Mayr (1988) has shown to be incompatible with selectionism.

In order to place this problem in some historical context I wish to refer to the origins of psychoanalysis, to consider, in greater detail,

Freud's relation to neuroscience and evolutionary biology. This bit of intellectual history has been subject to very different interpretations. There are those who would claim that Freud, in the "Project for a Scientific Psychology" and in his book "On Aphasia," used the language of neurophysiology to clothe his essentially psychological theories, that his theories were not primarily neurophysiological in the first place, and that he used neurophysiology only as a metaphor to shape his essentially psychological model of the mind (Grossman, 1992). I believe that the truth is otherwise. Although Freud appeared at times to accept a conventional mind/brain parallelism or dualism, a case can be made that he remained essentially a monist. This is an interpretation of Freud's neurological theory of mind offered by the philosopher Robert Solomon (1974). There is, I believe, convincing evidence that a significant portion of psychoanalytic theory remains, as Freud intended it to be, a theory of the brain. Whether it is an acceptable theory of the brain is another question. Considering the embryonic state of neuroscience at the close of the nineteenth century, Freud had to practically invent his own brain physiology. It is perhaps for this reason he never published "The Project" but nevertheless he did preserve much of it within his later theory of psychoanalysis.

As I have noted, it is unfortunate for psychoanalysis that biology can no longer consider instincts to be entities. Freud considered the instinct concept as the foundation on which his theory rested. For Freud, the "elementary" instincts were analogous to the physicist's elementary particles. Freud said (1923, p.255) "Psychoanalysis early became aware that *all mental occurrences must be regarded as built on the basis of an interplay of forces of the elementary instincts.*" Freud borrowed a classification of instinct from his interpretation of evolutionary biology. His original classification proceeded along conventional lines in that he divided instincts into what he called the ego instincts, the instinct for self-preservation, which included aggression and the sexual instinct. However, this classification was soon replaced with a less conventional duality, that of eros and thanatos. This later transcendent classification of instinct is perhaps more philosophy than science. Freud believed that eros represented a unifying force whereas thanatos, the death instinct, represented the tendency of all living things to revert back to an inanimate state. In this he was expressing a kind of Goethe-like romantic biological theorizing. Today, few psychoanalysts believe in Freud's death instinct, they dismiss it as metaphysics, but many psychoanalysts accept, what is in effect, a bowdlerized version of Freud's dual instinct theory. That is, they believe that sexuality and aggression are instinctual entities, the overriding elements of all human motivation.

But the problem does not rest here, for, as you know, there were on Freud's part additional erroneous beliefs and misunderstanding of Darwinian evolution that have contributed to the estrangement of psychoanalysis from contemporary evolutionary biology. Freud believed in a Lamarckian theory of evolution and did not understand Darwin's population theory. Furthermore, he uncritically accepted Haeckel's law that ontogeny recapitulates phylogeny. Freud asserted that experience over long periods of time could be inherited and that evolutionary processes effected primarily the fitness of the group rather than the individual. Freud said (1915, p.120) "There is naturally nothing to prevent our supposing that the instincts themselves are, at least in part, precipitates of the effect of external stimulation, which in the course of phylogenesis have brought about modifications in the living substance." I should add, as you also know, that Darwin had similar beliefs. For example in "The Expression of the Emotions in Man and Animals," Darwin (1872, p.103) believed that gestures and the expression of specific emotions can become habitual and after repeated generations can alter the nervous system and become innate. In some respects Freud's errors reflect the fact that he was a child of his time. His belief in Lamarckianism, his misunderstanding of Darwin's theory, and his uncritical acceptance of Haeckel's law were all commonplace in the late nineteenth and early twentieth century.

It is not surprising that Freud's instinct theory or drive theory, as it has come to be called, is the most divisive conceptual issue in psychoanalytic theory today. Those psychoanalysts who wish to preserve the Freudian instinct paradigm must do so by declaring that psychoanalysis is free standing and has no relation to evolutionary biology. For example, a very respected psychoanalytic theorist, Hans Loewald, asserted that the instinct concept in psychoanalysis is a psychological concept, and as such is a different concept entirely as compared to the biologic concept of instinct(Loewald, 1980). This was not Freud's view. Freud spoke of instincts as well as affects as concepts on the frontier between the mind and the body (Freud, 1915). There is in psychoanalysis as well as in cognitive science a strong impetus to remove biology from the mind.

I am not suggesting that TNGS can resolve the mind/brain problem or that the concept of value can be used as a substitute for a psychoanalytic theory of instincts. But *value* combined with *reentry* is a basic concept of the highest generality and as such it is not too far fetched to suggest that TNGS may assist in generating a theory of motivation based on selection. I have already tried to indicate how we can move from the concept of value to a concept of meaning that is relevant for psychoanalysis. Inasmuch as value plus reentry exerts a selective process on consciousness, it selects what is of *interest* to the animal, which is another way of referring to motivation. William James also spoke of interests as exerting as selective influence on consciousness. "Millions of items of the outward order are present to my senses which never properly enter into my experience. Why? Because they have no *interest* for me. My *experience is what I agree to attend to*. Only such items which I notice shape my mind—without selective interest, experience is an utter chaos" (James, 1890, p.402). James also referred to interests as a hot place in a man's consciousness; such interests can take the form of ideas or ideals, to which the individual is devoted and which become the habitual center of his personal energy.

What I am suggesting is that at the highest level of generality there is a congruence between TNGS as a global theory of brain function and psychoanalysis as a global theory of mind. If we move away from this highest level of generality into the domain of particularities, we should expect that this congruence will no longer pertain. For example, I am told that noninvasive scanning techniques make it possible to observe that the visual cortex will light up when a subject is asked to imagine that he is seeing an object. Such techniques will record the simultaneity of brain states and experience but it would not be possible to claim that such brain states are identical to experience. TNGS would not predict an identity between brain states and experience, for, as Edelman indicated in "The Remembered Present," the fact of degeneracy would argue against it.

Despite the congruence that I believe exists between TNGS and psychoanalytic theory and observation, the leap we take between the brain and the mind remains mysterious. I suspect that most of us here are monists with regard to the mind and brain and that we are not too troubled by what philosophers label as a problem of ontology: do brain and mind occupy identical or separate modes of existence? But nevertheless a problem remains. The philosopher John Searle argues in his paper "Consciousness, Unconsciousness and Intentionality" (1989) that some but not all unconscious neurophysiological processes are mental. As an experienced psychoanalyst I know of nothing that would counter Searle's claim that unconscious mental processes are neurophysiological. But if such processes are neurophysiological and outside of experience, by what right do we label them as mental? William James believed it to be illogical to refer to the unconscious as mental and preferred the term "subconscious." But Freud as well as Searle postulated that the unconscious contains latent meaning; it contains a potentiality to generate meaning.

As you know, philosophers have, for centuries, puzzled over the problem of the privacy of mental events. Some would claim that it is illogical to think that can I show you my sense data. A patient cannot show you their pain but some *aspect* of their pain can be communicated. If this were not true psychoanalysis and psychotherapy could not be possible. Searle asks the question what is meant when something is designated as mental? His answer is that to be designated as mental, an unconscious state must be a possible candidate for consciousness and must have a certain "aspectual shape." Searle's use of the term "aspectual" indicates that in defining subjective experience there are a multiplicity of aspects, a multiplicity of private meanings. Searle has, I believe, offered a solution to this problem of private mental states. He uses the example that an individual's desire for water is different from a desire for H_2O and that this difference cannot be *exhaustively* known to an outside observer. The term "exhaustively" is pertinent; experience is private, but *aspects* of experience can be known to an outside observer. A counterquestion would be "Can brain events be exhaustively known?" Paradoxically, the unconscious may turn out to be a less private domain compared to consciousness. This is something that Freud would not have predicted. The philosopher Herbert Feigl (1958), in the paper "The 'Mental' and the 'Physical'," raised a question for which there are still no answers. Can we move from states of the brain to states of experience by means of a translation, or should we resign ourselves to a twofold source of knowledge?

References

Darwin, C. (1872). "The Expression of the Emotions in Man and Animals." Univ. of Chicago Press, Chicago (reprinted, 1965).

Edelman, G. (1987). "Neural Darwinism: The Theory of Neuronal Group Selection." Basic Books, New York.

Edelman, G. (1989). "The Remembered Present: A Biological Theory of Consciousness." Basic Books, New York.

Edelman, G. (1992). "Bright Air, Brilliant Fire: On the Matter of the Mind." Basic Books, New York.

Edelson, M. (1988). "Psychoanalysis: A Theory in Crisis." Univ. of Chicago Press, Chicago.

Fairbairn, W. R. D. (1952). "Psychoanalytic Studies of the Personality." Tavistock, London.

Feigl, H. (1958). The "mental" and the "physical." *In* "Concepts, Theories and the Mind-Body Problem. Minnesota Studies in the Philosophy of Science," Vol. 2. Univ. of Minnesota Press, Minneapolis.

Freud, S. (1895). Project for a scientific psychology. *In* "The Standard Edition of the Complete Psychological Works of Sigmund Freud" (J. Strackey, ed. and trans.), Vol. 1. Hogarth Press, London.

Freud, S. (1915). Instincts and their vicissitudes. *In* "The Standard Edition of the Complete Psychological Works of Sigmund Freud" (J. Strackey, ed. and trans.), Vol. 14. Hogarth Press, London.

Freud, S. (1923). Two encyclopaedia articles. *In* "The Standard Edition of the Complete

Psychological Works of Sigmund Freud" (J. Strackey, ed. and trans.), Vol. 18. Hogarth Press, London.

Grossman, W. (1992). Hierarchies, boundaries and representation in the Freudian model of mental organization. *J. Am. Psychoanal. Assoc.* **40**(1), 27–62.

James, W. (1890). "The Principles of Psychology," Vol. 1. Dover, New York (reprinted 1950).

Johnson, M. (1987). "The Body in the Mind." Univ. of Chicago Press, Chicago.

Kernberg, O. (1976). "Object Relations: Theory and Clinical Psychoanalysis." Jason Aronson, New York.

Lakoff, G. (1987). "Women, Fire, and Dangerous Things." Univ. of Chicago Press, Chicago.

Loewald, H. (1980). Instinct theory, object relations and psychic structure formation. *In* "Papers on Psychoanalysis." Yale Univ. Press, New Haven, CT.

Masson, J., ed. and trans. (1985). "The Complete Letters of Sigmund Freud to Wilhelm Fliess." Harvard Univ. Press, Cambridge, MA.

Mayr, E. (1988). "Toward a New Philosophy of Biology." Harvard Univ. Press (Belknap), Cambridge, MA.

Modell, A. (1990). "Other Times, Other Realties toward a Theory of Psychoanalytic Treatment." Harvard Univ. Press, Cambridge, MA.

Modell, A. (1993). "The Private Self." Harvard Univ. Press, Cambridge, MA.

Rommetveit, R. (1985). Language acquisition as increasing linguistic structuring of experience and symbolic behavior control. *In* "Culture Communication and Cognition, Vygotskian Perspectives" (J. Wertsch, ed.). Cambridge Univ. Press, Cambridge, UK.

Sandler, J., and Joffe, W. (1969). Towards a basic psychoanalytic model. *Int. J. Psychoanal.* **50**(1), 79–90.

Searle, J. (1989). Consciousness, unconsciousness, and intentionality. *Philos. Top.* **17**(1), 193–209.

Solomon, R. (1974). Freud's neurological theory of mind. *In* "Freud: A Collection of Critical Essays," (R. Wollheim, ed.), Doubleday Anchor, New York.

Tomkins, S. (1988). "Affect Imagery Consciousness," Vol. 1. 1962. Springer, New York.

A NEW VISION OF THE MIND

Oliver Sacks

Albert Einstein College of Medicine
New York, New York 10014

Five years ago the concepts of "mind" and "consciousness" were virtually excluded from scientific discourse. Now they have come back, and every week we see the publication of new books on the subject. Reading most of this work, we may have a sense of disappointment, even outrage; beneath the enthusiasm about scientific developments, there is a certain thinness, a poverty and unreality compared to what we know of human nature, the complexity and density of the emotions we feel, and of the thoughts we have. We read excitedly of the latest chemical, computational, or quantum theory of mind, and then ask, "Is that all there is to it?"

I remember the excitement with which I read Norbert Wiener's "Cybernetics" when it came out in the late 1940s. And then, in the early 1950s, reading the work of Wiener's younger colleagues at MIT—a galaxy of some of the finest minds in America, including Warren McCulloch, Walter Pitts, and John von Neumann; reading about their pioneer explorations of logical automata and nerve nets, I thought, as many of us did, that we were on the verge of computer translation, perception, cognition, a brave new world in which ever more powerful computers would be able to mimic, and even take over, the chief functions of brain and mind. The very titles of the MIT papers were exalted and thrilling: "Machines that Think and Want," "The Genesis of Social Evolution in the Mindlike Behavior of Artifacts." [1]

During the 1960s, there was some faltering and questioning: it proved possible to put a man on the moon in this decade, but not possible for a computer to achieve a decent translation of a child's speech, much less a text of any complexity, or to achieve more than the most rudimentary mechanical perception (if indeed "perception" was a legitimate word here) (see Minsky, 1967). Or was it simply that one needed more computer power, and perhaps different programs or designs? Supercomputers emerged, and, soon, so-called neural networks, which do not consist

---

[1] The heady atmosphere of these days is vividly captured in "The Cybernetics Group" by Helms (1991), and many of the McCulloch papers were later collected in "Embodiments of Mind" (1965).

347

of actual neurons but computer simulations or models that attempt to mimic the nervous system. Though such networks start with random connections, and learn in a fashion—for example, how to recognize faces or words—they are always instructed what to do, even if they are not instructed how to do it. They are able to recognize in a formal, rule-bound way, but not in terms of context and meaning, the way an organism does.

Some of these networks have been developed on the West Coast, under the presiding genius of Francis Crick. And yet Crick has expressed fundamental reservations about them—can they, he has asked, really be said to think? Are they, in fact, like minds at all? We must indeed be very cautious before we allow that any artifact is (except in a superficial sense) "mindlike" or "brainlike" (Crick, 1989).

Thus if we are to have a model or theory of mind as this actually occurs in living creatures in the world, it may have to be radically different from anything like a computational one. It will have to be grounded in biological reality, in the anatomical and developmental and functional details of the nervous system; and also in the inner life or mental life of the living creature, the play of its sensations and feelings and drives and intentions, its perception of objects and people and situations, and, in higher creatures at least, the ability to think abstractly and to share through language and culture the consciousness of others.

Above all such a theory must account for the development and adaptation peculiar to living systems. Living organisms are born into a world of challenge and novelty, a world of significances, to which they must adapt or die. Living organisms grow, learn, develop, organize knowledge, and use memory—in a way that has no real analog in the nonliving.[2] Memory is characteristic of life. And memory brings about a change in the organism, so that it is better adapted, better fitted, to meet environmental challenges. The very "self" of the organism is enlarged by memory.

Such a notion of organic change as taking place with experience and learning, and as being an essential change in the structure and "being" of the organism, had no place in the classical theories of memory, which tended to portray it as a thing-in-itself, something *deposited* in the brain and mind—an impression, a trace, a replica of the original experience, like a photograph. (For Socrates, the brain was soft wax, imprinted with

---

[2] Though, increasingly, the term "adaptive systems" is used for automata or complex systems that can modify themselves in relation to assigned "tasks" or "challenges," and in a certain (but unbiological) sense be said to "adapt" or "learn." Such adaptive systems, of ever-increasing sophistication, are proving of major importance in many realms, and have been an especial concern of the researchers at the Santa Fe Institute.

impressions as with a seal or signet ring.) This was certainly the case with Locke and the empiricists, and has its counterpart in many of the current models of memory, which see it as having a definite location in the brain, something like the memory core of a computer.

The neural basis of memory, and of learning generally, the psychologist Donald Hebb hypothesized, lay in a selective strengthening or inhibition of the synapses between nerve cells and the development of groups of cells or "cell assemblies" embodying the remembered experience. His teacher Karl Lashley, however, who trained rats to do complex tasks after removing various parts of their brains, came to feel that it was impossible to localize memory or learning; that, with remembering and learning, changes took place throughout the entire brain. Thus, for Lashley, memory, and indeed identity, did not have discrete locations in the brain.[3] There seemed no possible meeting point between these two views: an atomistic or mosaic view of the brain as parceling memory and perception into small, discrete areas, and a global or "Gestalt" view, which saw them as being somehow spread out across the entire brain.

These disparate views of memory and brain function were only part of a more general chaos, a flourishing of many fields and many theories, independently and in isolation, a fragmentation of our approaches to, and views about, the brain. A comprehensive theory of brain function that could make sense of the diverse observations of a dozen different disciplines has been missing, and the enormous but fragmented growth of neuroscience in the past two decades has made the need for such a general theory more and more pressing. This was well expressed in a recent article in *Nature*, in which Jeffrey Gray spoke of the tendency of neuroscience to gather more and more experimental data, while lacking "a new theory . . . that will render the relations between brain events and conscious experience 'transparent'" (Gray, 1992; see Sacks, 1992, for my reply).

The needed theory, indeed, must do more: it must account for (or at least be compatible with) all the facts of evolution and neural development and neurophysiology, on the one hand, and all the facts of neurology and psychology, on the other. It must be a theory of self-organization and emergent order at every level and scale, from the scurrying of molecules and their micropatterns in a million synaptic clefts to the grand macropatterns of an actual lived life. Such a theory, Gray feels, "is at present unimaginable."

But just such a theory has been imagined, and with great force and originality, by Gerald Edelman, who, with his colleagues at the Neurosci-

---

[3] Lashley expressed this in a famous paper, "In Search of the Engram" (1950).

ences Institute at Rockefeller University over the past 15 years, has been developing a biological theory of mind, which he calls Neural Darwinism, or the Theory of Neuronal Group Selection (TNGS).[4]

Edelman's early work dealt not with the nervous system, but with the immune system, by which all vertebrates defend themselves against invading bacteria and viruses. It was previously accepted that the immune system "learned," or was "instructed," by means of a single type of antibody that molded itself around the foreign body, or antigen, to produce an appropriate, "tailored" antibody, and that these molds then multiplied and entered the bloodstream and destroyed the alien organisms. But Edelman showed that a radically different mechanism was at work; that we possess not one basic kind of antibody, but millions of them, an enormous repertoire of antibodies, from which the invading antigen "selects" one that fits. It is such a selection, rather than a direct shaping or instruction, that leads to the multiplication of the appropriate antibody and the destruction of the invader. Such a mechanism, which he called a "clonal selection," was suggested in 1959 by MacFarlane Burnet, but Edelman was the first to demonstrate that such a selectional mechanism actually occurs, and for this he shared a Nobel Prize in 1972.

Edelman then began to study the nervous system, to see whether this too was a selectional system, and whether its workings could be understood as evolving, or emerging, by a similar process of selection. Both the immune system and the nervous system can be seen as systems for recognition. The immune system has to recognize all foreign intruders, to categorize them, reliably, as "self" or "not self." The task of the nervous system is roughly analogous, but far more demanding: it has to classify, to categorize, the whole sensory experience of life, to build from the first categorizations, by degrees, an adequate model of the world; and in the absence of any specific programming or instruction to discover or create its own way of doing this. How does an animal come to recognize and deal with the novel situations it confronts? How is such individual development possible?

---

[4] Edelman first presented this in a relatively brief essay written in 1978. This essay was written, Edelman has said, in a single sitting, during a 13-hour wait for a plane in the Milan airport, and it is fascinating to see in this the germ of all his future thought—one gets an intense sense of the evolution occurring in *him*. Between 1987 and 1990 Edelman published his monumental and sometimes impenetrable trilogy "Neural Darwinism" (1987), "Topobiology" (1988), and "The Remembered Present: A Biological Theory of Consciousness" (1989), which presented the theory, and a vast range of relevant observations in a much more elaborate and rigorous form. He presents the theory more informally, but within a richer historical and philosophical discussion, in his most recent book, "Bright Air, Brilliant Fire" (1992).

The answer, Edelman proposes, is that an evolutionary process takes place—not one that selects organisms and takes millions of years, but one that occurs within each particular organism and during its lifetime, by competition among cells, or selection of cells (or, rather, cell groups) in the brain. This for Edelman is "somatic selection."

Edelman and his colleagues have been concerned not only to propose a principle of selection but to explore the mechanisms by which it may take place. Thus they have tried to answer three kinds of questions: Which units in the nervous system select and give different emphasis to sensory experience? How does selection occur? What is the relation of the selecting mechanisms to functions of brain and mind such as perception, categorization, and, finally, consciousness?

Edelman discusses two kinds of selection in the evolution of the nervous system—"developmental" and "experiential." The first takes place largely before birth. The genetic instructions in each organism provide general constraints for neural development, but they cannot specify the exact destination of each developing nerve cell, for these grow and die, migrate in great numbers, and in entirely unpredictable ways; all of them are "gypsies," as Edelman likes to say. Thus the vicissitudes of fetal development produce in every brain unique patterns of neurons and neuronal groups ("developmental selection"). Even identical twins with identical genes will not have identical brains at birth: the fine details of cortical circuitry will be quite different. Such variability, Edelman points out, would be a catastrophe in virtually any mechanical or computational system, wherein exactness and reproducibility are of the essence. But in a system in which selection is central, the consequences are entirely different; here variation and diversity are of the essence.

Now, already possessing a unique and individual pattern of neuronal groups through developmental selection, the creature is born, thrown into the world, there to be exposed to a new form of selection based on experience ("experiential selection"). What is the world of a newborn infant (or chimp) like? Is it a sudden incomprehensible (perhaps terrifying) explosion of electromagnetic radiations, sound waves, and chemical stimuli that make the infant cry and sneeze? Or an ordered, intelligible world, in which the infant discerns people, objects, events, and scenes?[5] We know that the world encountered is not one of complete meaning-

[5] In "To See and Not See" (Sacks, 1993), I describe not the personal world of an infant (of which we can never hope to get any report), but of a newly sighted adult. This man found himself deluged with raw visual sensations, and was at first wholly unable to recognize or discriminate people, objects, or even simple geometrical shapes. Nothing has shown me more clearly the crucial role of experience in the development of our perceptual capacities.

lessness and pandemonium, for the infant shows selective attention and preferences from the start.

Clearly there are some innate biases or dispositions at work; otherwise the infant would have no tendencies whatever, would not be moved to do anything, seek anything, to stay alive. These basic biases Edelman calls "values." Such values are essential for adaptation and survival; some have been developed through eons of evolution, and some are acquired through exploration and experience. Thus if the infant instinctively values food, warmth, and contact with other people (for example), this will direct its first movements and strivings. These "values"—drives, instincts, intentionalities—serve to weight experience differentially, to orient the organism toward survival and adaptation, to allow what Edelman calls "categorization *on* value" (e.g., to form categories such as "edible" and "nonedible" as part of the process of getting food). It needs to be stressed that "values" are experienced, internally, as feelings—without feeling there can be no animal life. "Thus," in the words of the late philosopher Hans Jonas, "the capacity for feeling, which arose in all organisms, is the mother-value of all values."

At a more elementary physiological level, there are various sensory and motor givens, from the reflexes that automatically occur (for example, in response to pain) to innate mechanisms in the brain, as, for example, the feature detectors in the visual cortex, which, as soon as they are activated, detect verticals, horizontals, boundaries, angles, etc., in the visual world.

Thus we have a certain amount of basic equipment; but, in Edelman's view, very little else is programmed or built in.[6] It is up to the infant animal, given its elementary physiological capacities, and given its inborn values, to create its own categories and to use them to make sense of, to *construct* a world—and it is not just a world that the infant constructs, but its own world, a world constituted from the first by personal meaning and reference.

Such a neuro-evolutionary view is highly consistent with some of the conclusions of psychoanalysis and developmental psychology—in particular, the psychoanalyst Daniel Stern's description of "an emergent self." "Infants seek sensory stimulation," writes Stern. "They have distinct biases or preferences with regard to the sensations they seek. . . . These

---

[6] And yet, clearly, much more complex capacities and dispositions may be "built in" to the genotype of the organism, although their development (or lack of development) may depend on experience. This is so for our species-specific linguistic capacity, our varied intellectual capacities (musical capacity is one of the most innate and specific), and many subtle dispositions and behavioral traits—this may be especially striking in identical twins who have been separated at birth.

are innate. From birth on, there appears to be a central tendency to form and test hypotheses about what is occurring in the world . . . [to] categorize . . . into conforming and contrasting patterns, events, sets, and experiences" (Stern, 1985). Stern emphasizes how crucial are the active processes of connecting, correlating, and categorizing information, and how with these a distinctive organization emerges, which is experienced by the infant as the sense of a self.

It is precisely such processes that Edelman is concerned with. He sees them as grounded in a process of selection acting on the primary neuronal units with which each of us is equipped. These units are not individual nerve cells or neurons, but groups ranging in size from about 50 to 10,000 neurons; there are perhaps a hundred million such groups in the entire brain. During the development of the fetus, a unique neuronal pattern of connections is created, and then in the infant, experience acts on this pattern, modifying it by selectively strengthening or weakening connections between neuronal groups, or creating entirely new connections.

Thus experience is not passive, a matter of impressions or sense data, but active, and constructed by the organism from the start. Active experience "selects," or carves out, a new, more complexly connected pattern of neuronal groups, a neuronal reflection of the individual experience of the child, of the procedures by which it has come to categorize reality.

But these neuronal circuits are still at a low level—how do they connect with the inner life, the mind, the behavior of the creature? It is at this point that Edelman introduces the most radical of his concepts—the concepts of "maps" and "reentrant signaling." A map, as he uses the term, is not a representation in the ordinary sense, but an interconnected series of neuronal groups that responds selectively to certain elemental categories—for example, to movements or colors in the visual world. The creation of maps, Edelman postulates, involves the synchronization of hundreds of neuronal groups. Some mappings, some categorizations, take place in discrete and anatomically fixed (or prededicated) parts of the cerebral cortex—thus color is "constructed" in an area called V4. The visual system alone, for example, has over 30 different maps for representing color, movement, shape, etc.

But where perception of *objects* is concerned, the world, Edelman likes to say, is not labeled, it does not come "already parsed into objects." We must *make* them, in effect, through our own categorizations: "Perception makes," Emerson said. "Every perception," says Edelman, echoing Emerson, "is an act of creation." Thus our sense organs, as we move about, take samplings of the world, creating maps in the brain. Then a sort of neurological "survival of the fittest" occurs, a selective strengthening of those mappings that correspond to "successful" perceptions—successful in that they prove the most useful and powerful for the building of "reality."

In this view, there are no innate mechanisms for complex personal recognition, such as the "grandmother cell" postulated by researchers in the 1970s to correspond to one's perception of one's grandmother.[7]

Nor is there any "master area," or "final common path," whereby all perceptions relating (say) to one's grandmother converge in one single place. There is no such place in the brain where a final image is synthesized, nor any miniature person or homunculus to view this image. Such images or representations do not exist in Edelman's theory, nor do any such homunculi. (Classical theory, with its concept of "images" or "representations" in the brain, demanded a sort of dualism, for there had to be a miniature "someone in the brain" to view the images; and then another, still smaller, someone in the brain of that someone; and so on, in an infinite regress. There is no way of escaping from this regress, except by eliminating the very concept of images and viewers, and replacing it by a dynamic concept of process or interaction.)

Rather, the perception of a grandmother or, say, of a chair, depends on the synchronization of a number of scattered mappings throughout the visual cortex: mappings relating to many different perceptual aspects of the chair (its size, its shape, its color, its "leggedness," its relation to other sorts of chairs—armchairs, kneeling chairs, baby chairs, etc.); and perhaps in other parts of the cortex as well (relating to the feel of sitting in a chair, the actions needed to do it, etc.). In this way the brain, the creature, achieves a rich and flexible percept of "chairhood," which allows the recognition of innumerable sorts of chairs as chairs (computers, by contrast, with their need for unambiguous definitions and criteria, are quite unable to achieve this). This perceptual generalization is dynamic and not static, and depends on the active and incessant orchestration of countless details. Such a correlation is possible because of the very rich connections between the brain's maps, connections that are reciprocal, and may contain millions of fibers.

These extensive connections allow what Edelman calls reentrant signaling, a continuous "communication" *between* the active maps, which enables a coherent construct such as "chair" to be made. This construct

---

[7] There may, however, be built-in mechanisms for certain generic recognition—such as the ability, which we share with all primates, to recognize the category of "snakes," even if we have never seen a snake before; or infants' ability to recognize the generic category of "faces" long before they recognize particular ones. There is now evidence for "face-detecting" cells in the cerebral cortex.

arises from the interaction of many sources. Stimuli from, say, touching a chair may affect one set of maps, stimuli from seeing it may affect another set. Reentrant signaling takes place between the two sets of maps and between many other maps as well, as part of the process of perceiving a chair.

This construct, it must be emphasized once again, is not comparable to a single image or representation—it is, rather, comparable to a giant and continually modulating equation, as the outputs of innumerable maps, connected by reentry, not only complement one another at a perceptual level but are built up to higher and higher levels. For the brain, in Edelman's vision, makes maps of its own maps, or "categorizes its own categorizations," and does so by a process that can ascend indefinitely to yield ever more generalized pictures of the world.

This reentrant signaling is different from the process of "feedback," which merely corrects errors.[8] Simple feedback loops are not only common in the technological world (as thermostats, governors, cruise controls, etc.), but are crucial in the nervous system, where they are used for control of all the body's automatic functions from temperature to blood pressure to the fine control of movement. (This concept of feedback is at the heart of both Wiener's cybernetics and Claude Bernard's concept of homeostasis.) But at higher levels, where flexibility and individuality are all-important, and where new powers and new functions are needed and created, one requires a mechanism that can construct, not just control or correct.

The process of reentrant signaling, with its thousands or hundreds of thousands of reciprocal connections within and between maps, may be likened to a sort of neural United Nations, in which dozens of voices are talking together, while including in their conversation a variety of constantly inflowing reports from the outside world, and giving them coherence, bringing them together into a larger picture as new information is correlated and new insights emerge. There is, to continue the metaphor, no secretary general in the brain; the very activity of reentrant signaling achieves the synthesis. How is this possible?

Edelman, who once planned to be a concert violinist, uses musical metaphors here. In a recent BBC radio broadcast, he said

> Think, if you had a hundred thousand wires randomly connecting four string quartet players and that, even though they weren't speaking words, signals were going back and forth in all kinds of hidden ways [as you usually get them by the

---

[8] Confusingly, the very term "reentrant" has occasionally been used in the past to denote such feedback loops. (It is used in this way by McCulloch in his early papers on automata.) Edelman gives the term "reentry" a radically new meaning.

subtle nonverbal interactions between the players] that make the whole set of sounds a unified ensemble. That's how the maps of the brain work by reentry.

The players are connected. Each player, interpreting the music individually, constantly modulates and is modulated by the others. There is no final or "master" interpretation—the music is collectively created. This, then, is Edelman's picture of the brain, an orchestra, an ensemble—but without a conductor, an orchestra that makes its own music.

The construction of perceptual categorizations and maps, the capacity for generalization made possible by reentrant signaling, is the beginning of psychic development, and far precedes the development of consciousness or mind, or of attention or concept formation—yet it is a prerequisite for all of these; it is the beginning of an enormous upward path, and it can achieve remarkable power even in relatively primitive animals like birds.[9] Perceptual categorization, whether of colors, movements, or shapes, is the first step, and it is crucial for learning, but it is not something fixed, something that occurs once and for all. On the contrary—and this is central to the dynamic picture presented by Edelman—there is then a continual recategorization, and this constitutes memory.

"In computers," Edelman writes, "memory depends on the specification and storage of bits of coded information." This is *not* the case in the nervous system. Memory in living organisms, by contrast, takes place through activity and continual recategorization.

> By its nature, memory . . . involves continual motor activity...in different contexts. Because of the new associations arising in these contexts, because of changing inputs and stimuli, and because different combinations of neuronal groups can give rise to a similar output, a given categorical response in memory may be achieved in several ways. Unlike computer-based memory, brain-based memory is inexact, but it is also capable of great degrees of generalization (Edelman, 1992, p. 102).

In the extended Theory of Neuronal Group Selection, which he has developed since 1987, Edelman has been able, in a very economical way, to accommodate all the "higher" aspects of mind–concept formation, language, consciousness itself—without bringing in any additional con-

---

[9] Thus if pigeons are presented with photographs of trees, or oak leaves, or fish, surrounded by extraneous features, they rapidly learn to "home in" on these, and to generalize, so that they can thereafter recognize any trees, or oak leaves, or fish straightaway, however distracting or confusing the context may be. It is clear from these experiments that perception selects, or rather creates, "defining" features (what counts as defining may be different for each pigeon), and cognitive categories, without the use of language, or being "told" what to do. Such category-creating behavior (which Edelman calls "noetic") is very different from the rigid, algorithmic procedures used by robots. [These experiments with pigeons are described in detail in "Neural Darwinism," (1987, pp. 247–251).]

siderations. Edelman's most ambitious project, indeed, is to try to delineate a possible biological basis for consciousness. He distinguishes, first, "primary" from "higher-order" consciousness:

> Primary consciousness is the state of being mentally aware of things in the world, of having mental images in the present. But it is not accompanied by any sense of [being] a person with a past and a future. . . . In contrast, higher-order consciousness involves the recognition by a thinking subject of his or her own acts and affections. It embodies a model of the personal, and of the past and future as well as the present. . . . It is what we as humans have in addition to primary consciousness (Edelman, 1992, p. 112).

The essential achievement of primary consciousness, as Edelman sees it, is to bring together the many categorizations involved in perception into a *scene*. The advantage of this is that "events that may have had significance to an animal's past learning can be related to new events." The relation established will not be a causal one, one necessarily related to anything in the outside world; it will be an *individual* (or "subjective") one, based on what has had value or meaning for the animal in the past.

Edelman proposes that the ability to create scenes in the mind depends on the emergence of a new neuronal circuit during evolution, a circuit allowing for continual reentrant signaling between, on the one hand, the parts of the brain where memory of value categories such as warmth, food, and light takes place and, on the other, the ongoing global mappings that categorize perceptions as they actually take place. This "bootstrapping process" (as Edelman calls it) goes on in all the senses, thus allowing for the construction of a complex scene. The scene, one must stress, is not an image, not a picture (any more than a map is), but a correlation between different kinds of categorization.

Mammals, birds, and some reptiles, Edelman speculates, have such a scene-creating primary consciousness, and such consciousness is "efficacious"; it helps the animal adapt to complex environments. Without such consciousness, life is lived at a much lower level, with far less ability to learn and adapt.

> Primary consciousness [Edelman concludes] is required for the evolution of higher-order consciousness. But it is limited to a small memorial interval around a time chunk I call the present. It lacks an explicit *notion* or a concept of a personal self, and it does not afford the ability to model the past or the future as part of a correlated scene. An animal with primary consciousness sees the room the way a beam of light illuminates it. Only that which is in the beam is explicitly in the remembered present; all else is darkness. This does not mean that an animal with primary consciousness cannot have long-term memory or act on it. Obviously, it can, but it cannot, in general, be aware of that memory or plan an extended future for itself based on that memory (Edelman, 1992, p. 122).

Only in ourselves—and to some extent in apes—does a higher order consciousness emerge. Higher order consciousness arises *from* primary consciousness—it supplements it, it does not replace it. It is dependent on the evolutionary development of language, along with the evolution of symbols, of cultural exchange; and with all this brings an unprecedented power of detachment, generation, and reflection, so that finally self-consciousness is achieved, the consciousness of being a self in the world, with human experience and imagination to call upon.

Higher order consciousness releases us from the thrall of the here and now, allowing us to reflect, to introspect, to draw on culture and history, and to achieve by these means a new order of development and mind. No other theorist I know of has even attempted a biological understanding of this step. To become conscious of being conscious, Edelman stresses, systems of memory must be related to representation of a self. This is not possible unless the contents, the scenes, of primary consciousness are subjected to a further process and are recategorized.

Though language, in Edelman's view, is not crucial for the development of higher order consciousness (there is some evidence of higher order consciousness and self-consciousness in apes), it immensely facilitates and expands this by making possible previously unattainable conceptual and symbolic powers. Thus two steps, two reentrant processes, are envisaged here: first, the linking of primary (or "value category") memory with current perception—a perceptual bootstrapping, which creates primary consciousness; second, a linking between symbolic memory and conceptual centers—the semantic boot-strapping necessary for higher consciousness. The effects of this are momentous: "The acquisition of a new kind of memory," Edelman writes, "leads to a conceptual explosion. As a result, concepts of the self, the past, and the future can be connected to primary consciousness. 'Consciousness of consciousness' becomes possible."[10]

At this point Edelman makes explicit what is implicit throughout his work—the interaction of "neural Darwinism" with classical Darwinism. What occurs explosively in individual development must have been equally critical in evolutionary development. Thus "at some transcendent moment in evolution," Edelman (1992) writes, there emerged "a variant

---

[10] This explosion normally occurs in the third year of life, and is spread over several months as language is acquired. But if through special circumstances—deafness, incarceration (as with Kaspar Hauser), or lack of contact with other human beings (as with "wild" children)—a child is denied contact with language at this age, and only develops it later, the development of higher order consciousness may be truly explosive, and may occur in a matter of hours or days, with the sudden, belated rushing-in of language (Sacks, 1984).

with a reentrant circuit linking value category memory" to current perception. "At that moment," Edelman continues, "memory became the substrate and servant of consciousness." And then, at another transcendent moment, by another, higher turn of reentry, higher order consciousness arose.

There is indeed much paleontological evidence that higher order consciousness developed in an astonishingly short space of time—some tens (perhaps hundreds) of thousands of years, not the many millions usually needed for evolutionary change. The speed of this development has always been a most formidable challenge for evolutionary theorists; Darwin could offer no detailed account of it, and Wallace was driven back to thoughts of a grand design.

The principles underlying brain development and the mechanisms outlined in the Theory of Neuronal Group Selection can, Edelman argues, account for this rapid emergence, because they allow for enormous changes in brain size over the relatively short evolutionary period in which *Homo sapiens* emerged. According to topobiology, relatively large changes in the structure of the brain can occur through changes in the timing of the genes that regulate the brain's morphology, changes that can come about as the result of relatively few mutations. And the premises of the Theory of Neuronal Group Selection allow for the rapid incorporation into existing brain structures of new and enlarged neuronal maps with a variety of functions.

New theories arise from a crisis in scientific understanding, an acute incompatibility between observations and existing theories. There are many such crises in neuroscience today. Edelman, with his background in morphology and development, speaks of the "structural" crisis, the now well-established fact that there is no precise wiring in the brain, that there are vast numbers of unidentifiable inputs to each cell, and that such a jungle of connections is incompatible with any simple computational theory. But, at the other extreme, he is also moved, as William James was, by the apparently seamless quality of experience and consciousness—the unitary appearance of the world to a perceiver, despite (as we have seen in regard to vision) the multitude of discrete and parallel systems for perceiving it; and the fact that some integrating or unifying or "binding" must occur, which is totally inexplicable by any existing theory.

Since the Theory of Neuronal Group Selection was first formulated, important new evidence has emerged suggesting how widely separated groups of neurons in the visual cortex can become synchronized and respond in unison when an animal is faced with a new perceptual task—a finding directly suggestive of reentrant signaling (Sacks, 1990). There is also much evidence of a more clinical sort, which one feels may be illuminated, and perhaps explained, by the Theory of Neuronal Group Selection.

I often encounter situations in day-to-day neurological practice that completely defeat classical neurological explanations, that cry out for explanations of a radically different kind, and that are clarified by Edelman's theory.[11] Thus if a spinal anesthetic is given to a patient—as used to be done frequently to women in childbirth—there is not just a feeling of numbness below the waist. There is, rather, the sense that one terminates at the umbilicus, that one's corporeal self has no extension below this, and that what lies below is not-self, not-flesh, not-real, not-anything. The anesthetized lower half has a bewildering nonentity, completely lacks meaning and personal reference. The baffled mind is unable to categorize it, to relate it in any way to the self. One knows that sooner or later the anesthetic will wear off, yet it is impossible to imagine the missing parts in a positive way. There is an absolute gap in primary consciousness that higher order consciousness can report, but cannot correct. Because human beings never experience their own primary consciousness "raw," but only as it has been transformed and enlarged by higher order consciousness, the terms in which we experience such a gap become conceptual—thus "alien" entails an explicit concept of "self" and "nothingness," an explicit concept of "being"; such experiences allow a sort of clinical ontology.[12]

This indeed is a situation I know well from personal no less than clinical experience, for it is what I experienced myself after a nerve injury to one leg, when for a period of 2 weeks, while the leg lay immobile and senseless, I found it alien, not mine, not me, not real. I was astonished when this happened, and was unassisted by my neurological knowledge—the situation was clearly neurological, but classical neurology has nothing to say about the relation of sensation to knowledge and to "self"; about how, normally, the body is "owned"; and how, if the flow of

---

[11] Some of these situations are discussed by Israel Rosenfield in his new book "The Strange, Familiar and Forgotten," wherein he speaks of "the bankruptcy of classical neurology."

[12] Animals without higher order consciousness or self-consciousness show no sign of recognizing self-absence or nothingness, and if the hindquarters of such an animal are anesthetized, the animal will simply ignore them, and go about it business, without showing any signs of bewilderment or that it perceives anything amiss. This is well described by the veterinarian James Herriott, in regard to a cow given a spinal anesthetic for obstructed calving; it became indifferent to the whole procedure as soon as the anesthetic took effect, and returned to munching its hay.

neural information is impaired, it may be lost to consciousness, and "disowned"—for it does not see consciousness as a process.[13]

Such body-image and body-ego disturbances can be fully understood, in Edelman's thinking, as breakdowns in local mapping, consequent upon nerve damage or disuse. It has been confirmed, further, in animal experiments, that the mapping of body image is not something fixed, but is plastic and dynamic, and dependent on a continual inflow of experience and use; and that if there is continuing interference with, say, one's perception of a limb or its use, there is not only a rapid loss of its cerebral map, but a rapid remapping of the rest of the body, which then excludes the limb.[14]

Stranger still are the situations that arise when the cerebral basis of body image is affected, especially if the right hemisphere of the brain is badly damaged in its sensory areas. At such times patients may show an "anosognosia," an unawareness that anything is the matter, even though the left side of the body may be senseless, and perhaps paralyzed, too. Or they may show a strange levity, insisting that their own left sides belong to someone else. Such patients may behave (as the eminent neurologist, M.-M. Mesulam, has written) "as if one half of the universe had abruptly ceased to exist . . . as if nothing were actually happening [there] . . . as if nothing of importance could be expected to occur there." Such patients live in a hemispace, a bisected world, but for them, subjectively, their space and world is entire. Anosognosia is unintelligible (and was for years misinterpreted as a bizarre neurotic symptom) unless we see it (in Edelman's term) as "a disease of consciousness," a total breakdown of high-level reentrant signaling and mapping in one hemisphere—the right hemisphere, which, Edelman suggests, may have only primary but no higher order consciousness—and a radical reorganization of consciousness in consequence.

Less dramatic than these complete disappearances of self or parts of the self from consciousness, but still remarkable in the extreme, are situations in which, following a neurological lesion, a dissociation occurs between perception and consciousness, or memory and consciousness, cases in which there remain only "implicit" perception or knowledge or

---

[13] A full discussion of such body-image or body-ego disturbances in relation to TNGS I can be found in a new afterword to the UK edition of my book *A Leg to Stand On* (Picador, 1992).

[14] Fundamental work showing the plasticity of the cerebral cortex, and the remarkable degree to which it can reorganize itself after injuries, amputations, strokes, etc., has been done by Michael Merzenich and his colleagues at the University of California in San Francisco (see, for example, Merzenich, *et al.*, 1988).

memory. Thus my amnesiac patient Jimmie ("The Lost Mariner") had no explicit memory of Kennedy's assassination, and would indeed say, "No president in this century has been assassinated, that I know of." But if asked, "hypothetically, then, if a presidential assassination had somehow occurred without your knowledge, where might you guess it occurred: New York, Chicago, Dallas, New Orleans, or San Francisco?" he would invariably "guess" correctly, Dallas.

Similarly, patients with visual agnosias, like Dr. P. ("The Man who Mistook his Wife for a Hat"), though not consciously able to recognize anyone, often "guess" the identity of people's faces correctly. And patients with total cortical blindness, from massive bilateral damage to the primary visual areas of the brain, while asserting that they can see nothing, may also mysteriously "guess" correctly what lies before them—so-called blindsight. In all these cases, then, we find that perception, and perceptual categorization of the kind described by Edelman, have been preserved, but have been divorced from consciousness.

In such cases it appears to be only the final process, in which the reentrant loops combine memory with current perceptual categorization, that breaks down. Their understanding, so elusive hitherto, seems to come closer with Edelman's "reentrant" model of consciousness.

Dissatisfaction with the classical theories is not confined to clinical neurologists; it is also to be found among theorists of child development, among cognitive and experimental psychologists, among linguists, and among psychoanalysts. All find themselves in need of new models. This has been abundantly clear at this conference on "Selectionism and the Brain." Particularly suggestive, for me, has been the work of Esther Thelen and her colleagues at the University of Indiana in Bloomington, who have for some years been making a minute analysis of the development of motor skills—walking, reaching for objects—in infants. "For the developmental theorist," Thelen writes, "individual differences pose an enormous challenge. . . . Developmental theory has not met this challenge with much success." And this is, in part, because individual differences are seen as extraneous, whereas Thelen argues that it is precisely such differences, the huge variation between individuals, that allow the evolution of unique motor patterns.

Thelen finds that the development of such skills, as Edelman's theory would suggest, follows no single programmed or prescribed pattern. Indeed there is great variability among infants at first, with many patterns of reaching for objects; but there then occurs, over the course of several months, a competition among these patterns, a discovery or selection of workable patterns, or workable motor solutions. These solutions, though roughly similar (for there are a limited number of ways in which an infant can reach), are always different and individual, adapted to the particular dynamics of each child, and they emerge by degrees, through exploration and trial. Each child, Thelen has shown, explores a rich range of possible ways to reach for an object and selects its own path, without the benefit of any blueprint or program. The child is forced to be original, to create its own solutions. Such an adventurous course carries its own risks—the child may evolve a *bad* motor solution—but sooner or later such bad solutions tend to destabilize, break down, and make way for further exploration, and better solutions (Thelen, 1990).[15]

When Thelen tries to envisage the neural basis of such learning, she uses terms very similar to Edelman's; she sees a "population" of movements being selected or "pruned" by experience. She writes of infants "remapping" the neuronal groups that are correlated with their movements, and "selectively strengthening particular neuronal groups." She has, of course, no direct evidence for this, and such evidence cannot be obtained until we have a way of visualizing vast numbers of neuronal groups simultaneously in a conscious subject, and following their interactions for months on end. No such visualization is possible at the present time, but it will perhaps become possible by the end of the decade. Meanwhile, the close correspondence between Thelen's observations and the kind of behavior that would be expected from Edelman's theory is striking.

If Esther Thelen is concerned with direct observation of the development of motor skills in the infant, Arnold Modell of Harvard has been concerned with psychoanalytical interpretations of early behavior; he too feels, like Thelen, that a crisis has developed, that it might also be resolved by the Theory of Neuronal Group Selection—indeed, the title of his paper is "Neural Darwinism and a Conceptual Crisis in Psychoanalysis." The particular crisis he spoke of was connected with Freud's concept of *Nachtraglichkeit*, the retranscription of memories that had become pathologically fixed, fossilized, but were now opened to consciousness, to new contexts and reconstructions, as a crucial part of the therapeutic process of liberating the patient from the past, allowing him to experience and move freely once again.

This process cannot be understood in terms of the classical concept of memory, in which a fixed record or trace or representation is stored in the brain—an entirely static or mechanical concept—but requires a

---

[15] Similar considerations arise with regard to recovery and rehabilitation after strokes and other injuries. There are no rules, there is no prescribed path of recovery; every patient must discover, or create, his own motor and perceptual patterns, his own solutions to the challenges that face him; and it is the function of a sensitive therapist to help him in this.

concept of memory as active and "inventive" (Rosenfield, 1991). That memory is essentially constructive (as Coleridge insisted, nearly two centuries ago)[16] was shown experimentally by the great Cambridge psychologist Frederic Bartlett. "Remembering," he wrote, "is not the re-excitation of innumerable fixed, lifeless and fragmentary traces. It is an imaginative reconstruction, or construction, built out of the relation of our attitude toward a whole mass of organized past reactions or experience."

It was just such an imaginative, context-dependent construction or reconstruction that Freud meant by *Nachtraglichkeit*—but this, Modell emphasizes, could not be given any biological basis until Edelman's notion of memory as recategorization. Beyond this, Modell as an analyst is concerned with the question of "self-creation"—how the self is created, its development and growth through finding, or making, personal meanings. Such a form of inner growth, so different from learning in the usual sense, he feels, may also find its neural basis in the formation of ever-richer but always self-referential maps in the brain, and their incessant integration through reentrant signaling, as Edelman has described it (Modell, 1990, 1993).

Others too—cognitive psychologists and linguists—have become intensely interested in Edelman's ideas, in particular by the implication of the extended Theory of Neuronal Group Selection, which suggests that the exploring child, the exploring organism, seeks (or imposes) meaning at all times, that its mappings are mappings of meaning, that its world and (if higher consciousness is present) its symbolic systems are *constructed* of meanings. When Jerome Bruner and others launched the cognitive revolution in the mid-1950s, this was in part a reaction to behaviorism and other "isms" that denied the existence and structure of the mind. The cognitive revolution was designed "to replace the mind in nature," to see the seeking of meaning as central to the organism. In a recent book,

---

[16] No one lived this distinction, or articulated it more eloquently, than Coleridge, who saw himself as "laying the foundation Stones of Constructive or Dynamic Philosophy in opposition to the merely mechanic" (in his letter to Brabant, July 21, 1815). This, for him, meant transforming the concepts of perception, memory, knowledge, and imagination, or, rather, seeing that these were of two sorts—which at various times he calls passive and active, dead and alive, false and true. In one of his notebooks (II:1509), he speaks of "mock" knowledge ("having no roots . . . no buds or twigs . . . but a dry stick of licorish") as opposed to true knowledge, which is rooted and grows and lives within one. And in his "Biographia Literaria," in a famous passage that might have served as an inspiration to Bartlett, he contrasts the constructive (Imagination) with the merely mechanic (Fancy): "The Imagination . . . dissolves, diffuses, dissipates, in order to recreate . . . it struggles to idealize and to unify. It is essentially *vital*, even as all objects (*as* objects) are essentially fixed and dead. Fancy, on the contrary, has no other counters to play with, but fixities and definites . . . [it] must receive all its materials ready made from the law of association."

"*Acts of Meaning*," Bruner (1990) describes how this original impetus was subverted, and replaced by notions of computation, information processing, etc., and by the computational (and Chomskian) notion that the syntax of a language could be separated from its semantics.

But, as Edelman writes, it is increasingly clear, from studying the natural acquisition of language in the child, and, equally, from the persistent failure of computers to "understand" language, its rich ambiguity and polysemy, that syntax cannot be separated from semantics. It is precisely through the medium of "meanings" that natural language and natural intelligence are built up. From George Boole, with his "Laws of Thought" in the 1850s, to the pioneers of artificial intelligence at the present day, there has been a persistent notion that one may have an intelligence or a language based on pure logic, without anything so messy as "meaning" being involved. That this is not the case, and cannot be the case, may now find a biological grounding in the Theory of Neuronal Group Selection.

None of this, however, can yet be proved—we have no way of seeing neuronal groups or maps or their interactions; no way of listening to the reentrant orchestra of the brain. Our capacity to analyze the living brain is still far too crude. Partly for this reason researchers in neuroscience have felt it necessary to simulate the brain, and the power of computers and supercomputers makes this more and more possible. One can endow simulated neurons with physiologically realistic properties, and allow them to interact in physiologically realistic ways.

Edelman and his colleagues at the Neurosciences Institute have been deeply interested in such synthetic neural modeling, and have devised a series of "synthetic animals" or artifacts designed to test the Theory of Neuronal Group Selection. Although these "creatures"—which have been named DARWIN I, II, III, and IV—make use of supercomputers, their behavior (if one may use the word) is not programmed, not robotic, but (in Edelman's word) "noetic." They incorporate both a selectional system and a primitive set of values—for example, that light is better than no light—which generally guide behavior but do not determine it or make it predictable. Unpredictable variations are introduced in both the artifact and its environment so that it is forced to create its own categorizations.

DARWIN IV or NOMAD, with its electronic eye and snout, has no goal, no agenda, but resides in a sort of pen, a world of varied simple objects (with different colors, shapes, textures, and weights). True to its name, it wanders around like a curious infant, exploring these objects, reaching for them, classifying them, building with them, in a spontaneous, idiosyncratic way (the movement of the artifact is exceedingly slow, and one needs time-lapse photography to bring home its creatural quality). No two "individuals" show identical behavior, and the details of their reachings and learnings cannot be predicted, any more than Thelen can predict the development of particular movement styles in her infants. If their value circuits are cut, the artifacts show no learning, no motivation, no convergent behavior at all, but wander around in an aimless way, like patients who have had their frontal lobes destroyed. Because the entire circuitry of these DARWINS is known, and can be seen functioning in detail on the screen of a supercomputer, one can continuously monitor their inner workings, their internal mappings, their reentrant signalings—one can see how they sample the environment, how the first, vague, tentative percepts emerge, and how, with hundreds of further samplings, they evolve and become recognizable, refined models of reality, following a process similar to that projected by Edelman's theory.[17]

Seeing the DARWINS, especially DARWIN IV, at work can induce a curious state of mind. Going to the zoo after my first sight of DARWIN IV, I found myself looking at birds, antelopes, lions, with a new eye: were they, so to speak, nature's DARWINS, somewhere up around DARWIN XII in complexity? And the gorillas, with higher order consciousness but no language—where would they stand? DARWIN XIX? And we, writing about the gorillas, where would we stand? DARWIN XXVII, perhaps? Edelman often wonders about the possibility of constructing a conscious artifact—he has no doubt of the possibility, but places it, mercifully, well on in the next century.

Neural Darwinism (or Neural Edelmanism, as Francis Crick has called it) coincides with our sense of "flow," that feeling we have when we are functioning optimally, of a swift, effortless, complex, ever-changing, but integrated and orchestrated stream of consciousness; (Csikszentmihalyi, 1990) it coincides with the sense that this consciousness is ours, and that all we experience and do and say is, implicitly, a form of self-expression, and that we are destined, whether we wish it or not, to a life of particularity and self-development; it coincides, finally, with our sense that life is a journey—unpredictable, full of risk and uncertainty, but, equally, full of novelty and adventure, and characterized (if not sabotaged by external

---

[17] Normally one is not aware of the brain's almost automatic generation of "perceptual hypotheses" (in Richard Gregory's term) and their refinement through a process of repeated samplings and testing. But under certain circumstances, as in recovery after acute nerve injury, one may become vividly aware of these normally unconscious (and sometimes exceedingly rapid) operations. I give a personal example of this in "A Leg to Stand On." One is much more aware of such hypothesizing when sensory information is scanty or ambiguous—as, for example, when driving in unfamiliar terrain at night.

constraints or pathology) by constant advance, an ever deeper exploration and understanding of the world.

Edelman's theory proposes a way of grounding all this in known facts about the nervous system and testable hypotheses about its operations. Any theory, even a wrong theory, is better than no theory; and this theory should at least stimulate a storm of experiment and discussion, for it is the first truly global theory of mind and consciousness, the first biological theory of individuality and autonomy.

References

Bartlett, F. C. (1932). "Remembering: A Study in Experimental and Social Psychology." Cambridge Univ. Pr., New York.

Bruner, J. (1990). "Acts of Meaning." Harvard Univ. Press, Cambridge, MA.

Burnet, F. M. (1959). "The Clonal Selection Theory of Acquired Immunity." Vanderbilt Univ. Press, Nashville, TN.

Crick, F. (1989). The recent excitement about neural networks. *Nature (London)* **337,** 129–132.

Csikszentmihalyi, M. (1990). "Flow: The Psychology of Optimal Experience." Harper Collins, New York.

Edelman, G. M. (1978). Group selection and phasic re-entrant signalling. *In* "The Mindful Brain" (G. M. Edelman and V. B. Mountcastle, eds.), pp. 51–100. MIT Press, Cambridge, MA.

Edelman, G. M. (1987). "Neural Darwinism: The Theory of Neuronal Group Selection." Basic Books, New York.

Edelman, G. M. (1988). "Topobiology: An Introduction to Molecular Embryology." Basic Books, New York.

Edelman, G. M. (1989). "The Remembered Present: A Biological Theory of Consciousness." Basic Books, New York.

Edelman, G. M. (1992). "Bright Air, Brilliant Fire: On the Matter of the Mind." Basic Books, New York.

Gray, J. (1992). *Nature (London)* **358,** 277.

Hebb, D. O. (1948). "The Organization of Behavior."

Helms, S. J. (1991). "The Cybernetics Group." MIT Press, Cambridge, MA.

Lashley, K. (1950). In search of the engram. *Symp. Soc. Exp. Biol.* **4.**

McCulloch, W. (1965). "Embodiments of Mind." MIT Press, Cambridge, MA.

Merzenich, M. M., Recanzone, G., Jenkins, W. M., Allard, T. T., and Nudo, R. J. (1988). Cortical representational plasticity. *In* "Neurobiology of the Neocortex" (P. Rakic and W. Singer, eds.), pp. 41–67. Wiley, New York.

Mesulam, M.-M. (1985). "Principles of Behavioral Neurology," pp. 259–88. Davis Co., Philadelphia.

Minsky, M. (1967). "Perceptrons." MIT Press, Cambridge, MA.

Modell, A. (1990). "Other Times, Other Realities." Harvard Univ. Press, Cambridge, MA.

Modell, A. (1993). "The Private Self." Harvard Univ. Press, Cambridge, MA.

Rosenfield, I. (1992). "The Strange, Familiar and Forgotten." Knopf, New York.

Rosenfield, I. (1991). "The Invention of Memory: A New View of the Brain." Basic Books, New York.

Sacks, O. (1989). "Seeing Voices," pp. 45–58. Univ. Calif. Press, Berkeley, CA.

Sacks, O. (1990). Neurology and the soul. *New York Review of Books,* November 22.

Sacks, O. (1992). Letter to the editor. *Nature (London)* **358,** 618.

Sacks, O. (1994). "A Leg to Stand On." Harper Collins, New York.

Sacks, O. (1993). To see and not see. *The New Yorker,* May 10.

Stern, D. (1985). "The Interpersonal World of the Infant: A View from Psychoanalysis and Developmental Psychology." Basic Books, New York.

Thelen, E. (1990). Dynamical systems and the generation of individual differences. *In* "Individual Differences in Infancy: Reliability, Stability, and Prediction" (J. Colombo and J. W. Fagen, eds.). Erlbaum, Hillsdale, NJ.

Wiener, N. (1961). "Cybernetics: Control & Communication in the Animal & the Machine," 2nd ed. MIT Press, Cambridge, MA.

SECTION V
DISCUSSION

Much has been learned about "normal" brain function through the study of illusory phenomena; several key examples can be found in the work of Ramachandran. Numerous visual illusions belonging to various classes have been described; they have always had a special appeal to scientists and nonscientists alike. New methods to generate stimuli using computer displays have led to a general proliferation of illusory phenomena. As it becomes easier and easier to generate new illusions, their sheer number and variety constitutes a serious challenge for any instructionist or information-processing approach to brain function. Instructionism is hard to reconcile with illusory phenomena of any kind, because such phenomena could only be considered as errors in performance. Indeed, why would an instructionist system be designed to experience illusions? On the other hand, what counts for a selectional system is the overall success of its performance. Stated somewhat loosely, given a high level of adaptation or survival, illusions may be allowed or even unavoidable. In fact, illusory phenomena may be a price that the system pays to achieve its global goals. Ramachandran's exploration of the perceptual correlates of somatosensory plasticity, culminating in his "remapping hypothesis" and neurobiological interpretation of Freudian repression, is a further example that "illusory" phenomena exist in all sensory modalities and can allow fruitful insight into cortical processes. Ramachandran observes that there is a strong connection to Darwinian and selectionist views of the brain.

Recent explorations of the underlying neurobiological mechanisms of illusions have revealed that they represent—at least in most cases—a manifestation of the same processes underlying normal perception. But what is "normal" and what is "illusory" in visual perception? Some functions of the visual system, such as color perception, are heavily dependent on the construction of new properties from relatively simple inputs. Color is not a property of the surrounding world (at least not in the sense that it exists as information ready to be sensed and assimilated), it is a construct of the brain. Is color therefore merely an illusion? Clearly, the boundary between illusory and nonillusory perception is not a sharp one, and one that can presumably be shifted by differences in developmental exposure to stimuli. The developmental foundations of perceptual illusions are largely unexplored and should provide further insight into what constitutes the neural bases for these phenomena.

It may seem surprising at first that a book on selectionism should have anything to do with psychoanalysis. It is true that Freud was significantly influenced by Darwin, but it is also widely accepted that his understanding of natural selection was seriously flawed. More generally, it is often assumed that psychoanalysis rests on rigid psychic determinism on one side, and insists on the other side on the ability of specific events that influence the unconscious to impress themselves or "instruct" psychic development, regardless of preexisting proclivities. Be it as it may, Modell argues in his chapter that both psychic development and the therapeutic setting are best interpreted in terms of the selectionist concept of memory as recategorization. At the origin of many intrapsychic conflicts Modell sees a failure of recategorization. Modell refers to Freud's view of memory as *Nachträglichkeit,* or retranscription. According to this view, value-laden experiences are reexperienced repeatedly at different developmental epochs and constantly modified in order to safeguard a coherent image of the self. Traumatic experiences would, through repression, interfere with this process and lead to various splittings or dissociations. The therapeutic setting can thus be seen as a situation in which such retranscription or recategorization is actuated in the presence of the analyst. Repetition compulsion, often experienced in the transference setting, would be both a symptom of the biological need to recategorize and a means to achieve that goal therapeutically. As Modell succinctly states, one might say that, through the retranscription of memory, the present can alter the past.

Another point of contact between psychoanalysis and selectionism discussed by Modell is that between Freud's instinct theory and Edelman's concept of value. Modell is highly critical of instinct theory. Rooted in outdated ideas of evolutionary biology, the vicissitudes of Freuds's notion of instinct are an example of how dangerous it was for psychoanalysis to lose track of its connections to evolutionary theory and to neurobiology. Recovering those connections, according to Modell, is the most urgent requirement for the survival of psychoanalytic insights. As with recategorization, it is another selectionist concept, value, that seems to be particularly well-suited to a fundamental application in psychoanalytic theory. The concept of value is founded in modern evolutionary biology, and at the same time it is being given specific structural and functional substrates in terms of selectionist neurobiology (see the introduction to Section I). The relationship of value to affect and personal meaning, and the interaction of value with recategorization, are discussed by Modell in a radical attempt to replace instinct theory by a theoretical edifice endowed with more solid biological foundations.

Though it is too early to judge whether such an operation will prove successful, it is perhaps useful to underline a specific aspect of the notion of value that seems to be particularly relevant to the interpretation of human behavior. Evolutionarily selected biases (innate values) are clearly required to explain the convergence of selectional systems toward adaptive behavior. They act as reference "pillars" around which selectional events are organized in the idiosyncratic history of each individual. Over time, however, other events may gain access to value systems and thereby reshape and refine the value landscape. These events become acquired values and may slowly gain control of many aspects of psychic and behavioral processes. One might conceptualize that some particular outcomes and distortions in the development of acquired values, triggered, for instance, by traumatic events, could lead to a warping of the value landscape and to various forms of psychopathology.

Since Freud's celebrated case histories were published, it has not been uncommon to find highly individual and remarkable psychopathological accounts in the analytic literature. It is somewhat surprising, however, to encounter clinical histories in neurology proper that display an equally striking degree of uniqueness. Despite attempts to systematize neuropsychological (and psychiatric) disorders, Sacks argues that it is clinically as well as scientifically mistaken to ignore their individual character. One is reminded of a central tenet of selectionist approaches, that individual variation is not just noise or error around an average; it has ontological dignity. More in this case than in any other, perhaps, it is the individual and not the average that is real, not unlike what happens with works of art: although similarities in style and genre may lead to useful generalizations, it would make little sense to listen to the average of the classical sonata, or to contemplate the average portrait of a man.

Another lesson from clinical neurology can be derived from the importance of interaction with the environment in a continuous circle of action and perception, and in a constant cycle of novelty and recategorization. There is an inevitable production of novelty (variation) inside the organism and outside it. These two sources of novelty are systematically tested against each other, in an incessant process of reciprocal adaptation. Given the immense dimensionality and the nonlinearities of the systems involved, coupled with their unpredictability, only selectional principles can account for neurological development, recovery, and reorganization. Most remarkable is the consistency between a selectionist view of the brain and the ability of an organism to react rapidly and adapt to dramatic alterations of its phenotypic organs or its nervous system. For instance, after a paralysis, both the phenotype and the brain rapidly adapt to a completely different set of internal as well as external constraints. In certain neuropsychological syndromes, e.g., hemineglect, the entire conscious self shrinks and readapts to a world that has been halved in extension. Mental dysfunction involves not just loss of function but also readaptation and adjustment of mental and brain organization.

The application of selectionism to clinical histories is also a strong reminder of a topic touched on in the discussion at the end of Section I. The triad "variation–selection–differential amplification" should never be considered *in abstracto,* but always in the context of a particular phenotype and of its previous history. In fact, variation never occurs in a vacuum, but it is constrained, at any given time, by the outcome of a long history of previous selectional events. In most cases variation is therefore *variation on a theme,* despite the fact that, depending on the relative strength of selectional events on one side and of intrinsic constraints on the other, even the theme may change. The interaction between long-range constraints with local variation, both in space and in time, can explain the coexistence of similarity and individuality, regularity and unpredictability, and conservation and change. Thus it is perhaps appropriate that the last chapter of this book devoted to "Selectionism and the Brain" is a lively account of a global view of brain function that, in the best vein of naturalistic description, tries to account for the endless variety of nature and of human experience.

INDEX

CONTENTS OF RECENT VOLUMES